Health in England 1996

What people know, what people think, what people do

A survey of adults aged 16–74 in England carried out by Social Survey Division of ONS on behalf of the Health Education Authority

Jacqui Hansbro, Ann Bridgwood,
with
Antony Morgan, Mary Hickman

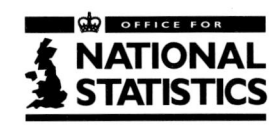

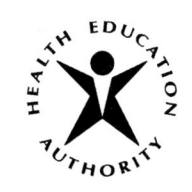

OFFICE FOR NATIONAL STATISTICS

HEALTH EDUCATION AUTHORITY

London: The Stationery Office

© *Crown copyright 1997*
First published 1997

ISBN 0 11 691672 9

Printed in the United Kingdom for The Stationery Office
4/97 C15 10170

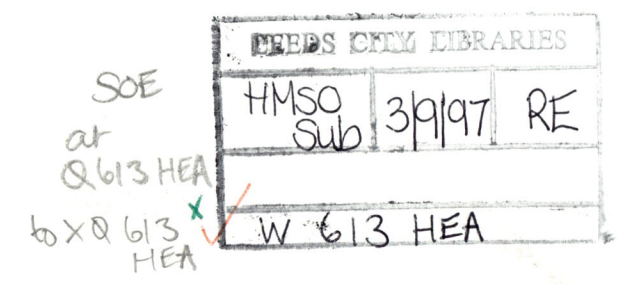

Contents

	Page
Foreword	vii
Project Team	viii
Authors' acknowledgements	ix
Notes to tables	ix
Summary of main findings	**1**

Part A - Chapters 1-9

1	**Background and aims of the survey**		**6**
	1.1	Background to the survey	6
	1.2	The role of the Health Education Authority	6
	1.3	Models of health behaviour change	7
	1.4	The aims and design of the survey	8
	1.5	Characteristics of the sample	8
	Annex	*Health of the Nation* objectives and targets	10

2	**Smoking and drinking**		**13**
	2.1	Introduction and background	14
	2.2	Prevalence of smoking and levels of consumption	14
	2.3	Giving up smoking	15
	2.4	Smoking and children	17
	2.5	Smoking in the workplace	17
	2.6	Consumption of alcohol	18
	2.7	Knowledge of alcohol units	19
	2.8	Attitudes to changes in 'sensible drinking levels'	20
	2.9	Characteristics of people most likely to smoke and drink heavily	21

3	**Physical activity**		**24**
	3.1	Introduction and background	25
	3.2	Recommended levels of physical activity	25
	3.3	Participation in physical activity	25
	3.4	Knowledge of recommended levels of physical activity	29
	3.5	Attitudes towards physical activity	29

4	**Nutrition**		**33**
	4.1	Introduction and background	34
	4.2	Knowledge of what constitutes a healthy diet	34
	4.3	What informants look for when shopping for food	35
	4.4	Eating habits	36
	4.5	Attitudes towards diet	38
	Annex	Methodological notes	41

			Page
5	**Drug use**		42
	by Antony Morgan, Mary Hickman, Christine Callum, Paige Sinkler,		
	Hilary Whent – *Health Education Authority*		
	5.1	Introduction and background	43
	5.2	Prevalence of drug use	43
	5.3	Knowing people who use drugs	48
	5.4	Intentions to stop using drugs	49
	5.5	Methods of taking drugs	49
	5.6	Taking drugs in combination	49
	5.7	Attitudes to drugs	50
6	**Sexual health**		52
	6.1	Introduction and background	53
	6.2	Number of sexual partners in the last year	53
	6.3	Perceptions of risk	54
	6.4	Use of condoms with a new partner	56
7	**Behaviour in the sun**		59
	7.1	Introduction and background	60
	7.2	Behaviour in the sun	60
	7.3	Attitudes towards a suntan	61
8	**General health and doctor consultations**		63
	8.1	Introduction and background	64
	8.2	Self-reported general health	64
	8.3	Self-reported morbidity	65
	8.4	Self-reported stress	66
	8.5	Respondents' assessments of whether they led a healthy life	67
	8.6	Respondents' assessments of which factors are good and bad for their health	67
	8.7	General attitudes towards health	67
	8.8	Consultations with GPs and other health professionals	68
	Annex	Methodological notes	71
9	**Conclusion: knowledge, attitudes and behaviour**		73
	9.1	Introduction	73
	9.2	Sex	73
	9.3	Age	73
	9.4	Social class	74
	9.5	Conclusion	74

Page

Part B - Reference section

    Reference tables

1	Characteristics of the sample	81
2	Smoking and drinking	82
3	Physical activity	115
4	Nutrition	130
5	Drug use	152
6	Sexual health	170
7	Behaviour in the sun	185
8	General health and doctor consultations	196
	Appendix A	222

Appendix A: **Sample design, response to the survey, weighting, characteristics of the responding sample and sampling errors**   **241**

A.1	Introduction	241
A.2	The sample design	241
A.3	Sampling individuals within households	242
A.4	Response to the survey	242
A.5	Non-response and weighting	242
A.6	Characteristics of the responding sample	243
A.7	The accuracy of the survey results	245

Appendix B: **Monitoring Frameworks and Health Promotion Indicators**   **247**
    by Antony Morgan and Mary Hickman, *Health Education Authority*

B.1	Introduction and background	247
B.2	Monitoring frameworks	247
B.3	Other related work	248

Appendix C: **Physical activity - Energy intensity categories and frequency measures for different types of activity**   **249**
    by Alison Walker

C.1	The indicators of participation in physical activity	249
C.2	Energy intensity categories and frequency measures by activity type	249
C.3	Reference period	250
C.4	Changes to the physical activity questions between 1995 and 1996	250
C.5	Effect of the changes	250

Appendix D: **Technical appendix**   **252**

D.1	Logistic regression	252
D.2	Age standardisation	253

Appendix D: **Fieldwork documents**   **254**

E.1	The questionnaire	254
E.2	The proxy questionnaire	278
E.3	The prompt cards	283

List of figures   303

List of tables   305

Health in England 1996 : What people know, what people think, what people do   **v**

Foreword

This report is the second in a series of annual surveys set up to monitor trends in health-related knowledge, attitudes and behaviour in the adult population in England.

Knowledge and expertise in performance indicators for health promotion are scarce. To redress this balance the HEA have been working for several years to produce a series of health promotion indicators that would enable it to demonstrate the impact of *The Health of the Nation* and other health promotion policies upon the health-related behaviours of individuals. The Health Education Monitoring Survey (HEMS) was established as a way of monitoring these health promotion indicators for adults.

I welcome this report and the contribution it makes to the HEA's knowledge base for health promotion in England. It will be of great interest to all those working in this field, both nationally and at a local level.

PROFESSOR PAMELA GILLIES
Director of Research
Health Education Authority

Project team

Health Education Authority

Antony Morgan	**Head of Effectiveness and Monitoring Research**
Mary Hickman	**Research Manager**
Christine Callum	**Statistician**
Paige Sinkler	**Research Officer**
Hilary Whent	**Research Officer**

ONS

Jil Matheson	**Research Director**
Jacqui Hansbro	**Project Manager**
Ann Bridgwood	**Principal Social Survey Officer**
Dev Marway	**Computing Officer**
Anne Klepacz	**Field Officer**
Theresa Parker	**Assistant Field Officer**
Nigel Hudson	**Administrative Officer**

Consultant

Alison Walker	**Consultant on physical activity**

Authors' acknowledgements

We would like to thank everybody who contributed to the Survey and the production of this report. We were supported by our specialist colleagues in ONS who carried out the sampling, fieldwork, computing and coding stages, and by our colleagues who helped us with the administrative duties. Thanks are due to the interviewers who showed commitment and enthusiasm throughout the Survey. We would also like to thank colleagues at the Health Education Authority, especially Christine Callum, Paige Sinkler and Hilary Whent, for their contribution to the Survey and also Alison Walker, for her contribution as consultant on physical activity. Thanks also to Iain Noble for his contribution in setting up the initial survey.

Most importantly, we would like to thank all those people who gave up their time to take part in this Survey, and showed such an interest in its aims.

Notes to tables

1. Where the base number is less than 30, numbers rather than percentages are shown in italics in square brackets.

2. The column percentages may add to 99% or 101% because of rounding.

3. A percentage may be quoted in the text for a single category that is identifiable in the tables only by summing two or more component percentages. In order to avoid rounding errors, particularly as the data were weighted, the percentage has been recalculated for the single category and may therefore differ by one percentage point from the sum of the percentages derived from the tables.

4. The following conventions have been used within tables :

    -    no observations (zero value)
    0   less than 0.5%
    []   numbers on a base of less than 30

5. Unless otherwise stated, changes and differences mentioned in the text have been found to be statistically significant at the 95% confidence level.

6. Values for means, medians, percentiles and standard errors (SE) are shown to an appropriate number of decimal places.

7. Non-response and missing information: the information from an individual who co-operated in the survey may be incomplete, either because of a partial refusal or because the individual did not understand, did not know the answer or refused to answer a particular question.

   Respondents who did not co-operate at all are omitted from all analysis; those who did not co-operate with a particular section (e.g. the self-completion schedule) are omitted from the analysis of that section. The 'no answers' arising from the omission of particular items have been excluded from the base numbers shown in the tables and from the bases used in percentaging.

8. Data relating to the HEA suggested health promotion indicators are shaded on the tables.

Summary of main findings '96

1. Background and aims of the survey (Chapter 1)

The Health Education Monitoring Survey (HEMS) 1996 is the second in a series of studies designed to monitor trends in the health-related knowledge, attitudes and behaviour of adults aged 16–74 living in private households in England. The survey was commissioned by the Health Education Authority (HEA) and carried out by the Social Survey Division (SSD) of the Office for National Statistics (ONS); the first survey was carried out in 1995[1].

In 1992, the Government published the *Health of the Nation* White Paper[2]. Subtitled 'A strategy for health in England', the White Paper identified five Key Areas where there was both the greatest need and the greatest scope for making cost-effective improvements in the overall health of people in England. These were: coronary heart disease and stroke; cancers; mental illness; HIV/AIDS and sexual health; and accidents. For each Key Area, the White Paper set out overall objectives for improved health, and specific targets to be met by set dates. In addition, it published targets for risk factors associated with the five Key Areas, including smoking, alcohol, diet and nutrition, obesity, blood pressure, and HIV/AIDS.

Since the publication of the White Paper, the government has developed a number of other initiatives for areas not covered by the *Health of the Nation*, such as drug use and environmental issues[3,4].

Many *Health of the Nation* targets aim for improvements in mortality and morbidity figures, which can only be measured in the long term. Because of this the HEA has been developing a series of health promotion indicators which are designed to measure intermediate progress. These range from indicators relating to individual knowledge, attitudes and behaviour to institutional health-related policies. The HEMS was established as a way of monitoring these health promotion indicators.

2. Smoking and drinking (Chapter 2)

Prevalence of smoking

- Thirty one per cent of men and 29% of women were current cigarette smokers (that is, they smoked at least one cigarette a day); prevalence was highest among the 16–24 age-group and decreased with age. The mean number of cigarettes smoked per day was 12.9 for women and 15.3 for men.

Giving up smoking

- Sixty five per cent of current smokers said they would like to give up smoking, but 56% would find it 'very difficult' or 'fairly difficult' to give up and 45% said they were unlikely to do so.

- Just over three quarters (77%) of current smokers had tried to give up smoking; almost half (48%) of those who had given up had done so for less than a month and another 27% for less than a week.

- The most common reason given for stopping smoking was 'health reasons', mentioned by 55% of ex-smokers. Both current smokers who had tried to give up and ex-smokers were asked what methods they had used to give up: 'will-power' was the method most commonly used by those who had successfully stopped smoking.

Smoking and children

- Over three quarters (78%) of parents with children aged under 16 living in the household thought the health of their child was affected by people smoking in the home.

- The overwhelming majority (92%) of parents with children aged 9–15 did not want their children to smoke.

Smoking in the workplace

- Seventy seven per cent of adults aged 16–74 who had a job worked for an employer who operated a no-smoking policy. Women were more likely than men to work for an employer with a no-smoking policy.

Consumption of alcohol

- Alcohol consumption was highest in the 16–24 age-group. The mean weekly number of units of alcohol consumed by women was 7.7, compared with an average of 18.0 units consumed by men.

Health in England 1996 : What people know, what people think, what people do

Respondents' assessment of their drinking

- Seventeen per cent of adults who drank at least once or twice a week said they would like to drink less.

- Almost a half (45%) of respondents who would like to drink less thought they were unlikely to cut down, while a fifth (20%) intended to cut down in the next month.

Knowledge of alcohol units

- Eighty four per cent of men and 81% of women had heard about measuring alcohol in units. Among this group 43% were able to give the correct number of units in a glass of wine and in a pint of beer and 34% correctly identified the number of units in a single pub measure of spirits.

Attitudes to changes in 'sensible drinking levels'

- Twenty six per cent of respondents had not heard about the changes to a daily benchmark of 2–3 units or less a day for women and 3–4 units or less a day for men, and another 38% said the changes were of no interest. Only a small proportion (14%) said they felt confused about the changes and 22% did not feel confused.

3 Physical activity (Chapter 3)

Participation in physical activity

- A quarter of respondents participated less than once a week in 30 minutes or more of moderate-intensity activity. The likelihood of being inactive increased with age; 42% of men and 46% of women aged 65–74 were defined as 'sedentary', compared with 9% of men and 20% of women in the 16–24 age-group.

- Men and younger respondents were most likely to have engaged in at least moderate-intensity activity lasting at least 30 minutes on five or more days a week, and in vigorous-intensity activity lasting at least 20 minutes on three or more days a week in the four weeks before interview.

Knowledge of recommended levels of physical activity

- The majority of men (73%) and women (69%) thought that, on each of the days someone engages in physical activity, the activity should last at least 30 minutes.

- A quarter of respondents said that physical activity should be undertaken for at least 30 minutes on at least five days a week, the recommended guidelines for frequency and duration of moderate-intensity activity.

Attitudes towards physical activity

- Seventy six per cent of men and 71% of women said they were 'very' or 'fairly' physically active compared with others of the same age.

- About half of men (54%) and women (49%) thought they were getting enough exercise to keep fit.

- Over two thirds (68%) of respondents wished to take more exercise; the proportion saying this declined with age, particularly after the age of 55.

- A quarter of respondents intended to take more exercise in the next month, while another fifth said they would do more in the next six months. Just over two fifths (41%) said they were unlikely to do more.

- Lack of time (52%), not being the sporty type (15%), having an injury or disability (14%), and poor health (9%) were the most commonly mentioned barriers to exercise.

4 Nutrition (Chapter 4)

Knowledge of what constitutes a healthy diet

- When respondents were asked to describe a healthy diet, the four most commonly given answers were: eating lots of fruit, vegetables and salad; cutting down on fat; eating lots of fibre; and eating lots of starchy carbohydrates.

What informants look for when shopping for food

- Almost two thirds (65%) of men and just over one third (36%) of women either never shopped for food or never looked at the ingredients.

- Among those who did shop for food, there were some differences between men and women in what they looked for: 40% of women compared with 24% of men looked at the fat content and 16% of women, but only 9% of men, looked at the sugar content.

Eating habits

- Thirty eight per cent of adults aged 16–74 reported eating bread; fruit, vegetables or salad; and potatoes, rice or pasta daily.

- Twenty two per cent of respondents reported using semi-skimmed or skimmed milk; no fat, low- or reduced-fat spread; and eating chips less than once a week.

- A third (33%) of adults said they ate confectionery less than once a week and just over a quarter (26%) said they ate biscuits or cakes less than once a week.

- Almost a fifth (19%) respondents thought their diet was healthy, and almost three quarters (73%) thought it was quite good but could improve.

- Of those who thought their diet was not as healthy as it could be, 36% did not want to change; 30% wanted to change but did not think it was likely they would; 11% intended to change in the next month; 15% in the next six months and 7% in the next year.

Attitudes towards diet

- Almost a third (32%) of respondents agreed with the statement 'I get confused over what's supposed to be healthy and what isn't'; 68% agreed that 'experts never agree about what foods are good for you'; 37% thought that 'eating healthy food is expensive'; 75% agreed that 'healthy foods are enjoyable'; and 38% agreed with the statement 'the tastiest foods are the ones that are bad for you.'

Drug use (Chapter 5)

Prevalence of drug taking

- Respondents aged 16–54 were asked whether they had used any drugs which had not been prescribed by a doctor; they were asked about their use of amphetamines, cannabis, cocaine, crack, ecstasy, heroin, LSD, magic mushrooms, methadone, amyl nitrate, glues and solvents, anabolic steroids and tranquillisers. Thirty eight per cent of men and 26% of women reported ever having taken one or more drugs listed; 17% of men and 11% of women had taken at least one in the past year and 12% of men and 6% of women had done so in the past month.

- The most common drug taken was cannabis; 28% of respondents aged 16–54 had ever taken cannabis, 13% had ever taken amphetamines and 9% had ever taken amyl nitrates.

- Drug use was less prevalent among older than among younger respondents. For example, 42% of respondents aged 16–29 had ever taken cannabis, compared with 21% of those aged 30–54.

- Among those who had ever used a drug, 56% of those aged 19–21 had used a drug in the past month, compared with 16% of those aged 30–54.

Knowing people who use drugs

- Those aged 16–19 were most likely to know someone who had used drugs (85% did so, compared with 26% of those aged 45–54).

Intentions to stop using drugs

- One in ten of those who had used drugs in the past month did not see the need ever to stop using drugs.

Methods of taking drugs

- Respondents who had ever used drugs were asked by which method they had taken them: over four fifths (84%) had smoked drugs, just over one third (34%) had swallowed them, one fifth (20%) had sniffed drugs, just over one in ten (11%) had inhaled them. Only 1% had injected them.

Taking drugs in combination

- About one in twenty (6%) respondents had taken two or more drugs in the past year; among this group about half (49%) had taken two or more drugs in combination on one occasion.

Attitudes to drugs

- Seventy per cent of respondents agreed that 'all use of drugs is wrong unless with a doctor's prescription or bought from a chemist'.

- Just over half (55%) of respondents disagreed with the statement 'I don't mind other people using drugs'. Older respondents were more likely to disagree with the statement than younger respondents, for example 71% of those aged 45–54 disagreed with the statement compared with 32% of those aged 16–19.

Sexual health (Chapter 6)

Number of sexual partners in the last year

- Sixteen per cent of men and 10% of women aged 16–54 reported two or more sexual partners in the 12 months before interview.

Perceptions of risk

- Thirty per cent of men and 31% of women thought they had 'no risk' of being infected with HIV, while 33% of men and 34% of women made the same assessment of their risk of contracting another sexually transmitted disease (STD). Older respondents were less likely than younger ones to see themselves as at risk.

Use of condoms with a new partner

- Only a minority (18%) of respondents thought it would be 'difficult to raise the subject of using a condom with a new partner'.

- More than two thirds of women (67%), and almost three fifths of men (58%) said they would always use a condom 'if in the near future they did have sex with a new partner', while 17% of women and 31% of men said 'it would depend'. Only 1% of respondents stated that they would never use a condom.

- Among those who reported a new partner in the last year, 60% of men and 63% of women used a condom the first time they had intercourse with their most recent partner.

7 Behaviour in the sun (Chapter 7)

Behaviour in the sun

- Just over a quarter (29%) of men and women (23%) had been sunburnt in the last 12 months.

- The proportion of people saying they had been sunburnt decreased with age from 41% of those aged 16–24 to only 8% of those aged 65–74.

- Over two thirds (68%) of adults used a suncream; women were more likely than men to have done so (74% compared with 61%).

- Suncreams were most commonly used when sunbathing either abroad or in this country.

Attitudes towards a suntan

- Women were more likely than men to think that having a suntan was important; 31% said it was, compared with 20% of men.

- Forty five per cent of respondents agreed that having a suntan made them feel healthier and 45% thought that a suntan made them look more attractive. Women were more likely than men to agree with each of these statements.

8 General health and doctor consultations (Chapter 8)

Self-reported general health and morbidity

- Eighty per cent of men and 78% of women said that their general health was 'very good' or 'good'.

- Women were slightly more likely than men to report a long-standing illness or disability, 37% did so, compared with 35% of men.

Self-reported stress

- Sixty nine per cent of women and 62% of men said they had experienced a 'moderate' or 'large' amount of stress in the 12 months prior to interview. More than two fifths (41%) of men and more than half (53%) of women had experienced stress which they felt was harmful to their physical or mental health.

Respondents' assessments of which factors are good and bad for their health

- When asked to choose which, if any, of a list of factors were currently good for their health, respondents were most likely to cite relationships and family (mentioned by 59%), what they ate (56%), and exercise (47%). Pollution, lack of exercise and 'my weight' were most often seen by respondents as currently bad for their health; 29%, 27% and 27% respectively mentioned these.

General attitudes towards health

- When asked for their general opinions about health, 88% of respondents agreed that to have good health is the most important thing in life and 67% that it is sensible to do exactly what the doctors say. Only 25% agreed with the statement that generally health is a matter of luck.

Consultations with GPs and other health professionals

- Almost three quarters (73%) of women and three fifths (60%) of men had talked to a GP at his or her surgery in the last year. An additional 3% of men and 4% of women had spoken to another health professional, such as a nurse or health visitor, at the surgery or health centre.

- Thirty per cent of male and 36% of female current and ex-smokers who had given up smoking in the last year had discussed smoking with a GP or other health professional; 13% of male and 6% of female current and ex-drinkers had discussed drinking.

Notes and references

1. Bridgwood A et al. *Health in England 1995: what people know, what people think, what people do.* HMSO (London 1996).

2. Department of Health. *The Health of the Nation: a strategy for health in England.* HMSO (London 1992).

3. Central Drugs Coordination Unit. *Tackling drugs together: a strategy for England 1995-1998.* HMSO (London 1995). Drug use was discussed in the *Health of the Nation* White Paper, but mainly in relation to HIV/AIDS.

4. Department of Health/Department of the Environment. *UK Environmental Action Plan Cm 3323.* HMSO (London 1996).

Part A - Chapters 1 – 9

1 Background and aims of the survey

The Health Education Monitoring Survey (HEMS) 1996 is the second in a series of studies designed to monitor trends in the health-related knowledge, attitudes and behaviour of adults aged 16-74 living in private households in England. The survey was commissioned by the Health Education Authority (HEA) and carried out by the Social Survey Division (SSD) of the Office for National Statistics (ONS); the first survey was carried out in 1995[1].

The main aim of the 1995 HEMS Survey was to collect baseline data against which future change could be measured; the 1996 survey is the first to monitor change. In both years, the interview included questions on behaviour in the sun, smoking, drinking, physical activity, nutrition, and socio-demographic characteristics. The 1995 survey showed that there were high levels of knowledge of ways of avoiding skin cancer, which foods contained saturated fats and the causes of lung cancer, heart disease and stroke. These questions were omitted from the 1996 survey, as it was not felt necessary to ask them every year. New questions were added to the 1996 interview on attitudes towards having a suntan, respondents' assessment of the effect of stress on their health, and attitudes towards children's smoking. In addition, the 1995 interview included a self-completion module on sexual health; in 1996, this was shortened considerably and respondents were also asked about their use of and attitudes towards drugs. The topics covered by the two years of the survey are summarised in Figure 1.1. **(Figure 1.1)**

Respondents to the 1996 survey will be interviewed for a second time in 1997, a year after their initial interview. The aims of the follow-up interview are to monitor any changes between 1996 and 1997 and to examine the relationship between intentions expressed in the initial interview and any reported changes in behaviour.

Although this report is part of a series, it is designed to be used as an independent volume. This chapter therefore repeats some background information which was included in the 1995 report.

1.1 Background to the survey

In 1992, the Government published the *Health of the Nation* White Paper[2]. Subtitled 'A strategy for health in England', the White Paper identified five Key Areas where there was both the greatest need and the greatest scope for making cost-effective improvements in the overall health of people in England. These were: coronary heart disease and stroke; cancers; mental illness; HIV/AIDS and sexual health; and accidents. For each Key Area, the White Paper set out overall objectives for improved health, and specific targets to be met by set dates. In addition, it published targets for risk factors associated with the five Key Areas, including smoking, alcohol, diet and nutrition, obesity, blood pressure, and HIV/AIDS.

The White Paper emphasised that the *Health of the Nation* strategy and targets needed to be underpinned by adequate systems for:

- monitoring and appraising the health of the population, and progress towards meeting the targets

- research into the effectiveness and cost effectiveness of actions taken

- the measurement of health outcomes

In support of these aims, the Department of Health has published annual progress reports[3] and established a number of initiatives, including the development of the Public Health Common Data Set[4] and the Central Health Monitoring Unit's *Epidemiological Overviews*, the most recent of which is about health-related behaviour[5]. The Health Survey for England is also used for monitoring progress towards the achieving the HON targets[6]. The data collected by HEMS complement those collected annually by the Health Survey for England.

Since the publication of the White Paper, the government has developed a number of other initiatives for areas not covered by the *Health of the Nation*, such as drug use and environmental issues[7,8].

1.2 The role of the Health Education Authority

The *Health of the Nation* White Paper recognises the contribution of health promotion to achieving its targets. As a result, the HEA has been considering complementary strategies to support the monitoring process. In 1993 it established the HEA Targets Project, drawing on extensive experience of collecting information about the population's knowledge, attitudes and behaviour about health and related subjects.

Many *Health of the Nation* targets aim for improvements in mortality and morbidity figures, which can only be measured in the long term. Because of this the HEA has been developing a series of health promotion indicators (see Appendix B) which are designed to measure intermediate progress. These range from indicators relating to individual knowledge, attitudes and

Figure 1.1 Health of the Nation Key Areas and Risk Factors and topics covered in the HEMS questionnaire in 1995 and 1996

Key Area	Questionnaire topics and year of inclusion in the survey
Coronary heart disease	Knowledge of the causes of coronary heart disease and stroke (1995)
Cancer	Knowledge of the causes of lung cancer (1995) Knowledge of ways of avoiding skin cancer (1995) Avoiding exposure to the sun (1995 and 1996) Attitudes towards having a suntan (1995 and 1996)
Mental Illness	Self-reported stress (1995 and 1996) and its perceived effect on health (1996)
HIV/AIDS & sexual health	Age of first sexual intercourse (1995) Use of contraception on occasion of first sexual intercourse (1995) Use of condoms (1995) Use of condoms with a new partner (1995 and 1996) Perception of own risk of HIV infection (1995 and 1996) Knowledge of groups at risk of HIV infection (1995) Attitudes towards condom use (1995)
Accidents	(Not covered)

Risk factor	Questionnaire topics
Smoking	Smoking prevalence and consumption (1995 and 1996) Giving up smoking (1995 and 1996) Workplace policies on smoking (1995 and 1996) Attitudes towards smoking in the home (1995 and 1996) Attitudes towards children's smoking (1996) Exposure of non-smokers to cigarette smoke (1995) Discussing smoking with a GP or other health professional (1995 and 1996)
Nutrition	Knowledge of the constituents of a balanced diet (1995 and 1996) Knowledge of foods containing saturated fats (1995) Attitudes towards healthy eating (1995 and 1996) Eating habits (1995 and 1996) Alcohol consumption (1995 and 1996) Cutting down alcohol consumption (1995 and 1996) Knowledge of alcohol units (1995 and 1996) Discussing nutrition and alcohol consumption with a GP or other health professional (1995 and 1996)
Blood pressure	Knowledge of recommended levels of activity (1996) Whether taking sufficient exercise to keep fit (1995 and 1996) Intentions to take more exercise (1995 and 1996) Barriers to physical activity (1995 and 1996) Level and intensity of physical activity (1995 and 1996) Discussing physical activity with a GP or other health professional (1995 and 1996)
HIV/AIDS	Number of sexual partners (1995 and 1996) Unprotected sexual intercourse (1995) Use of non-prescribed drugs (1996) Giving up drugs (1996) Injecting drug users (1996) Attitudes towards drug use (1996)

behaviour to institutional health-related policies. To date, these indicators have been presented in a series of monitoring frameworks which the HEA is using to set out:

- the organisation's *overall* objective in relation to particular *Health of the Nation* targets and other government initiatives

- a series of more *specific* objectives which will secure the achievement of the overall objective

- the interventions that are necessary to achieve the specific objectives

- the information, in the form of health promotion indicators, which can be used as proxy measures of success in the achievement of objectives

Monitoring frameworks do not encompass all of the information required to evaluate health promotion programmes. They do, however, provide a context for health promotion work. By using data relating to the chosen indicators in conjunction with other information, they support management information systems in assessing and evaluating the effectiveness of health promotion strategies.

The HEA does not see these frameworks as definitive; they are dynamic and will continue to evolve over time.

1.3 Models of health behaviour change

The White Paper argues that all of the main risk factors which it identified can be influenced by changes in behaviour. For those who smoke, for example, stopping smoking is the single most effective way of reducing the risk of coronary heart disease and stroke. Similarly, avoiding excessive exposure to the sun can reduce the risk of skin cancer, while safer sexual practices are seen as a key method of reducing the risk of infection by HIV and other sexually transmitted diseases. An integral part of the White Paper's strategy is helping individuals to be more aware of risk factors and of how to make the lifestyle changes necessary to avoid them.

The design and analysis of the HEMS survey were informed by two psychological models of health behaviour change, which explore the relationships between attitudes, knowledge and behaviour – the Theory of Planned Behaviour and the Stages of Change Model. These represent two different types of theoretical approach, continuum models and stage models, and are briefly outlined here.

Ajzen's Theory of Planned Behaviour[9], an extension of Fishbein and Azjen's Theory of Reasoned Action[10], argues that a person's intention to perform a given behaviour is a function of three basic determinants: attitude towards the behaviour, subjective norms and perceived behavioural control. Each of these three constructs is held to be a function of beliefs; respectively, behavioural beliefs, normative beliefs and control beliefs. According to the model, it is necessary to change these underlying beliefs if behaviour is to change.

Prochaska's Stages of Change Model[11] has three dimensions: the stages through which people pass when changing their behaviour, the processes which they utilise to make changes, and the levels at which change occur. The most recent version of the model postulates five stages of change: precontemplation (not seriously thinking about change); contemplation (seriously thinking about change); preparation (ready to change); action (attempting to change) and maintenance (change achieved). Successful change involves progressing through these stages, from precontemplation to maintenance. Movement through the stages is a cyclical rather than a linear process and relapse is the rule rather than the exception. Most individuals do not, however, give up after relapsing, but cycle back into the precontemplation stage; a study of smokers cited by Prochaska and DiClemente[12] found that, on average, self-changers made three serious revolutions through the stages of change before they exited into a life relatively free from temptations to smoke. Others get stuck at a particular stage of change.

This report examines the links between knowledge, attitudes and behaviour, but it was not the intention formally to test models. They are, however, referred to when appropriate during discussion of the various health topics in subsequent chapters. Results from the follow-up interviews in 1997 will make it possible to measure any changes in behaviour, and to explore how these relate to intentions expressed in 1996. That analysis will be informed by the models of change.

1.4 The aims and design of the survey

The HEMS was established as one method of monitoring progress towards HON targets in the area of health and health-related knowledge, attitudes and behaviour among the adult population in England. It builds on previous health and lifestyle surveys carried out by the HEA. The aim of the 1995 HEMS survey was to collect data which would provide a benchmark for the measurement of trends from 1995 to 2000 and beyond, and many of the suggested health promotion indicators were measured for the first time by the 1995 survey. They have been modified, not only in the light of the HEMS findings, but also as a result of work being undertaken simultaneously by specialist project teams within the HEA to develop and update the suggested framework in their own areas of specialism.

The target population for the survey was adults aged 16–74 living in private households in England. A probability sample of addresses was selected from the Postcode Address File (PAF). Interviewers contacted each address and identified all residents aged 16–74. Adults within this age-range were listed in order of age, eldest first, and one adult in the household was selected at random to be interviewed. A more detailed description of the sample design and selection procedure is given in Appendix A.

All those who agreed to take part in the survey were interviewed for about an hour about their health-related knowledge, attitudes and behaviour. The interviews were carried out using lap-top computers. Respondents aged 16–54 were asked to do a self-completion module asking about their use of and attitudes towards drugs. The module also included a few questions on sexual health. For this part of the interview, the interviewer handed the lap-top to the respondent, who keyed in the answers him or herself.

Proxy interviews were carried out where the selected person was unable to be interviewed or was absent from home for the entire field period. These interviews lasted 10–15 minutes and concentrated on health-related behaviour.

Fieldwork was carried out in May and June 1996. Seventy four per cent of those eligible to do so agreed to take part in the survey, making a total of 4,645 interviews. An additional 2% (145 selected persons) were interviewed by proxy. Among informants aged 16–54, 98% did the self-completion module. More details of response are given in Appendix A.

In order to allow comparison with other sources of data, questions from relevant surveys, such as the Health and Lifestyles Survey, the Health Survey for England, the General Household Survey, the British Crime Survey and the Wellcome Trust Survey of Sexual Attitudes and Lifestyles, were used where possible. The *Health of the Nation* Key Areas and risk factors, and the related questionnaire topics are shown in Figure 1.1; the full and proxy questionnaires are included in Appendix E.

1.5 Characteristics of the sample

The characteristics of the sample are described only briefly here; they are discussed in more detail in Appendix A. A higher proportion of men than of women were defined on the basis of their own current or last job as belonging to the professional and managerial social classes. Men were also more likely than women to be qualified to a higher level, to be in paid employment in the week prior to interview, and to report a gross annual household income of £30,000 or more. The tables and charts in the rest of the report usually show topics analysed by sex, age and social class. The other characteristics listed in Table 1.1 are discussed only when they are of particular interest. **(Table 1.1)**

Notes and references

1. Bridgwood A et al. *Health in England 1995: what people know, what people think, what people do*. HMSO (London 1996).

2. Department of Health. *The Health of the Nation: a strategy for health in England*. HMSO (London 1992).

3. Department of Health. *The Health of the Nation one year on: a report on the progress of the Health of the Nation*. HMSO (London 1994). Department of Health. *Fit for the future: a second report on the progress of the Health of the Nation*. HMSO (London 1995).

4. An initial set of *Population Health Outcome Indicators* was published in 1993 by the Department of Health. They are now produced annually, with new indicators added each year.

5. Department of Health. *Health-related behaviour: an epidemiological overview*. HMSO (London 1996). *Epidemiological Overviews* present data on recent trends in specific areas of health. Overviews on coronary heart disease and stroke were published in 1994 and one on asthma in 1995. The latest in the series, on health-related behaviour, was published in 1996. All were published by HMSO.

6. White A et al. *Survey for England 1991*. HMSO (London 1993); Breeze E et al. *Health Survey for England 1992*. HMSO (London 1994); Bennett N et al. *Health Survey for England 1993*. HMSO (London 1995); Colhoun H et al. *Health Survey for England 1994*. HMSO (London 1996).

7. Central Drugs Coordination Unit. *Tackling drugs together: a strategy for England 1995-1998*. HMSO (London 1995). Drug use was discussed in the *Health of the Nation* White Paper, but mainly in relation to HIV/AIDS.

8. Department of Health/Department of the Environment. *UK Environmental Action Plan Cm 3323*. HMSO (London 1996).

9. Ajzen I. The theory of planned behaviour. *Organisational Behaviour and Human Decision Processes*, 1991, vol. 50, pp. 179–211.

10. Fishbein M and Ajzen I. *Belief, attitudes, intentions and behaviour: an introduction to theory and research*. Addison-Wesley (Boston 1975).

11. Prochaska J O. Strong and weak principles for progressing from precontemplation to action on the basis of twelve problem behaviours. *Health Psychology*, 1994, vol. 13, pp. 46–51.

12. Prochaska J O and DiClemente C C. Towards a comprehensive model of change. In Miller W R and Heather N (eds). *Treating addictive behaviours*. Plenum Press (New York 1986).

Annex to Chapter 1

Health of the Nation Objectives and Targets

The *Health of the Nation* key areas which are referred to in the HEMS report are listed below together with the objectives and targets.

Key area: Coronary heart disease

Objective:

To reduce the level of ill-health and death caused by coronary heart disease and stroke, and the risk factors associated with them.

Main targets
Coronary heart disease and stroke

A: To reduce death rates for both CHD and stroke in people under 65 by at least 40% by the year 2000 (from 58 per 100,000 population in 1990 to no more than 35 per 100,000 for CHD, and from 12.5 per 100,000 population in 1990 to no more than 7.5 per 100,000 for stroke).

B: To reduce the death rate for CHD in people aged 65–74 by at least 30% by the year 2000 (from 899 per 100,000 population in 1990 to no more than 629 per 100,000).

C: To reduce the death rate for stroke in people aged 65–74 by at least 40% by the year 2000 (from 265 per 100,000 population in 1990 to no more than 159 per 100,000).

Smoking

D: To reduce the prevalence of cigarette smoking in men and women aged 16 and over to no more than 20% by the year 2000 (a reduction of at least 35% in men and 29% in women, from a prevalence in 1990 of 31% and 28% respectively).

Diet and Nutrition

E: To reduce the average percentage of food energy derived by the population from saturated fatty acids by at least 35% by 2005 (from 17% in 1990 to no more than 11%).

F: To reduce the average percentage of food energy derived by the population from total fat by at least 12% by 2005 (from about 40% in 1990 to no more than 35%).

Obesity

G: To reduce the percentage of men and women aged 16–64 who are obese by at least 25% for men and at least 33% for women by 2005 (from 8% for men and 12% for women in 1986/87 to no more than 6% and 8% respectively).

Blood Pressure

H: To reduce mean systolic blood pressure in the adult population by at least 5mm Hg by 2005.

Alcohol

I: To reduce the proportion of men drinking more than 21 units of alcohol per week from 28% in 1990 to 18% by 2005, and the proportion of women drinking more than 14 units of alcohol per week from 11% in 1990 to 7% by 2005.

Key area: Cancer

Objectives:

To reduce ill-health and death caused by breast and cervical cancer.

To reduce ill-health and death caused by skin cancers – by increasing awareness of the need to avoid excessive skin exposure to ultra-violet light.

To reduce ill-health and death caused by lung cancer – and other conditions associated with tobacco consumption throughout the population.

Main targets
Breast cancer

A: To reduce the death rate for breast cancer in the population invited for screening by at least 25% by the year 2000 (from 95.1 per 100,000 population in 1990 to no more than 71.3 per 100,000).

Cervical cancer

B: To reduce the incidence of invasive cervical cancer by at least 20% by the year 2000 (from 15 per 100,000 population in 1986 to no more than 12 per 100,000).

Skin cancer

C: To halt the year-on-year increase of skin cancer by 2005.

Lung cancer

D: To reduce the death rate for lung cancer by at least 30% in men under 75 and 15% in women under 75 by 2010 (from 60 per 100,000 for men and 24.1 per 100,000 for women in 1990 to no more than 42 and 20.5 respectively).

E: To reduce the prevalence of cigarette smoking in men and women aged 16 and over to no more than 20% by the year 2000 (a reduction of at least 35% in men and 29% in women, from a prevalence in 1990 of 31% and 28% respectively).

F: In addition to the overall reduction in prevalence, at least a third of women smokers to stop smoking at the start of their pregnancy by the year 2000.

G: To reduce the consumption of cigarettes by at least 40% by the year 2000 (from 98 billion manufactured cigarettes per year in 1990 to 59 billion).

H: To reduce smoking prevalence among 11–15 year olds by at least 33% by 1994 (from about 8% in 1988 to less than 6%).

Health in England 1996 : What people know, what people think, what people do

Key area: HIV/AIDS and sexual health

Objectives:

To reduce the incidence of HIV infection.

To reduce the incidence of other sexually transmitted diseases.

To develop further and strengthen monitoring and surveillance.

To provide effective services for diagnosis and treatment of HIV and other STDs.

To reduce the number of unwanted pregnancies.

To ensure the provision of effective family planning services for those people who want them.

Main targets
HIV/AIDS and Sexual Health

A: To reduce the incidence of gonorrhoea among men and women aged 15–64 by at least 20% by 1995 (from 61 new cases per 100,000 population in 1990 to no more than 49 new cases per 100,000).

B: To reduce the rate of conceptions amongst the under 16s by at least 50% by the year 2000 (from 9.5 per 1,000 girls aged 13–15 in 1989 to no more than 4.8).

C: To reduce the percentage of injecting drug-misusers who report sharing injecting equipment in the previous four weeks by at least 50% by 1997, and by at least a further 50% by the year 2000 (from 20% in 1990 to no more than 10% by 1997 and no more than 5% by the year 2000).

2 Smoking and drinking

Summary of main findings

- Thirty one per cent of men and 29% of women were current cigarette smokers. The mean number of cigarettes smoked per day was 12.9 for women and 15.3 for men. (Section 2.2).

- Sixty five per cent of current smokers said they would like to give up smoking, but 56% would find it 'very difficult' or 'fairly difficult' to give up and 45% said they were unlikely to give up. (Sections 2.3.1, 2.3.2 and 2.3.5).

- 'Will-power' was the method most commonly used by those who had successfully stopped smoking. (Section 2.3.4).

- Over three quarters of parents thought the health of their child was affected by people smoking in the home. (Section 2.4).

- The overwhelming majority of parents (92%) did not want their children to smoke. (Section 2.4).

- Seventy seven per cent of adults aged 16–74 who had a job worked for an employer who operated a no-smoking policy. (Section 2.5).

- Alcohol consumption was highest in the 16–24 age-group. The mean weekly number of units of alcohol consumed by women was 7.7 compared with 18.0 consumed by men. (Section 2.6.1).

- Reported levels of consumption were higher in 1996 than in 1995 for two groups; men aged 65–74 and women aged 16–24. (Section 2.6.1).

- Seventeen per cent of adults who drank at least once or twice a week would like to drink less. (Section 2.6.2).

continued

- **Eighty four per cent of men and 81% of women had heard about measuring alcohol in units. Forty three per cent of respondents who had heard about measuring alcohol in units were able to give the correct number of units in a glass of wine and in a pint of beer and 34% in a single pub measure of spirits. (Section 2.7).**

- **Twenty six per cent of respondents had not heard about the changes to a daily benchmark of between 2 and 3 units or less a day for women and between 3 and 4 units or less a day for men and 38% said the changes were of no interest. Only a small proportion (14%) said they did feel confused about the changes and 22% did not feel confused. (Section 2.8).**

2.1 Introduction and background

Smoking and drinking were both identified in the *Health of the Nation* White Paper[1] as risk factors for coronary heart disease (CHD) and stroke. Smoking was identified as a risk factor in its own right while drinking is a risk factor in that it contributes to raised blood pressure level. Smoking is an important cause of ill-health and mortality and imposes significant costs on society, for example in terms of health care cost and human suffering. Those who smoke are at greater risk than non-smokers of lung cancer, coronary heart disease, chronic bronchitis and emphysema, stroke, atherosclerotic peripheral vascular disease and cancers of the oral cavity, larynx and oesophagus [2,3].

While it is generally agreed that smoking is bad for health, the links between drinking and health are not so clear cut and there has been a lot of debate about the risks and benefits of drinking. The *Health of the Nation* White Paper stated that drinking fewer than 21 units per week by men and 14 units per week by women is unlikely to cause health problems[1]. However, prolonged heavy drinking is associated with raised blood pressure[4], cirrhosis of the liver, increased risk of some forms of cancer [5], and psychological and social problems[5].

In 1994 the government set up an Inter-Departmental group to look at sensible drinking levels, and at the end of 1995 changed the recommendations for 'sensible drinking' from 21 units per week for men and 14 for women to a recommended daily benchmark of between 3 and 4 units or less per day for men and between 2 and 3 units or less per day for women[6]. The *Health of the Nation* targets have not yet been changed in accordance with this and the questions on HEMS still reflect the old 'sensible' drinking levels.

Men over the age of 40 and post-menopausal women who drink a moderate[7] amount of alcohol have been found to have a lower risk of cardiovascular disease and ischaemic stroke than both heavy drinkers and non-drinkers[5]. The Sensible Drinking report[6] concluded that, for people in these age-groups, alcohol does give protection against the development of coronary heart disease; the maximum benefit is gained from drinking between 1 and 2 units of alcohol per day and there is no additional benefit in drinking more than 2 units a day.

The *Health of the Nation* targets aim to reduce the prevalence of smoking and harmful alcohol consumption. Reducing the prevalence of smoking means both reducing the proportion of people who start smoking and persuading current smokers to give up. This chapter looks at respondents' current behaviour and attitudes towards smoking and drinking. To be successful health promotion campaigns need to be properly targeted and the chapter finishes by looking at the characteristics of people who drink and smoke heavily.

2.2 Prevalence of smoking and levels of consumption

Over the last few decades smoking prevalence has been decreasing among adults[8] although the proportion of teenage girls who start smoking has recently appeared to increase[9]. HEMS 1996 measures smoking prevalence using the same questions as many other surveys, such as the General Household Survey (GHS) and the Health Survey for England; smokers are asked how many cigarettes they smoke a day at weekends and on week days.

Figure 2.1 shows the prevalence of smoking by age and sex and compares the overall prevalence with that reported on the 1995 HEMS survey. Thirty one per cent of men and 29% of women were current cigarette smokers; prevalence was highest among the 16–24 age-group and decreased with age, while the proportion of ex-regular smokers increased with age. There was no significant difference between 1995 and 1996 in the overall proportion of people aged 16–74 who smoked. (**Figure 2.1 and Tables 2.1–2.3**)

Figure 2.1 Prevalence of cigarette smoking by age and sex: adults aged 16–74

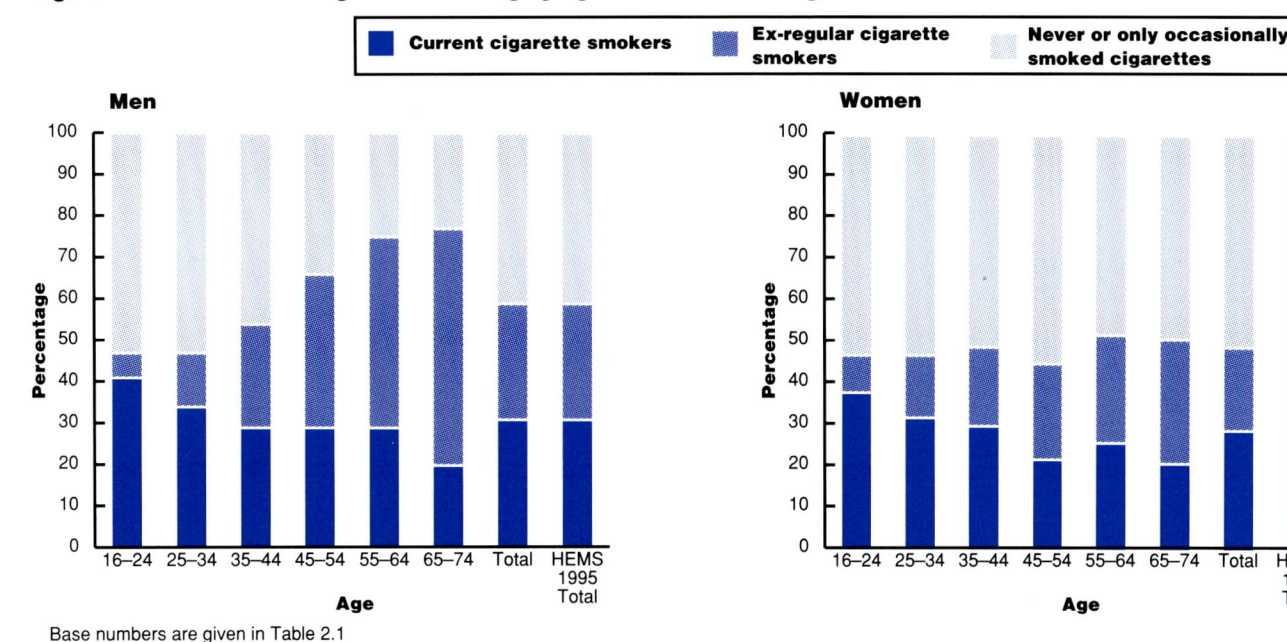

Base numbers are given in Table 2.1

The mean number of cigarettes smoked per day was lower for women than it was for men: 12.9 compared with 15.3. Ex-smokers were asked how many cigarettes a day they used to smoke; just over half (52%) used to smoke 20 or more cigarettes per day compared with 31% of current smokers. Ex-smokers may overestimate the number of cigarettes they used to smoke while current smokers may underestimate the number they now smoke. There was no significant difference in the mean number of cigarettes smoked per week between 1995 and 1996. (**Tables 2.4–2.5**)

2.3 Giving up smoking

2.3.1 Wanting to give up smoking

HEA suggested health promotion indicator: The proportion of regular smokers who want to give up smoking

One aspect of reducing the prevalence of smoking is to persuade current smokers to give up smoking, and a lot of health promotion work involves trying to help smokers quit. Both Fishbein and Ajzen's Theory of Reasoned Action and Prochaska and DiClemente's Stages of Change model have been used successfully in health promotion, particularly with regard to smoking, to devise strategies to help people to change their behaviour[10]. The contemplation stage described in Prochaska and DiClemente's model involves thinking about changing behaviour, while Fishbein and Ajzen say that people need to have the desire to change their behaviour in order to succeed. Sixty five per cent of current smokers said that they would like to quit, not significantly different from the 1995 survey. As in 1995, smokers aged 25–44 were more likely than smokers in other age-groups to say that they would like to give up smoking, possibly because younger smokers feel they will have time to give up later and the older smokers may be the ones who have already tried to give up and failed. (**Figure 2.2 and Tables 2.6–7**)

People who smoked fewer than 10 cigarettes per day were less likely than those who smoked more to say they would like to give up smoking: 57% compared with 70% of those who smoked 10–19 cigarettes per day and 69% of those who smoked 20 or more per day. (**Table 2.8**)

2.3.2 Perceived dependence on smoking

HEMS included a question designed to measure perceived dependence on smoking. Smokers were asked how easy they would find it to go without smoking for a whole day and over half (56%) would find it 'fairly difficult' or 'very difficult', not significantly different from 1995. Smokers aged 16 to 24 were more likely than older smokers to say that they would find it easy to go without smoking for a whole day. This lower perceived dependence on smoking may explain why smokers in this age-

Figure 2.2 Percentage of current smokers who would like to give up smoking by age: current smokers aged 16–74

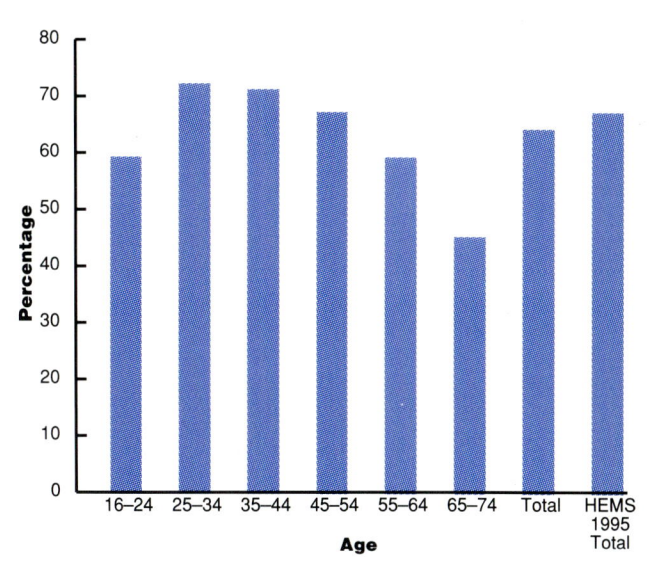

Base numbers are given in Table 2.6

Health in England 1996 : What people know, what people think, what people do 15

Figure 2.3 How easy or difficult smokers would find it to go without smoking for a whole day by number of cigarettes smoked per day: current smokers aged 16–74

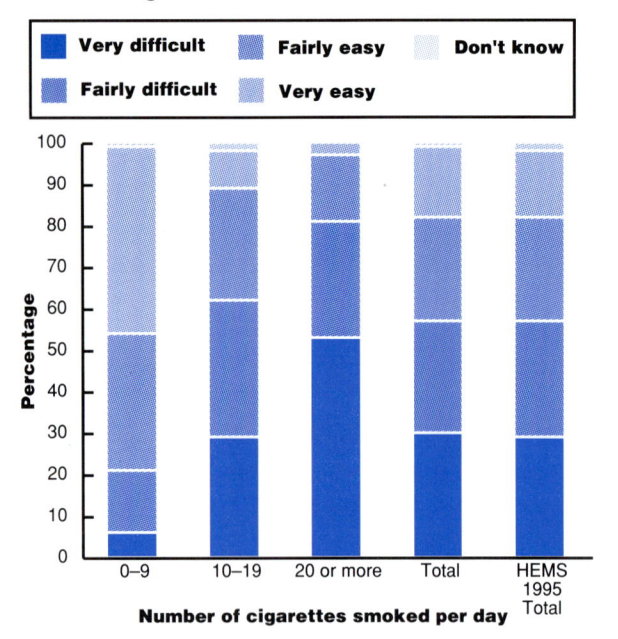

Base numbers are given in Table 2.10

Figure 2.4 Percentage of current smokers who have tried to give up smoking by age: current smokers aged 16–74

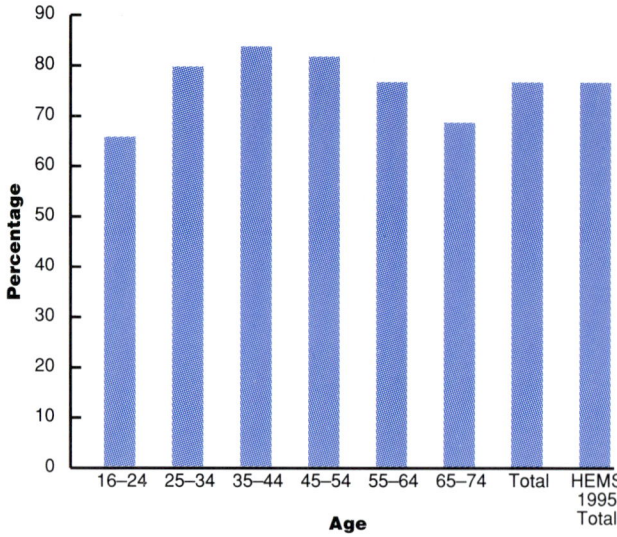

Base numbers are given in Table 2.11

group were less likely to want to give up smoking. Those smoking fewer than 10 cigarettes per day were much more likely than heavier smokers to say they would find it 'very easy' or 'fairly easy'; 78% did so compared with only 19% of those who smoked 20 or more cigarettes a day. **(Figure 2.3 and Tables 2.9–2.10)**

2.3.3. Attempting to give up smoking

> HEA suggested health promotion indicator: The proportion of smokers who have tried to give up in the last 12 months

According to Prochaska and DiClemente's Stages of Change model, smokers who would like to give up smoking may try to give up several times before finally succeeding. Smokers were asked if they had ever tried to give up smoking and just over three quarters (77%) said they had; those in the 16–24 and in the 65–74 age-groups were less likely than other smokers to say they had. Those who smoked fewer than 10 cigarettes per day (69%) were less likely than other smokers (80%) to have tried to give up. Table 2.7 shows that smokers who had previously tried to give up smoking were more likely than those who had never tried to say they would like to give up. **(Figure 2.4 and Tables 2.7 and 2.11)**

Almost half (48%) of current smokers who had tried to give up had done so for less than a month, 27% for less than a week. At the other extreme, 21% of smokers had given up for a year or more before starting again. Smokers who currently smoked 10 or more cigarettes per day were more likely than those who smoked fewer than 10 a day to have given up for less than a month while just over a third (34%) of smokers who smoked fewer than 10 cigarettes per day had previously given up for a year or more. **(Figure 2.5 and Tables 2.12–2.13)**

2.3.4 People who have succeeded in stopping smoking

As well as looking at smokers who had tried to give up, HEMS looked at people who had succeeded in giving up smoking. Almost three quarters (74%) of ex-smokers had given up five years or more ago. This does not differ significantly from the findings in the HEMS 1995 report. Ex-smokers were asked to give the main reasons why they had stopped smoking. The most common reason, mentioned by 55% of ex-smokers, was 'health reasons'. Those aged 35–44 were most likely to cite 'family reasons' for giving up; 21% of men and 19% of women in this age group did so. In addition, 18% of women of this age gave pregnancy as a reason for stopping smoking. The oldest age-group was most likely to mention cost; almost a quarter (23%) gave this as the main reason. **(Tables 2.14–2.16)**

Figure 2.5 Length of time smokers gave up for: current smokers aged 16–74 who had previously tried to give up

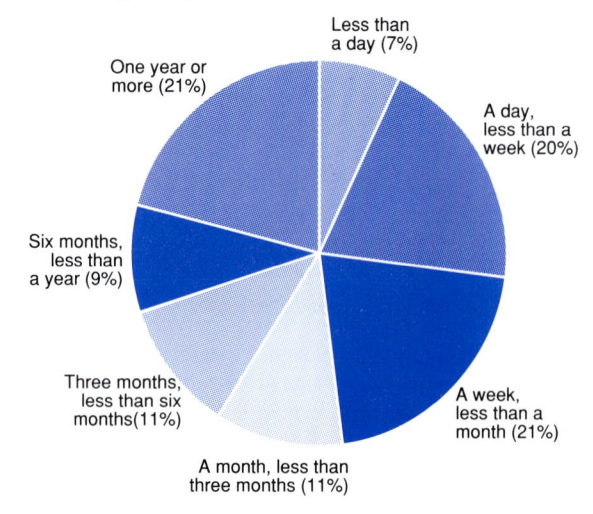

- Less than a day (7%)
- A day, less than a week (20%)
- A week, less than a month (21%)
- A month, less than three months (11%)
- Three months, less than six months (11%)
- Six months, less than a year (9%)
- One year or more (21%)

Base numbers are given in Table 2.12

Both ex-smokers and current smokers who had tried to give up were asked what methods they had used to help them. Will-power was the method most commonly mentioned both by those who had successfully given up and those who were still smokers; over 80% of both groups cited this. Prochaska and DiClemente said that it was important that people felt they had control and so will-power is an important aspect of giving up smoking. Over a quarter of current smokers who had tried to give up and who smoked 20 or more cigarettes per day had tried using either nicotine chewing gum (25%) or a nicotine patch (27%) but only 7% and 6% respectively of ex-smokers who had smoked more than 20 a day had used these methods. This may, of course, be a cohort effect as methods such as nicotine chewing gum and nicotine patches were probably not so widely available at the time when some ex-smokers gave up smoking. **(Table 2.17).**

2.3.5 Intentions to stop smoking

According to Fishbein and Azjen's Theory of Reasoned Action intentions play an important part in changing people's behaviour, as they indicate how much people are willing to try to change. Fishbein and Azjen claim that the stronger the intention to change the more likely it is that a person will change his or her behaviour[11]. In order to assess smokers' intentions, the interviewer showed them a card and asked which of the following statements applied to them:

- I intend to give up smoking within the next month
- I intend to give up smoking within the next six months
- I intend to give up smoking within the next year
- I intend to give up smoking but not in the next year
- I'm unlikely to give up smoking[12]

Forty five per cent of smokers said that they were unlikely to give up smoking. It is not possible to make direct comparisons with the HEMS 1995 data as the question wording changed between the two years.[13]

Almost a quarter (23%) of smokers said that they 'intended to give up but not in the next year'. The proportion of smokers who said they were unlikely to give up smoking increased with age from only a quarter (24%) of those aged 16–24 to over three quarters (77%) of those aged 65–74. A higher proportion (55%) of people who smoked 20 or more cigarettes per day than of people who smoked fewer than 10 cigarettes per day (37%) said that they were unlikely to give up smoking. **(Tables 2.18–2.19)**

Given that the majority of smokers said they would like to give up, the high proportion saying they are unlikely to do so suggests that they may be being realistic. Amost half (45%) of smokers who said they would like to give up did intend to do so within the next year, although almost a third (32%) thought they would be unlikely to give up. A large majority of those who did not want to give up smoking (94%) either thought that they were unlikely to give up smoking at all or that they would give up but not in the next year. The follow-up survey in 1997 will allow exploration of the association between intentions and attempts to give up. **(Table 2.20)**

2.4 Smoking and children

> HEA suggested health promotion indicator: The proportion of parents with children aged under 16 living in the household who are aware that passive smoking is harmful to children

The *Health of the Nation* White Paper stated that 'exposure to environmental tobacco smoke has been linked with respiratory illness in infants and young children' and the HEA have developed an indicator to reflect this. Respondents with a child under 16 in the household who had previously said that they, another household member, or visitors, smoked in the house were asked how much they thought the health of their child was affected by this. Over three quarters of parents with children aged under 16 living in the household thought that the health of their child was affected by smoking in the home; 15% thought it was affected 'a great deal'; 28% 'quite a lot'; and 35% 'a little'. The proportion of parents who thought smoking did affect the health of their children decreased with age; among 16–24 year-olds, 87% thought that smoking affected the health of their children, compared with 73% of people aged 45 or over. Current smokers were more likely than people who had never smoked (87%, compared with 68%) to think that smoking in the home affected the health of their children. **(Tables 2.21–2.23)**

Respondents who had children aged 9–15 were asked which of the following two statements described how they felt about their children smoking:

- I don't want them to smoke
- It's up to them whether they smoke

The majority (92%) of parents did not want their children to smoke; there was no significant difference by age and sex. Parents in Social Classes IV and V were slightly less likely than parents in Social Class I and II to say they did not want their children to smoke. Eighty five per cent of parents who were smokers themselves did not want their children to smoke. **(Tables 2.24–2.26)**

2.5 Smoking in the workplace

> HEA suggested health promotion indicator: The proportion of the working population whose workplace operates a smoking policy

The *Health of the Nation* states that a large majority of employees should be covered by a no-smoking policy by 1995. In 1996, 77% of HEMS respondents who were working worked for employers who operated such a policy. Women were more likely than men to work for an employer who operated a no-smoking policy. This probably reflects the difference in the type of work men and women do. Men in non-manual occupations were more likely than those in manual occupations to have a no-smoking policy. Among women it was those in Social Classes IV and V who were least likely to have a no-smoking policy. Employees working in a large establishment (89%) were most likely and the self-employed with no employees least likely (33%) to have a no-smoking policy. The findings on workplace no-smoking policy were not significantly different from those reported in 1995. **(Tables 2.27– 2.29)**[14]

2.6 Consumption of alcohol

2.6.1 Consumption of alcohol

Measuring the consumption of alcohol in units is much more difficult than measuring the consumption of cigarettes. The methodology used by HEMS is the same as that used on the GHS and on the Health Survey for England. Respondents were asked about six types of alcoholic drink, how often they consumed each type of drink and how much they usually drank on any one day. This information was used to estimate the number of units consumed per week[15]. It is known, however, that surveys which rely on reported behaviour underestimate the amount of alcohol consumed when compared to estimates based on alcohol sales[16]. People are particularly likely to underestimate the amount they drink at home and may genuinely find it difficult to remember the amount they have drunk on any one occasion.

As would be expected from other survey research on drinking, Figure 2.6 shows that women's consumption of alcohol was much lower than men's: the mean weekly number of units consumed by women was 7.7 compared with 18.0 for men. Twenty seven per cent of women but only 14% of men were non-drinkers or drank less than one unit per week. Almost a third of men reported drinking more than 21 units a week compared with just under a fifth (17%) of women who reported drinking 15 units or more. Drinking consumption for both men and women was higher in the 16–24 age group than it was in the other age-groups. The mean consumption in this age-group was 22.4 units a week for men and 14.4 for women. **(Figure 2.6 and Table 2.34)**

Figure 2.6 Mean weekly consumption of alcohol in units by age: adults aged 16–74

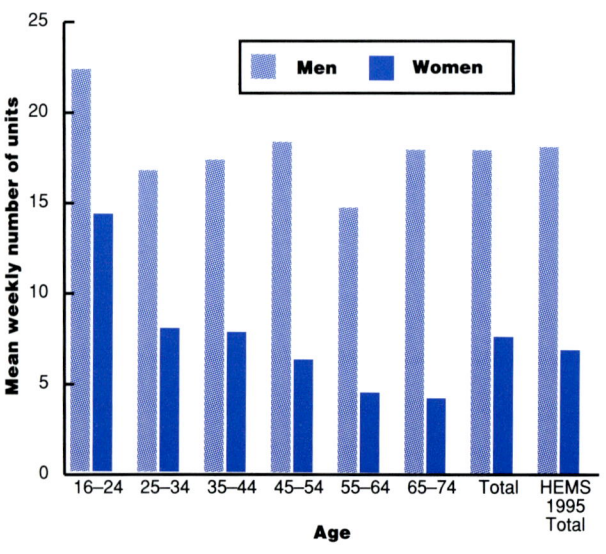

Base numbers are given in Table 2.34

For men there were differences in the pattern of alcohol consumption in different social classes; those in Social Classes IV and V had a mean weekly alcohol consumption of 20.9 units compared with 15.1 units for those in Social Class III (Non-Manual). There were no significant differences for women. **(Table 2.35)**

The general pattern of consumption reported in 1996 was the same as in 1995 but there were significant differences between the two years for two groups; among men aged 65–74 the mean weekly number of units reported was 11.7 in 1995 and 18.0 in 1996 while women aged 16–24 reported a mean consumption of 9.9 in 1995 and 14.4 in 1996.

As there is a wide variation on the amounts people drink the mean number of units consumed per week is derived from a skewed distribution, that is, a high proportion of people consume a small number of units per week while a few people drink a lot. This is illustrated by the difference between the mean and the median weekly number of units shown in Table 2.34. Means of alcohol consumption should generally be treated with some caution but particularly in the case of HEMS 1996 data where there were a few very high reported consumption rates for women aged 16–24 and men aged 65–74[17] which have resulted in a high mean for these groups. If these cases are removed from the data and the means recalculated, the mean for women aged 16–24 is 12.4 units while for men aged 65–74 it is 15.8 units. These are still significantly higher than the means reported in 1995 for these groups. **(Table 2.34)**

HEMS 1996 included separate questions on consumption of 'alcopops'; these questions were not asked on the 1995 survey. This change in the question wording could account for some of the difference in consumption between the two years, especially among the younger age-group. It is important to note that the proportion of drinkers in this age-group has not increased significantly between the two years so it cannot be concluded from this data that the availability of 'alcopops' has encouraged more young people to start drinking.

The proportions drinking 'alcopops' decreased with age; 62% of those aged 16–24 reported drinking them in the last 12 months compared to only 6% of those aged 45–74. Women aged 16–24 were more likely than men in the same age-group to have drunk them (72% compared with 55%). Sixteen per cent of women aged 16–24 said they had drunk 'alcopops' at least once or twice a week, another 16% drunk them once or twice a month and 23% had only drunk them once or twice in the last 12 months. Figure 2.8 compares the percentage of people aged 16–24 who had consumed different types of alcoholic drink in the last 12 months. Although 'alcopops' were a commonly consumed drink amongst this age-group, higher proportions reported drinking beer, spirits and wine. 'Alcopops' accounted for as much as a fifth (21%) of total alcohol consumption of women aged 16–24 compared with only 12% of alcohol consumed by men in this age-group. **(Figures 2.7–2.8 and Tables 2.36–2.38)**

2.6.2 Respondents' assessment of their drinking

As stated earlier, the models of change state that people need to have the desire to change their behaviour in order to change it successfully. Respondents who drank at least once or twice a week were asked to say whether they thought they drank:

- about the right amount
- or would you like to drink less?[18]

The majority of adults thought that they drank about the right amount; 83% of respondents gave this answer, compared with 17% who said they would like to drink less. There was no difference between the proportions of men and women choosing each option but a higher proportion of people aged 16–24 (26%) than of people in the older age-groups said that they would like to

18 Health in England 1996 : What people know, what people think, what people do

Figure 2.7 Percentage consuming alcoholic soft drinks in the last 12 months by age and sex: adults aged 16–74

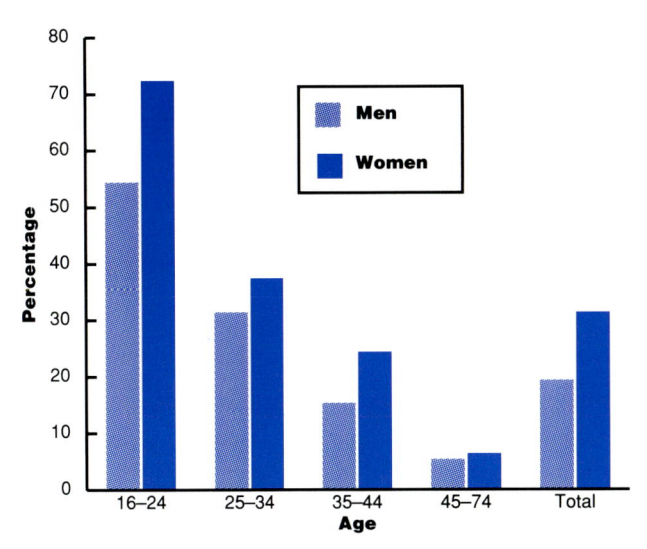

Base numbers are given in Table 2.36

Figure 2.8 Percentage consuming different types of alcoholic drinks in the last 12 months: adults aged 16–24

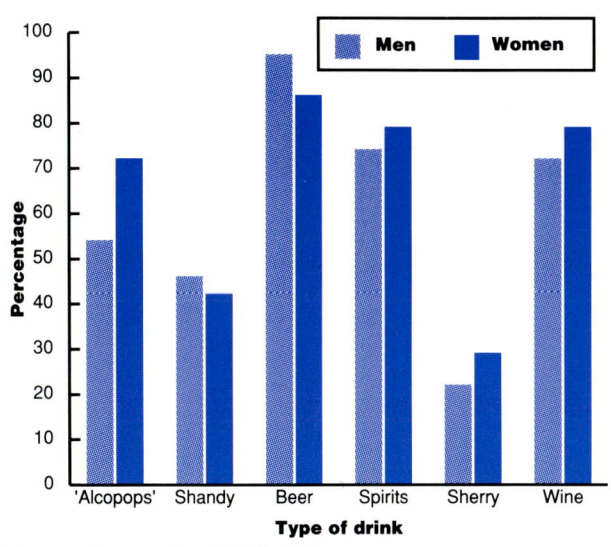

Base numbers are given in Table 2.38

drink less. This probably reflects the higher consumption levels among this age-group. The heaviest drinkers were most likely to say they would like to drink less; 45% of men consuming 51 units per week or more and 54% of women consuming 36 units per week or more did so, compared with 13% of men who drank 11–21 units and 13% of women who drank 8-14 units a week. (**Figure 2.9, Tables 2.39–2.40**)

Respondents who said they would like to drink less were asked whether and when they intended to cut down on their drinking and were shown a card with a similar set of answers to those used for the smoking section of the interview:

- I intend to cut down on my drinking within the next month
- I intend to cut down on my drinking within the next six months

Figure 2.9 Percentage who would like to drink less by the amount of alcohol consumed per week and sex: adults aged 16–74

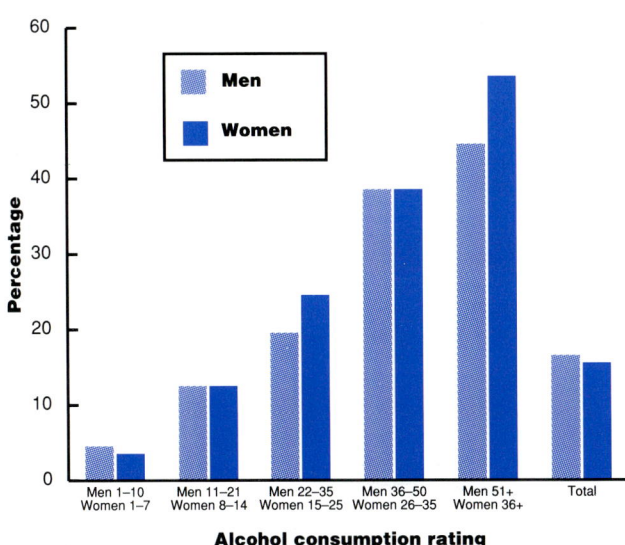

Base numbers are given in Table 2.40

- I intend to cut down on my drinking within the next year
- I intend to cut down on my drinking, not in the next year
- I'm unlikely to cut down on my drinking

Almost half of respondents who would like to drink less thought they were unlikely to cut down, while a fifth intended to cut down in the next month. Respondents aged 45–74 were more likely than younger respondents to say they were unlikely to cut down on their drinking; perhaps because they feel it is too late to change or too difficult. (**Tables 2.41– 2.43**)

2.7 Knowledge of alcohol units

> HEMS suggested health promotion indicator: The proportion of people who have heard of units that can correctly state the number of units in a glass of wine, pint of beer and a single pub measure of spirits

In order for people to monitor their levels of drinking and follow the recommended daily benchmarks of between 2 and 3 units or less per day for women and between 3 and 4 units or less per day for men they need to understand what is meant by a unit of alcohol and how many units different drinks contain. The majority of men (84%) and women (81%) had heard about measuring alcohol in units. Among women, there was a slight increase in the proportion who had heard about measuring alcohol in units from 77% in 1995 to 81% in 1996 and this was the case for all age groups. (**Table 2.44**)

Having heard of measuring alcohol in units did not necessarily mean that the respondent knew how many units there were in different types of drink. Over a third of those who had heard of units did not know how many there were in a glass of wine, a pint of beer or a single pub measure of spirits and over a fifth gave the incorrect answers. Forty three per cent correctly said that there was one unit in a glass of wine, 43% said that there were two units in a pint of beer and 34% that there was one unit in a single pub

Health in England 1996 : What people know, what people think, what people do

Figure 2.10 Percentage who had heard of units of alcohol and correctly indentified the number in specified drinks by sex: adults aged 16–74 who had heard of units of alcohol

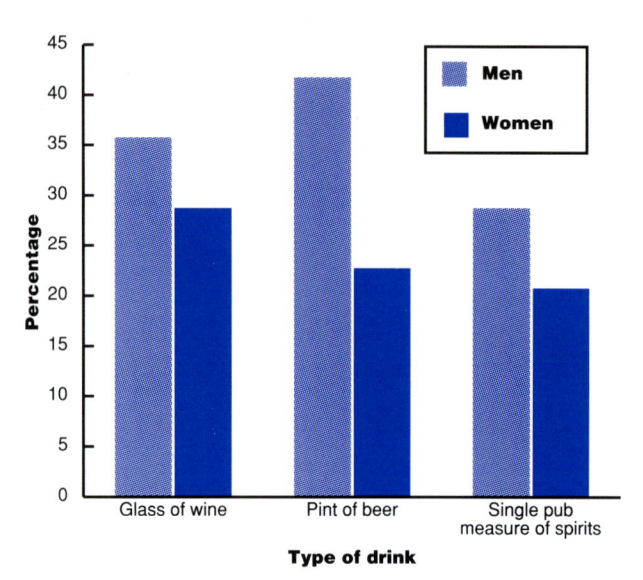

Base numbers are given in Table 2.45

measure of spirits. Men were more likely than women, respondents in the younger age-groups (16–44) more likely than those in the older age-groups, and respondents in Social Classes I and II more likely than those in the other social classes to give the correct number of units in each drink. **(Figure 2.10 and Tables 2.45–2.47)**

Respondents consuming fairly high levels of alcohol were more likely to know how many units were contained in different types of drink. Sixty one per cent of men who drank between 22 and 35 units per week stated correctly the number of units in a pint of beer compared with 34% of male non-drinkers. Knowledge of alcohol units per drink was lowest among non-drinkers and among men drinking fewer than ten units per week and women drinking fewer than seven per week. **(Figure 2.11 and Table 2.48)**

2.8 Attitudes to changes in 'sensible drinking levels'

As stated earlier, the Inter-Departmental working group on sensible drinking suggested a daily benchmark of between 2 and 3 units of alcohol or less per day for women and between 3 and 4 units or less per day for men. Respondents were asked what their attitude was to the changes; they were shown a card and asked to say which one of the following statements applied to them:

- I haven't heard anything about the changes
- I feel confused about the changes
- I don't feel confused about the changes
- It is of no interest to me

Twenty six per cent of respondents had not heard about the changes and 38% said the changes were of no interest. Only a small proportion (14%) said they did feel confused about the changes and 22% did not feel confused. Respondents in the 16–24 age-group were more likely than older respondents to say they had not heard anything about the changes, while respondents aged 45–

Figure 2.11 Percentage who had heard of units of alcohol and correctly indentified the number in specified drinks, by alcohol consumption and sex: adults aged 16–74 who had heard of units of alcohol

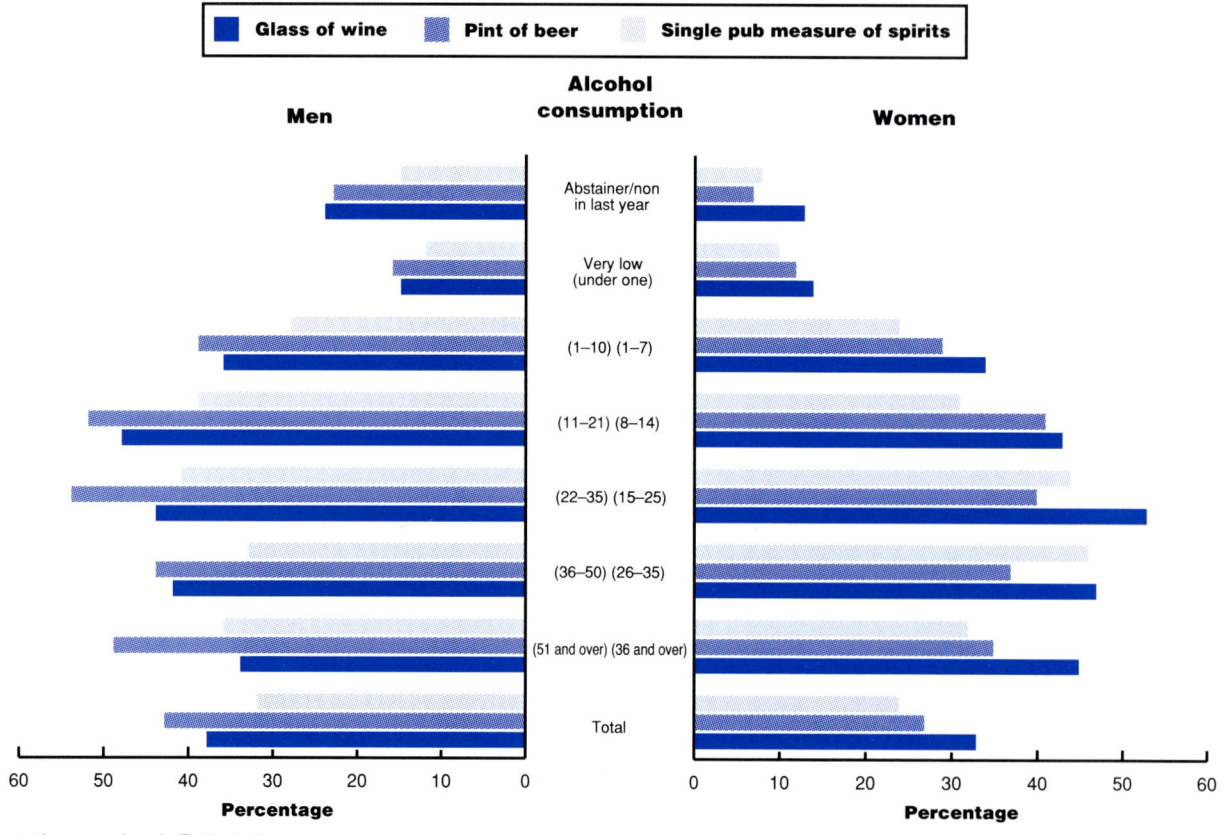

Base numbers are given in Table 2.48

20 Health in England 1996 : What people know, what people think, what people do

Figure 2.12 Attitudes to changes in sensible drinking levels: adults aged 16–74

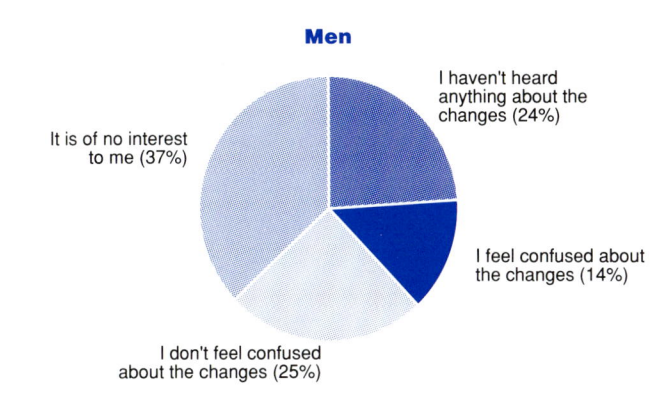

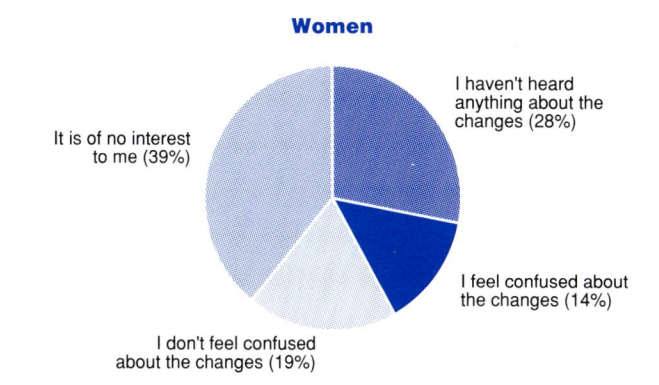

Men
- I haven't heard anything about the changes (24%)
- I feel confused about the changes (14%)
- I don't feel confused about the changes (25%)
- It is of no interest to me (37%)

Women
- I haven't heard anything about the changes (28%)
- I feel confused about the changes (14%)
- I don't feel confused about the changes (19%)
- It is of no interest to me (39%)

Base numbers are given in Table 2.49

54 were the least likely to give this answer. Respondents in the older age-groups were more likely than younger respondents to say it was of no interest to them; 57% of women and 42% of men aged 65–74 said this compared with 27% of women and 30% of men aged 16–24. **(Figure 2.12 and Table 2.49)**

Respondents in Social Classes I and II were most likely not to feel confused about the changes, while respondents in Social Classes IV and V were most likely not to have heard about the changes. **(Table 2.50)**

Respondents who did not drink at all or who drank less than one unit per week were much more likely than other respondents to say the changes were of no interest to them. Men who drank 36–50 units per week and women who drank 26–35 units per week were more likely than other respondents to say they did not feel confused. The majority of respondents who had not heard about measuring alcohol in units said they had not heard anything about the changes (42%) or it was of no interest to them (45%). **(Table 2.51 and Table 2.52)**

2.9 Characteristics of people most likely to smoke and to drink heavily

In health promotion work it is essential to target campaigns to try to persuade people to adopt a more healthy lifestyle; it may be useful to target campaigns at people who are likely to engage in behaviour with a high health risk. Smoking can be identified as a 'high risk' behaviour, as can heavy drinking[19]. People may take part in more than one 'high risk' behaviour; a third of smokers also drank heavily. **(Table 2.53)**

The analysis in both the 1995 and 1996 HEMS looked separately at the characteristics associated with smoking and drinking heavily using cross-tabulation techniques. It is not always easy to see if there are interactions between variables, for example, drinking consumption was highest among people aged 16–24 but the cross-tabulation does not show how much age interacts with other characteristics such as social class or marital status. It is, therefore, interesting to look at how these factors interrelate and this can be done using logistic regression[20], a multivariate statistical technique which can be used to predict the odds of behaviour occurring for different combinations of independent variables (odds refers to the ratio of the probability that the event will occur to the probability that the event will not occur).

The data from the 1995 and 1996 surveys were combined and a logistic regression was carried out to look at the odds of people smoking and drinking heavily. Having run cross-tabulations on the data it was decided to include the following independent variables in the regression:

- sex
- age
- marital status
- economic activity status
- social class
- tenure
- region
- income
- self-reported stress
- whether the respondents had any children aged under 16 in the household

The logistic regression found that, controlling for the other independent variables, region and income did not have a significant effect on whether a person engaged in 'high risk' behaviour but the other variables did.

For each of the variables included in the regression a coefficient is produced which represents the factor by which the odds of a person smoking and drinking heavily increases if the person has that characteristic. One of the categories of the independent variable is defined as a reference category (with a value of 1.00) and the odds are given in comparion to this[21]. If the values of all the variables in the model are the same except for sex, men are 1.73 times more likely (i.e. the odds ratio is 1.73) to smoke and drink heavily than women. Another example would be age where people aged 16–24 are 5.36 times more likely than those aged 65–74 to smoke and to drink heavily assuming all the other variables are held constant. Figure 2.13 shows that age was the most important factor in predicting whether a person smoked and drank heavily. **(Figure 2.13)**

Health in England 1996 : What people know, what people think, what people do

Figure 2.13 Odds of an individual smoking and drinking more than 21 units a week (men) or more than 14 units a week (women)
Adults aged 16–74 (HEMS 1995 and HEMS 1996)

Characteristics	Multiplying factors	95% Confidence intervals
Sex		
Male	1.73*	1.46–2.06
Female	1.00	
Age		
16–24	5.36*	3.47–8.27
25–34	4.17*	2.78–6.26
35–44	3.20*	2.12–4.83
45–54	2.81*	1.89–4.17
55–64	1.54*	1.03–2.31
65–74	1.00	
Marital status		
Married/cohabiting	1.00	
Widowed/divorced/separated	1.83*	1.47–2.28
Single	1.57*	1.26–1.95
Economic activity status		
Working	1.12	0.89–1.40
Unemployed	1.77*	1.25–2.51
Economically inactive	1.00	
Social Class		
I & II	1.00	
III (NM)	1.04	0.82–1.31
III (M)	1.59*	1.28–1.97
IV & V	1.27*	1.02–1.59
Tenure		
Owner occupied	1.00	
Rented from Local Authority or Housing Association	1.22	0.97–1.53
Privately rented	1.50*	1.21–1.86
Self-reported stress		
Completely free of stress or small amount of stress	1.00	
Moderate or large amount of stress	1.37*	1.16–1.63
Parent		
Has children aged under 16 living in household	1.00	
Does not have children aged under 16 living in household	1.35*	1.10–1.66
Number of cases in the model	**8414**	
Baseline odds	**0.009**	

* Significant at the 95% level

Notes and references

1. Department of Health. *The Health of the Nation: A strategy for health in England*. HMSO (London 1992).

2. Health Education Authority. *Health Update 2 Smoking*. HEA (1995).

3. Health Education Authority. *The smoking epidemic: counting the cost in England*. HEA (London 1991), cited in Health Education Authority, *Health Update 2 Smoking*, HEA (1995).

4. Shaper A G. *Coronary Heart Disease Risks and reasons*. Current Medical Literature (1988).

5. Health Education Authority. *Alcohol Health Update*. HEA (1997).

6. Department of Health. *Sensible drinking: The report of an inter-departmental working group*. (1995).

7. The definition of 'moderate' and 'heavy' drinking varies slightly between different studies. 'Moderate' drinking usually refers to people who drink up to 2 units of alcohol per day while 'heavy' drinking refers to those who drink more than three units per day.

8. Bennett N et al. *Living in Britain: Results from the General Household Survey 1994*. HMSO (London 1996).

9. Diamond A and Goddard E. *Smoking among secondary school children in 1994*. HMSO (1996).

10. Cole A. The persuaders....... *Healthlines,* December 1995–January 1996.

11. Azjen I. The theory of planned behaviour. *Organizational behaviour and human decision processes,* vol. 50, 1991, 179–211.

12. These statements were presented to the respondent on a card and the order differed depending on whether or not the respondent had said that he or she would like to give up smoking.

13. In 1995 respondents were only given three possible answer categories:

    - I intend to give up smoking within the next month
    - I intend to give up smoking within the next year
    - I'm unlikely to give up smoking

    A higher proportion (57%) of HEMS 1995 respondents said that they were unlikely to give up smoking than respondents to HEMS 1996 but as there was the option to say 'Intend to give up but not in the next year' in 1996 it is possible that respondents may have given this answer instead of 'unlikely to give up smoking'.

14. Tables 2.30–2.33 are not commented on in the text.

15. The method used to calculate the alcohol consumption rating is to multiply the number of units of each type of drink consumed on a usual occasion by the frequency with which it was drunk, using the factors shown below, and totalling across all drinks.

    Multiplying factors for converting drinking frequency and number of units consumed on a usual occasion into number of units consumed per week.

Drinking frequency	*Multiplying factor*
Almost every day	7.0
5 or 6 days a week	5.5
3 or 4 days a week	3.5
Once or twice a week	1.5
Once or twice a month	0.375
Once every couple of months	0.115
Once or twice a year	0.029

    The number of units of each type of drink consumed on a 'usual' occasion is multiplied by the factor corresponding to the frequency with which the drink was consumed. In all except the first category, the factors are averages of the range of frequencies shown in the category, for example where a drink was consumed '3–4 days a week', the amount drunk was multiplied by 3.5.

16. Goddard E. Detailed recall of drinking behaviour over seven days. *Survey Methodology Bulletin,* vol. 31, 1992.

17. There were three cases of women aged 16–24 who reported consuming 116, 162 and 150 units per week and two cases of men aged 65–74 who reported drinking 234 and 166 units per week. The pattern of answers these people gave to the drinking questions was consistent and believable so there was no justification for excluding them from the data but the means reported should be treated with caution.

18. This was a change from the question which was asked in 1995 when respondents were asked if they would like to cut down on their drinking so it is not possible to make direct comparisons between the two years.

19. The definition of heavy drinking used in HEMS is men drinking more than 21 units per week and women drinking more than 14 units per week. This definition reflects the current *Health of the Nation* targets rather than the new recommended daily benchmarks.

20. An explanation of logistic regression is given in Appendix D.

21. The odds of engaging in 'high risk' behaviour for people with different characteristics can be calculated by multiplying the baseline odds shown at the bottom of the table by the appropriate factors. So, for example, a single male aged 16–24 who is working, in Social Class III (Non-Manual), privately renting with no or a small amount of self-reported stress and no children aged under 16 would have odds calculated as shown below:

    0.009 x 1.73 x 5.36 x 1.57 x 1.12 x 1.04 x 1.50 x 1.00 x 1.35 = 0.31

    This would give odds of 0.31 to one that a person with these characteristics would smoke and drink heavily.

3 Physical activity

Summary of main findings

- A quarter of respondents participated less than once a week in 30 minutes or more of moderate-intensity activity. The likelihood of being inactive increased with age; 42% of men and 46% of women aged 65–74 were defined as 'sedentary', compared with 9% of men and 20% of women in the 16–24 age-group. (Section 3.3).

- Men and younger respondents were most likely to have engaged in at least moderate-intensity activity lasting at least 30 minutes on five or more days a week, and in vigorous-intensity activity lasting at least 20 minutes on three or more days a week in the four weeks before interview. (Section 3.3).

- The majority of men (73%) and women (69%) thought that, on each of the days someone engages in physical activity, the activity should last at least 30 minutes. (Section 3.4).

- A quarter of respondents said that physical activity should be undertaken for at least 30 minutes on at least five days a week, the recommended guidelines for frequency and duration of moderate-intensity activity. (Section 3.4).

- Seventy six per cent of men and 71% of women said they were 'very' or 'fairly' physically active compared with others of the same age. (Section 3.5.1).

- About half of men (54%) and women (49%) thought they were getting enough exercise to keep fit. (Section 3.5.1).

- Over two thirds of respondents wished to take more exercise; the proportion saying this declined with age, particularly after the age of 55. (Section 3.5.2).

- A quarter of respondents intended to take more exercise in the next month, while another fifth said they would do more in the next six months. Just over two fifths (41%) said they were unlikely to do more. (Section 3.5.3).

- Lack of time (52%), not being the sporty type (15%), having an injury or disability (14%), and poor health (9%) were the most commonly-mentioned barriers to exercise. (Section 3.5.4).

3.1 Introduction and background

Physical activity was identified by the *Health of the Nation* White Paper as a risk factor for the Key Area of coronary heart disease (CHD) and stroke. The relative risk of coronary heart disease and stroke resulting from inactivity appears to be similar in magnitude to that from smoking, raised plasma cholesterol and raised blood pressure[1]. Physical activity and nutrition together have an indirect effect on the likelihood of CHD and stroke in that obesity, which results from a dietary energy intake chronically in excess of energy expenditure, contributes to both raised plasma cholesterol and raised blood pressure.

Participation in physical activity may also contribute indirectly to the achievement of HON targets in the Key Areas of accidents and mental health. There is evidence that weight-bearing exercise helps to maintain bone mass, and active men and women are less likely than those who are sedentary to experience osteoporotic fractures. It is not yet clear whether this is due to the direct effect of exercise on bone density or whether improved muscular strength, balance and co-ordination prevent accidents by reducing the likelihood of falling. Regular exercise is also associated with raised self-esteem and decreased levels of moderate depression and anxiety[2]. By contributing to feelings of well-being, physical activity can also enhance people's quality of life, thus contributing to the HON aim of adding 'life to years'.

Respondents were asked about their participation in and attitudes towards physical activity, and about their knowledge of recommended levels of activity.

3.2 Recommended levels of physical activity

Physical activity refers to any bodily movement produced by skeletal muscles that results in energy expenditure. It therefore includes activities undertaken as part of day-to-day living and during the course of work, as well as leisure time activities such as exercise and sport.

There has been considerable discussion over the last two decades about the level of physical activity required for health gain. Guidelines developed by the American College of Sports Medicine in 1978, revised in 1992, recommended that for maximum protection against CHD, people should engage in three or more sessions of at least 20 minutes of vigorous-intensity activity a week. Research studies, including the 1995 HEMS, have shown, however, that only a small proportion of the population is active at this level[3,4,5]. In addition, this degree of activity is seen as an unrealistic and possibly inappropriate goal for high risk, inactive sections of the population[6].

At least three weekly sessions of vigorous activity remains the ideal, but there is accumulating epidemiological evidence that increasing participation in moderate exercise can result in health gain at both the individual and the population level. For individuals, moderate exercise, such as walking instead of driving short distances, can increase physical fitness and result in improvements in several health and clinical variables; this is especially true for individuals who are initially inactive and unfit[7]. There appears to be an inverse association between the amount of physical activity and the risk of CHD and stroke, with some evidence of a 'dose-response' relationship[8]. At a population level it has been argued that, given the current low levels of participation in physical activity, greater health gain would result from persuading inactive people to engage in moderate activity than from moving moderately-active people to the vigorous-intensity level[9]. Health promotion is also more likely to be successful if it focuses on attainable goals[6].

In the United States, the Centers for Disease Control and the American College of Sports Medicine have recommended that every US adult should accumulate 30 minutes or more of at least moderate-intensity activity on most, preferably all, days of the week. Although sustained periods of 30 minutes confer the greatest benefit, even intermittent activity totalling 30 minutes over the day is believed to be beneficial if carried out at the intensity of brisk walking[9]. In the UK, the Department of Health set up a Physical Activity Task Force in September 1993. An international symposium was organised by the HEA in April 1994 to support the Task Force; it endorsed three national objectives:

- to reduce the proportion of the population who are sedentary[10]
- to increase the proportion of the population who take a minimum of 30 minutes of at least moderate physical activity on five days a week
- to increase the proportion of the population who take on average three periods of vigorous physical activity of 20 minutes duration a week[11]

3.3 Participation in physical activity

> HEA suggested health promotion indicators:
>
> The proportion of people aged 16–74 active at 'moderate' or 'vigorous' level for 30 minutes or more, five days a week
>
> The proportion of people aged 16–74 active at a 'vigorous' level for 20 minutes three days a week

Physical activity as measured by HEMS includes activity at work; activity at home, both heavy housework, and DIY and gardening; walks of 1–2 miles or more; and sports and exercise activities (including cycling). Stair climbing, light housework and caring activities are not included.

Two summary measures of physical activity were calculated: one based on occasions of moderate- or vigorous-intensity activity lasting at least 30 minutes, the other on vigorous-intensity activity lasting at least 20 minutes. Moderate-intensity activity included brisk or fast walking, heavy housework, gardening or DIY, swimming or cycling (if it did not make the respondent out of breath or sweaty), and some specified occupations. Vigorous intensity activity included running, swimming or cycling (if they made the participant out of breath or sweaty), and some specified occupations.

The reference period for both these summary measures was the four weeks prior to interview. Appendix C explains in detail how information on type of activity, duration, frequency and intensity are combined to produce the two summary measures.

As noted in the previous section, the international symposium hosted by the HEA in 1994 developed three national objectives; to reduce the proportion of the population which is sedentary, to increase the proportion who engage in at least moderate-intensity activity lasting 30 minutes or more on at least five days a week, and to increase the proportion who undertake at least three sessions a week of vigorous activity lasting for 20 minutes or more. Tables 3.1–3.4 show the proportion of HEMS respondents in each of those categories.

A quarter of respondents were classed as 'sedentary'; that is, they participated less than once a week in 30 minutes or more of moderate-intensity activity. With the exception of the 16–24 age-group, there was no significant difference in the proportion of men and women, or of respondents from different social classes in this category, but the likelihood of being sedentary increased with age; 42% of men and 46% of women aged 65–74 were defined as inactive, compared with 9% of men and 20% of women in the 16–24 age-group. Men, the younger age-groups and respondents in the manual social classes were most likely to be participating in at least moderate-intensity activity lasting at least 30 minutes on five or more days a week.

Because of the strong association between participation in physical activity and age, it is important to take age into account when investigating the relationship between physical activity and other social characteristics such as social class; this can be done by calculating age-standardised ratios[12]. A ratio of more than 100 indicates a greater likelihood of participation in at least moderate-intensity activity on five or more days a week than would be expected in that group on the basis of age distribution alone. Conversely, a ratio of less than 100 indicates that the members of the group are less likely to be active at this level than would be expected from the age composition of the group. Age-standardised ratios confirm the relationship between social class and participation in at least moderate-intensity activity on five or more days a week. With the exception of women in Social Classes I and II, respondents in non-manual social classes had lower than expected ratios and those in manual social classes higher than expected ratios when age was taken into account. **(Figure 3.1 and Tables 3.1–3.3)**

Men and younger respondents were also more likely to have engaged in vigorous-intensity activity lasting at least 20 minutes on three or more days a week in the four weeks before interview, but the relationship between levels of vigorous activity and social class was not as straightforward. Men in Social Classes III (Non-Manual), IV and V and women in Social Classes I and II were most likely to have been active at this level. Activity at work accounts for a proportion of moderate-intensity activity, but is less likely to be counted towards vigorous-intensity activity. **(Table 3.4)**

There were some changes in question wording between 1995 and 1996, mainly to reflect the symposium's objectives. In 1995, respondents were asked on how many *occasions* they had participated in sports and activities; this was changed to *days* in 1996. As Appendix C shows, this made no difference to the proportions participating in at least moderate-intensity activity. Information was collected in 1995 on walks of two miles or more lasting 40 minutes; in 1996, this was changed to walks of 1-2 miles, lasting at least 30 minutes. The proportion of respondents who engaged in at least moderate-intensity activity on five or more days a week was slightly higher in 1996 than in 1995, although the difference was only significant among women. Walking accounts for a proportion of moderate activity, and reducing the length of qualifying walks appears to have resulted in an increase in the proportion reaching the recommended levels; this probably accounts for the difference between the two years. This would seem to be confirmed by the lack of a significant difference in the proportions engaging in vigorous-intensity activity in 1995 and 1996; walking does not count towards this summary measure (see Appendix C for a more detailed discussion).

Tables 3.1–3.2 and 3.4 are based on cross-tabulation techniques, and look at sex, age and social class separately. They do not show how much these attributes interact with each other and with other characteristics such as highest qualification level. As noted in Chapter 2, it is possible to look at how different factors interrelate by using logistic regression[13], a multivariate statistical technique which can be used to predict the odds of a behaviour (for example, being sedentary or not sedentary) occurring for people

Figure 3.1 Level of physical activity by age and sex: adults aged 16–74

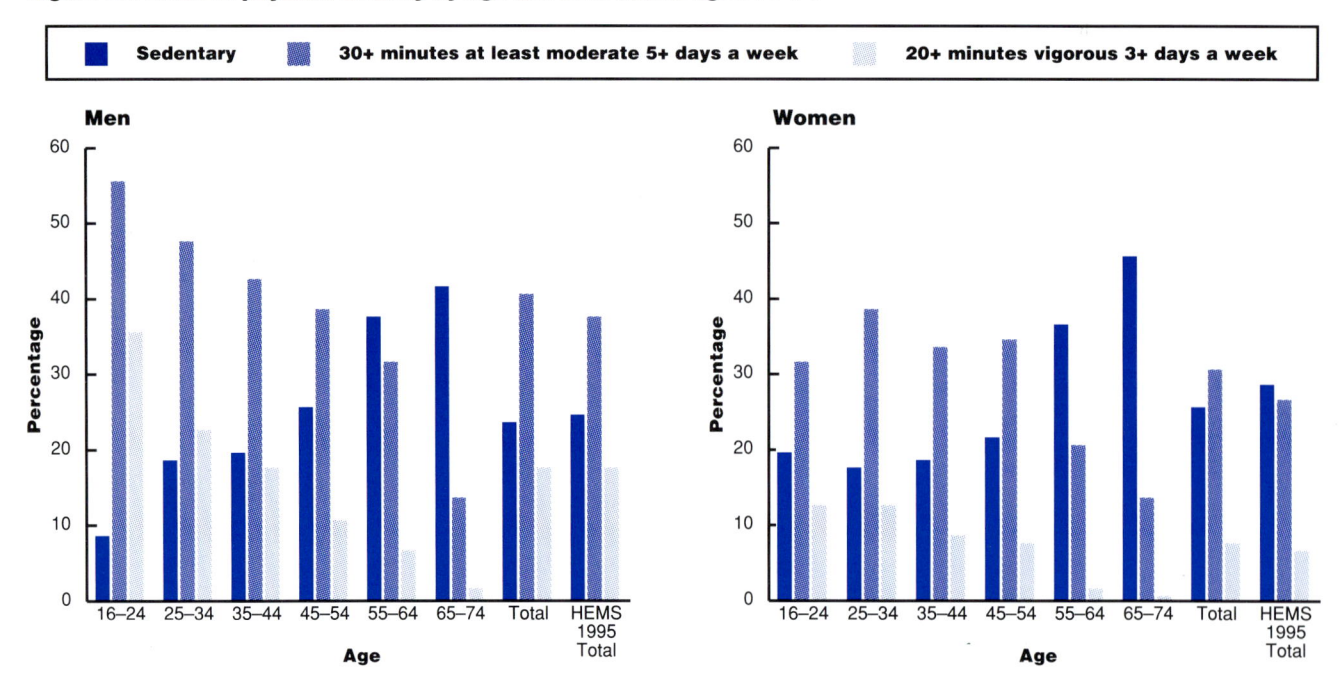

with different combinations of the characteristics under consideration (odds refers to the ratio of the probability that the event will occur to the probability that the event will not occur). The regression looks at the effect of each of the independent variables on the dependent variable, which has just two categories (for example, being sedentary or not sedentary) while holding all the others constant.

Data from the 1995 and 1996 surveys were combined and three logistic regression models were run to look at the odds of being sedentary, of participating in at least moderate-intensity activity lasting at least 30 minutes on five or more days a week, and of engaging in at least 20 minutes of vigorous-intensity activity on three or more days a week. The independent variables used in the models were characteristics which the literature had shown to be associated with participation in physical activity; for all three models, they were:

- sex
- age
- marital status
- highest qualification level
- economic activity status
- social class
- tenure
- income
- whether the respondent had any children aged under 16 in the household

The results are shown in Figures 3.2–3.4. The figures in the columns headed 'Multiplying factors' can be thought of as 'weights'; they represent the factor by which the odds of a respondent engaging in the relevant behaviour (for example, being sedentary) increase with the attribute shown compared to a reference category[14]. For each characteristic shown, the reference category (shown with a value of 1.00) was taken to be the group of respondents least likely to engage in the relevant level of activity. The characteristics are listed in order of importance.

Age, social class and economic activity status proved to be significant in all three models, but their relative importance varied with the level of activity under consideration. The most important factor in predicting whether someone was sedentary or not was age; the odds of being sedentary rose with increasing age, with those aged 65–74 having more than twice the odds as the 16–24 age-group. Being economically inactive, having no qualifications and belonging to a non-manual social class also increased the odds of being classed as sedentary. Sex and gross weekly household income were rejected by the model as not significant factors. **(Figure 3.2)**

Economic activity status was the most important factor predicting participation in at least moderate-intensity activity lasting at least 30 minutes on five or more days a week. Respondents who were working had almost two and a half times the odds of being in this category as those who were economically inactive. This probably reflects the contribution which occupational activity makes to this summary measure of physical activity; it will be recalled that moderate-intensity activity includes brisk or rapid walking, activity at home, activity at work for some specified occupations and some sports and exercise activities. The effect of occupation appears to be confirmed by social class being the second most important factor, with respondents belonging to a manual social class having twice the odds of those in non-manual classes of achieving this level of activity. Age and sex were the third and fourth most important factors. **(Figure 3.3)**

Figure 3.2 Odds of an individual being sedentary
Adults aged 16–74 (HEMS 1995 and HEMS 1996)

Characteristics	Multiplying factors	95% Confidence intervals
Age		
16–24	1.00	
25–34	1.21	0.95–1.54
35–44	1.41*	1.10–1.81
45–54	1.55*	1.20–2.00
55–64	2.12*	1.63–2.76
65–74	2.44*	1.85–3.21
Marital status		
Married/cohabiting	1.14	0.97–1.34
Widowed/divorced/separated	0.94	0.78–1.13
Single	1.00	
Economic activity status		
Working	1.00	
Unemployed	1.16	0.87–1.54
Economically inactive	1.77*	1.55–2.01
Highest qualification level		
'A' level or above	1.00	
Other qualifications	1.03	0.90–1.18
No qualifications	1.50*	1.28–1.75
Social Class		
I & II	1.28*	1.10–1.49
III (NM)	1.27*	1.09–1.49
III (M)	1.00	
IV & V	1.02	0.87–1.19
Tenure		
Owner occupied	0.97	0.82–1.15
Rented from Local Authority or Housing Association	1.18	0.97–1.43
Privately rented	1.00	
Parent		
Has children aged under 16 living in household	1.00	
Does not have children aged under 16 living in household	1.29*	1.11–1.50
Number of cases in the model	**8498**	
Baseline odds	**0.105**	

* Significant at the 95% level

Occupational activity makes only a small contribution to the summary measure of vigorous-intensity activity, and economic activity status and social class were the least important factors retained by this model. This summary measure is more narrowly defined than the moderate-intensity summary measure; walking and activity at home do not count towards it, and a much smaller range of occupations is eligible. Sports and exercise make a relatively larger contribution to vigorous-intensity activity than they do to moderate-intensity activity. Age was the most important factor in predicting whether respondents undertook vigorous-

Figure 3.3 Odds of an individual participating in moderate-intensity activity lasting at least 30 minutes on five or more days a week
Adults aged 16–74 (HEMS 1995 and HEMS 1996)

Characteristics	Multiplying factors	95% Confidence intervals
Economic activity status		
Working	2.45*	2.11–2.83
Unemployed	1.88*	1.45–2.45
Economically inactive	1.00	
Social Class		
I & II	1.19*	1.03–1.37
III (NM)	1.00	
III (M)	2.12*	1.81–2.49
IV & V	2.14*	1.85–2.48
Age		
16–24	3.68*	2.83–4.78
25–34	3.12*	2.51–3.89
35–44	2.40*	1.85–2.90
45–54	2.32*	1.92–2.99
55–64	1.87*	1.50–2.33
65–74	1.00	
Sex		
Male	1.22*	1.10–1.6
Female	1.00	
Marital status		
Married/cohabiting	0.79	0.69–0.92
Widowed/divorced/separated	1.00	
Single	0.76	0.64–0.92
Gross weekly household income		
Less than £5,000	1.00	
£5,000–£9,999	1.22*	1.01–1.49
£10,000–£19,999	1.25*	1.02–1.53
£20,000 or more	1.12	0.90–1.39
Number of cases in the model	**8498**	
Baseline odds	**0.072**	

* Significant at the 95% level

intensity activity lasting 20 minutes or more on at least three days a week; the odds of engaging in this level of activity were raised by a factor of 17 for those aged 16–24, compared with the 65–74 age-group, and more than doubled for men compared with women. Gross weekly household income was the third factor highlighted by the model, with the odds rising with increasing income. **(Figure 3.4)**

Figure 3.4 Odds of an individual participating in vigorous-intensity activity lasting at least 20 minutes on three or more days a week
Adults aged 16–74 (HEMS 1995 and HEMS 1996)

Characteristics	Multiplying factors	95% Confidence intervals
Age		
16–24	17.02*	9.07–31.95
25–34	14.25*	7.76–26.16
35–44	9.72*	5.26–17.94
45–54	6.28*	3.42–11.54
55–64	3.62*	1.94–6.73
65–74	1.00	
Sex		
Male	2.16*	1.84–2.54
Female	1.00	
Gross weekly household income		
Less than £5,000	0.81	0.56–1.15
£5,000–£9,999	1.00	
£10,000–£19,999	1.40*	1.07–1.83
£20,000 or more	1.88*	1.42–2.47
Marital status		
Married/cohabiting	0.67	0.53–0.86
Widowed/divorced/separated	1.00	
Single	0.92	0.70–1.20
Highest qualification level		
'A' level or above	1.72*	1.33–2.21
Other qualifications	1.44*	1.13–1.83
No qualifications	1.00	
Parent		
Has children aged under 16 living in household	1.00	
Does not have children aged under 16 living in household	1.29*	1.07–1.56
Economic activity status		
Working	1.13	0.88–1.45
Unemployed	1.73*	1.19–2.50
Economically inactive	1.00	
Social Class		
I & II	0.90	07.3–1.12
III (NM)	1.00	
III (M)	1.06	0.83–1.34
IV & V	1.27*	1.00–1.60
Number of cases in the model	**8498**	
Baseline odds	**0.004**	

* Significant at the 95% level

3.4 Knowledge of recommended levels of physical activity

> HEA suggested health promotion indicator: The proportion of adults aged 16–74 who say that the recommended time to be spent on physical activity is at least 30 minutes on five or more days a week

The levels of activity recommended in the HEA symposium's second and third objectives are based on a combination of frequency, duration and intensity (see Appendix C for full details). HEMS respondents were asked two questions to measure their awareness of the recommended levels of frequency and duration: on how many days a week people should undertake physical activity and for how long on each day. They were not asked about intensity.

Just over a fifth (21%) of respondents thought people should be physically active on fewer than three days a week, 33% said 3–4 days a week and 39% five or more. There were no significant differences in the proportion of men and women giving each answer. The majority of men (73%) and women (69%) thought that, on each of the days someone engages in physical activity, it should last 30 minutes or more, almost equal proportions saying exactly 30 minutes (36%) and more than 30 minutes (35%). The proportion choosing 30 minutes or more declined with age, from over three quarters of those aged 16–24 to just over two thirds of the 65–74 age-group, and was higher among the manual than the non-manual social classes, although the difference was only significant among men. More than three quarters of men in Social Classes IV and V, for example, thought activity should be undertaken for at least 30 minutes, compared with just over two thirds of men belonging to Social Classes I and II. **(Tables 3.5-3.6)**

Table 3.7 suggests that there is a trade-off between frequency and duration; almost nine out of ten of those who thought people should be physically active on fewer than three days a week said activity should last at least half an hour, compared with just over six out of ten respondents who opted for five or more days a week. Among those who thought that the number of days 'depends on the person', 39% were unable to say how long activity should last. **(Table 3.7)**

The information on frequency and duration was combined and the results are shown in Tables 3.8–3.9. A quarter of respondents said that physical activity should be undertaken for at least 30 minutes on at least five days a week (the recommended guidelines for frequency and duration), while over three fifths said that people should be physically active on at least three days a week for at least 20 minutes[15]. Just under a third thought activity was necessary on fewer than three days a week or for less than 20 minutes at a time.

There were no significant differences in the proportions of men and women, or of respondents in each social class choosing five days and 30 minutes, but the likelihood of doing so increased with age, from 15% of those aged 16–24 to 37% of the 65–74 age-group. There was no age difference in the proportions saying people should be active for at least 20 minutes on three or more days a week. **(Figure 3.5 and Tables 3.8–3.9)**

Figure 3.5 Percentage saying people should be physically active for 30+ minutes on 5+ days a week by age and sex: adults aged 16–74

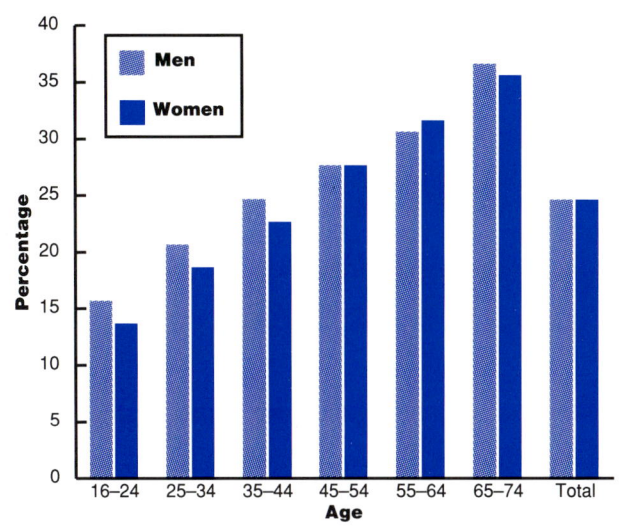

Base numbers are given in Table 3.8

3.5 Attitudes towards physical activity

> HEA suggested health promotion indicators:
>
> The proportion of people aged 16–74 claiming to be 'fairly' or 'very' physically active
>
> The proportion of people aged 16–74 claiming enough exercise to keep fit
>
> The proportion of people aged 16–74 who would like to do more exercise
>
> The proportion of people aged 16–74 who intend to do more exercise in the next 6–12 months

3.5.1 Assessment of own level of physical activity

The Theory of Reasoned Action (TRA)[16] and the later Theory of Planned Behaviour[17] argue that intentions and behaviour are predicted by two pathways; the 'attitudinal component' comprises individual beliefs and attitudes, while the 'normative component' is concerned with the beliefs of significant others and the extent to which people wish to comply with such beliefs. Godin applied the Theory of Reasoned Action to exercise; he found that exercise intentions are good predictors of actual exercise involvement, and about 30% of the variance in intentions is explained by the attitudinal and normative components of the TRA, with nearly all studies showing that the attitudinal component is dominant[18].

HEMS respondents were asked a number of questions to explore their attitudes towards physical activity, whether they intended to be more active and perceived barriers to exercise. As in 1995, respondents were asked how physically active they were 'compared with others of the same age'; 76% of men and 71% of women said they were 'very' or 'fairly' physically active, not significantly different from 1995. Respondents in manual social classes were more likely than those in non-manual groups to feel they were more active, but the difference was only significant among men. Men (84%) and women (80%) aged 65–74, the least active group, were most likely to think of themselves as very or fairly physically active, but the proportions assessing themselves in this way were high in all age-groups. As discussed in Chapter 8, research has shown that questions on self-reported long-standing illness which refer to 'people of your age' tend to yield lower estimates of the prevalence of chronic sickness than questions without an age reference; it appears that elderly people, in particular, regard limitations in their daily activities, especially difficulties with eyesight and hearing, as a normal part of growing old, not as evidence of illness or disability[19]. Similarly, people who perceive that their peers are not very active are perhaps more likely to assess themselves as relatively active, even when their actual participation in physical activity is low compared with recommended levels and with that of people in other age-groups. **(Tables 3.10–3.11)**

Respondents were asked whether they were getting enough exercise to keep fit; about half of men (54%) and women (49%) said they were, which was not significantly different from 1995. This is lower than the proportion claiming to be very or fairly physically active compared with others of the same age, suggesting that more respondents are using absolute rather than relative criteria when answering this question, but it is still at odds with evidence on actual participation; the proportion who feel they exercise enough is about twice as high as the proportion actually participating at the recommended level for at least moderate-intensity activity. Those belonging to the manual social classes were most likely to feel that they took sufficient exercise, which reflects the data on participation, but the oldest age-group (which is the least active) were most likely to feel they exercised enough. Qualitative research has shown that one of the reasons people tend to overestimate their level of activity and fitness is because they feel 'fit' enough for a sedentary lifestyle[6,20]; older people, in particular, may feel that less exercise and lower levels of fitness are required at their age. **(Tables 3.12–3.13)**

3.5.2 Wish to take more exercise

With the exception of those who said they could not take exercise, respondents were asked if they would like to take more; 66% of men and 69% of women said they would[21]. The proportion saying this declined with age, particularly from the age of 55, while those in the non-manual social classes were more likely than respondents belonging to manual groups to want to take more exercise. Among those aged 16–24, a higher proportion of women (83%) than of men (69%) said they wanted to do more. **(Figure 3.6 and Table 3.14)**

3.5.3 Intentions to take more exercise

As noted earlier, intentions have been shown to be good predictors of actual participation in exercise. As in the smoking and drinking sections of the interview, respondents were asked about their future intentions, in this case, to take more exercise. Biddle[22] outlines a classification based on Prochaska and DiClemente's transtheoretical model of behaviour change[23,24]; individuals at the pre-contemplation stage are those not currently exercising and not intending to exercise in the near future, while 'contemplators' are non-exercisers who intend to start exercising in the near future. Those in the 'action' stage have recently begun to exercise, while those in the maintenance stage have been exercising for some time[22].

Figure 3.6 Percentage who would like to take more exercise by age and sex: adults aged 16–74

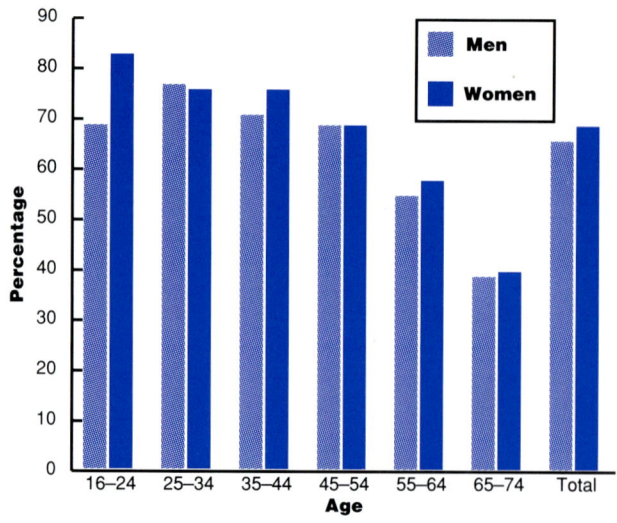

Base numbers are given in Table 3.14

HEMS does not have information on how long respondents have been exercising, so it is not possible to reproduce Biddle's schema exactly, but Tables 3.15–3.18 show respondents' intentions by age, sex, social class and level of activity. A quarter of respondents intended to take more exercise in the next month, while another fifth said they would do more in the next six months. Just over two fifths (41%) said they were unlikely ever to do more. There was no difference in the proportions of men and women saying they would increase their participation in the next month or next six months, but a slightly higher proportion of men (43%) than of women (39%) said they were unlikely to take more exercise. Among both men and women, more than half of those in manual social classes were not intending to increase their level of exercise, either at all or in the next year. Men in Social Class III (Non-Manual) and women in Social Classes I and II were most likely to say they would take more exercise within the next month or next six months. **(Figure 3.7 and Tables 3.15–3.16)**

Figure 3.7 Percentage who intend to take more exercise in the next six months by age and sex: adults aged 16–74

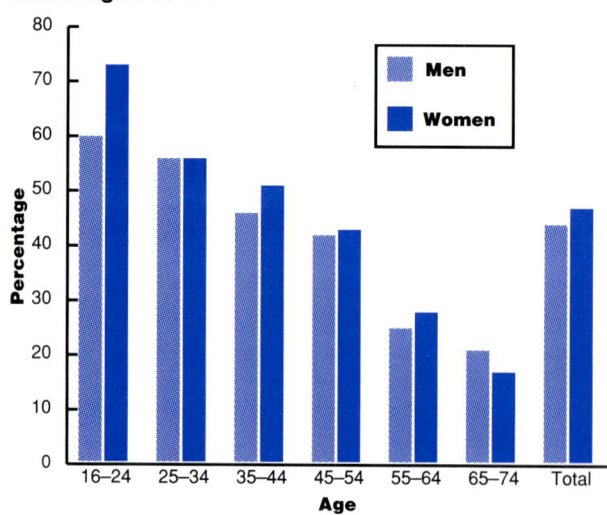

Base numbers are given in Table 3.15

Not unexpectedly, there was an association between intentions and whether respondents wanted to take more exercise. Among those who said they did not want to do more, 83% of men and 81% of women thought they were unlikely to do so. Interestingly, however, more than a fifth of those who wanted to take more exercise thought it was unlikely they would do so. Conversely, more than one in ten of those who did not want to do more thought they would do so within the next six months; this could be an indication of 'extrinsic' motivation, the 'okay, I'll exercise if I really must' approach, which Biddle[22] argues is more difficult to maintain in the long term than an approach based on enjoyment. Respondents engaging in at least moderate-intensity activity for at least 30 minutes on 3–4 days a week were most likely to say they would do more in the next month or six months; this group is already close to the recommended level for moderate-intensity activity and would only require a small increase in participation to attain it. **(Tables 3.17–3.18)**

3.5.4 Barriers to exercise

Some of the most common barriers to exercise have been well-documented in previous surveys; they include lack of time, lack of enjoyment, feeling uncomfortable or incompetent when exercising, and a concern about perceived poor physique[3,22]. People defined as 'sedentary' are particularly likely to express negative views about physical activity[20]. HEMS respondents were shown a list of things which 'people say stops them getting more exercise' and asked which, if any, applied to them. The reasons were:

- I don't have the time
- I have an injury or disability that stops me
- My health is not good enough
- I don't enjoy physical activity
- I'm not the sporty type
- Other
- None of these

As in other surveys, lack of time was the most commonly cited reason, mentioned by more than half of respondents. There was no significant difference in the proportion of men and women choosing this answer, but the likelihood of doing so declined with age, with only about a fifth of the oldest age-group giving this reason. Respondents in Social Classes I and II were most, and those in Social Classes IV and V least likely, to mention lack of time. Making time for structured exercise sessions is seen by people as a major obstacle to increasing participation in physical activity; for this reason, health promotion practitioners have been advised to emphasise activity which can be fitted into daily routines[25]. This includes activities such as walking instead of driving short distances or using the stairs instead of taking the lift. **(Figure 3.8 and Tables 3.19–3.20)**

The second most commonly mentioned reason, cited by a higher proportion of women (18%) than of men (12%) was 'I'm not the sporty type'. Women aged 45–64 were particularly likely to give this reason for not taking more exercise; Killoran et al[20] note that women tend to feel that exercise is more accessible to men, who are more easily able to carry on with sports such as football which they played at school. The proportions citing an injury or disability, or poor health increased with age. Biddle[22] has argued that enjoyment is essential if people are to maintain regular exercise; fewer than one in ten cited lack of enjoyment as a barrier to exercise.

In 1995, this question was only addressed to respondents who said they would like to take more exercise, so it is not possible to compare proportions; the *pattern* of responses was, however, similar in the two years.

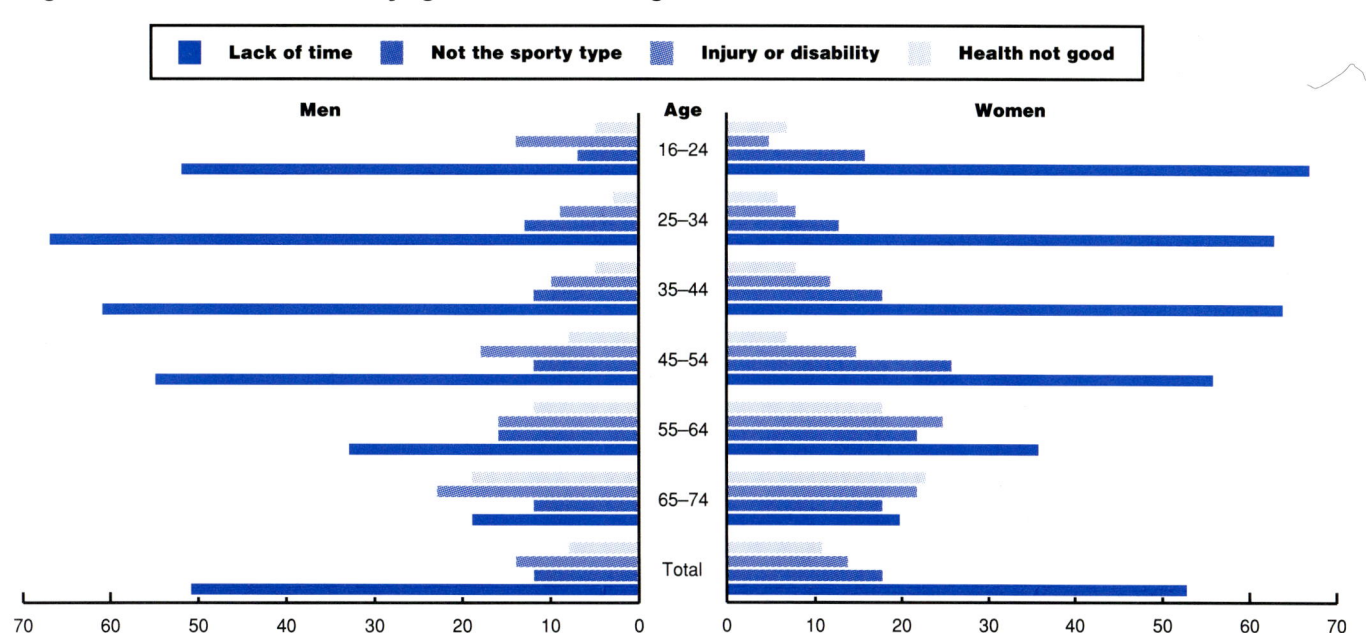

Figure 3.8 Barriers to exercise by age and sex: adults aged 16–74

Base numbers are given in Table 3.19

Health in England 1996 : What people know, what people think, what people do

Notes and references

1. Powell K E et al. Physical activity and the incidence of coronary heart disease. *American Review of Public Health,* vol. 8, 1987, pp. 253-287.

2. Health Education Authority. *Health Update 5: Physical Activity.* (London 1995).

3. *Allied Dunbar National Fitness Survey.* Sports Council (London 1992).

4. Colhoun H et al. *Health Survey for England 1994.* HMSO (London 1996).

5. Bridgwood A et al. *Health in England 1995: what people know, what people think, what people do.* HMSO (London 1996).

6. Wimbush E. A moderate approach to promoting physical activity: the evidence and implications. *Health Education Journal,* vol. 53, 1994, pp. 322-336.

7. Blair S N and Connelly J C. How much physical activity should we do? The case for moderate amounts and intensities of physical activity. In Killoran A et al (eds). *Moving on: international perspectives on promoting physical activity.* Health Education Authority (London 1994).

8. Marmot M and Thorogood M. Physical activity and coronary heart disease: gaps in knowledge. In Killoran A et al (eds). *Moving on: international perspectives on promoting physical activity.* Health Education Authority (London 1994). The authors warn, however, that there is a genetic element in CVD, which means that the relationship between physical activity and reduced risk is not straightforward.

9. Pate R R et al. Physical activity and public health: a recommendation from the centers for disease control and prevention and the American College of Sports Medicine. *Journal of the American Medical Association,* vol. 273, 1995, No. 5, pp. 402-407.

10. 'Sedentary' people are those who do not engage in 30 minutes or more moderate-intensity activity on at least one day a week.

11. Killoran A et al (eds). *Moving on: international perspectives on promoting physical activity.* Health Education Authority (London 1994).

12. See Appendix D.2 for a full explanation of age standardisation.

13. An explanation of logistic regression is given in Appendix D.1.

14. The odds of engaging in the behaviour in question for people with different characteristics can be calculated by multiplying the baseline odds shown at the bottom of the tables by the appropriate factors. So, for example, someone aged 65–74 who has no qualifications and is economically inactive, in Social Class III (Non-Manual), privately renting and no children aged under 16 would have odds calculated as shown below:

    $0.105 \times 2.44 \times 1.50 \times 1.77 \times 1.27 \times 1.00 \times 1.29 = 1.29$

    This would give odds of 1.29 that a person with these characteristics would be sedentary.

    The odds can be converted into a probability using the following formula:

    $$p = \frac{\text{odds}}{1 + \text{odds}}$$

    so odds of 1.29 can be converted to a probability of 56%, meaning that the model predicts 56% of people with the given combination of characteristics would be sedentary.

15. Respondents who said that physical activity should be undertaken for at least 30 minutes on five or more days a week are included in this group.

16. Fishbein M and Ajzen I. *Belief, attitudes, intentions and behaviour: an introduction to theory and research.* Addison-Wesley (Boston 1975).

17. Ajzen I. The theory of planned behaviour. *Organisational Behaviour and Human Decision Processes,* vol. 50, 1991, pp. 179-211.

18. Godin G. The theories of reasoned action and planned behaviour: overview of findings, emerging research problems and usefulness for exercise promotion. Journal of Applied Sport Psychology, vol. 5, pp. 141-157, cited in Biddle S. What helps and hinders people from becoming more physically active? in Killoran A et al (eds). *Moving on: international perspectives on promoting physical activity.* Health Education Authority (London 1994).

19. Goddard E. Measuring morbidity and some of the factors associated with it. *Health and Lifestyle surveys: towards a common approach: report of a workshop held on 7 November 1989 organised by the HEA and OPCS.* HEA and OPCS (London 1991).

20. Killoran A et al. Who needs to know what? An investigation of the characteristics of the key target groups for the promotion of physical activity in England. In Killoran A et al (eds). *Moving on: international perspectives on promoting physical activity.* Health Education Authority (London 1994).

21. It is not possible to compare the results from the 1995 and 1996 surveys, as this question was only addressed to those who thought they were not getting enough exercise in 1995.

22. Biddle S. What helps and hinders people from becoming more physically active? In Killoran A et al (eds). *Moving on: international perspectives on promoting physical activity.* Health Education Authority (London 1994).

23. Prochaska J O and DiClemente C C. Towards a comprehensive model of change. In Miller W R and Heather N (eds). *Treating addictive behaviours.* Plenum Press (New York 1986).

24. Prochaska J O. Strong and weak principles for progressing from precontemplation to action on the basis of twelve problem behaviours. Health Psychology, vol. 13, 1994, pp. 46–51.

25. Fentem P and Walker A. Setting targets for England: challenging, measurable and achievable. In Killoran A et al (eds). *Moving on: international perspectives on promoting physical activity.* Health Education Authority (London 1994).

4 Nutrition

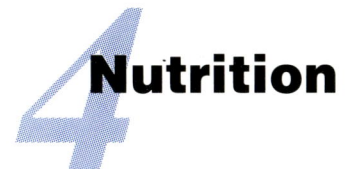

Summary of main findings

- When respondents were asked to describe a healthy diet, the four most commonly given answers were eating lots of fruit, vegetables and salad; cutting down on fat; eating lots of fibre; and eating lots of starchy carbohydrates. (Section 4.2).

- Almost two thirds of men (65%) and just over one third of women (36%) either never shopped or never looked at the ingredients. (Section 4.3).

- Among those who did shop for food, there were some differences between men and women in what they looked for; 40% of women looked at the fat content compared with 24% of men and 16% of women but only 9% of men looked at the sugar content. (Section 4.3).

- Thirty eight per cent of adults aged 16–74 reported eating bread; fruit, vegetables or salad; and potatoes, rice or pasta daily. (Section 4.4.1).

- Twenty two per cent of adults aged 16–74 reported using semi-skimmed or skimmed milk; no fat, low- or reduced-fat spread; and eating chips less than once a week. (Section 4.4.2).

- A third (33%) of adults aged 16–74 said they ate confectionery less than once a week and just over a quarter (26%) said they ate biscuits or cakes less than once a week. (Section 4.4.3).

- Almost a fifth (19%) of adults aged 16-74 thought their diet was healthy and almost three quarters thought it was quite good but could improve (73%). (Section 4.4.4).

- Of those who thought their diet was not as healthy as it could be, 36% did not want to change; 30% wanted to change but did not think it was likely they would; 11% intended to change in the next month; 15% in the next six months and 7% in the next year. (Section 4.4.4).

continued

> ■ Almost a third (32%) of respondents agreed with the statement 'I get confused over what's supposed to be healthy and what isn't'; 68% agreed with the statement 'experts never agree about what foods are good for you'; 37% agreed that 'eating healthy food is expensive'; 75% agreed that 'healthy foods are enjoyable'; and 38% agreed with the statement 'the tastiest foods are the ones that are bad for you'. (Section 4.5).

4.1 Introduction and background

The *Health of the Nation* White Paper identifies the dietary targets which are key to achieving a reduction in cardiovascular disease. It also notes that there is some evidence that a diet low in saturated fatty acids and high in starchy carbohydrates, fruit and vegetables reduces the risk of some cancers.

The three targets are: to reduce the average percentage of food energy derived from fat and saturated fat by the year 2005 and to reduce the number of people who are obese. To achieve these targets it states that a whole diet approach is crucial[1]. It is important that people eat a balanced diet chosen from a variety of foods. There are five main food groups:

- bread, other cereals and potatoes
- fruit and vegetables
- milk and dairy food
- meat, fish and alternatives
- foods containing fat, foods containing sugar

It is recommended that in order to have a healthy diet people should eat food from the first four groups daily and try to cut down on the amount of foods containing fat and foods containing sugar which they eat. The foods in the first group contain starch and fibre and should make up the main part of most meals[2].

4.2 Knowledge of what constitutes a healthy diet

> HEA suggested health promotion indicator: The proportion of the population who are able to state correctly three of the following ways of achieving a healthier diet – eat less fat; eat more fruit, vegetables and salad; eat more starchy carbohydrates (potatoes, pasta or rice); eat more fibre

The White Paper stated that in order for the *Health of the Nation* targets to be achieved it was necessary to disseminate information about healthy eating and encourage changes in eating habits. To find out what respondents knew about healthy eating interviewers used an open question asking them to describe a healthy diet; the answers given were coded in the interview. Interviewers were instructed not to prompt the respondents as we were interested in their spontaneous answers.

Figure 4.1 Percentage of respondents knowing what constitutes a healthy diet: adults aged 16–74

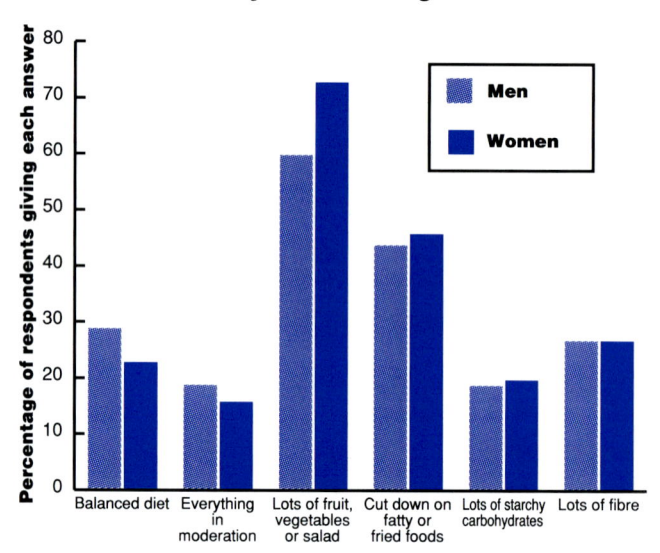

Base numbers are given in Table 4.1
Respondents were able to give more than one answer

Stockley[3] reported that nutritional knowledge has been found to be highest among younger and middle-aged people and among those in higher socio-economic groups; the findings from HEMS support this. When asked to describe a healthy diet the four most common answers given were eating lots of fruit, vegetables or salad, which was mentioned by 67% of respondents; cutting down on fat, which was mentioned by 45%; eating lots of fibre (27%) and eating lots of starchy carbohydrates (20%). Eating a 'balanced diet' was mentioned by 26% of respondents and 18% said that eating 'everything in moderation' was important. Sixteen per cent of respondents said avoiding red meat and eating white meat and fish was part of a healthy diet and 12% said that cutting down on sugar, cakes and confectionery was important. (Figure 4.1 and Table 4.1)

There was little difference in the answers given by men and women except that a higher proportion of women than of men mentioned eating lots of fruit, vegetables or salad (73% compared with 60% of men) and cutting down on confectionery (14% compared with 9%).

Respondents in the older age-groups were less likely than younger respondents to say that a healthy diet should include lots of starchy carbohydrates; only 11% of adults aged 65–74 gave this answer compared with 25% of adults aged 16–24. Sheiham et al[4] reported that in the late 1960s starchy foods such as potatoes were seen as 'bad' as they were thought to be fattening; this difference between the age-groups may reflect the possibility that older people still have this belief.

Men and women in Social Classes I and II were more likely than respondents in other social classes to include eating lots of fibre, cereals and wholemeal food in their answer; for example, 36% of women and 32% of men in Social Classes I and II did so, compared with 20% of men and 23% of women in Social Classes IV and V. **(Table 4.2)**

The table also shows the proportion of people who were able to state correctly at least three ways of moving towards a healthy diet. Although respondents seemed to have a broadly accurate view of a healthy diet the proportion who mentioned three out of the four items included in the suggested health promotion indicator was low; only 16%. Women were more likely than men to mention at least three of the ways of achieving a healthier diet (17%, compared with 14%) and women aged 25-34 were more likely than women in any other age-group to do so. Respondents in Social Classes I and II were more likely than respondents in the other social classes to mention at least three ways (20% compared with 13% of respondents in Social Classes IV and V). **(Tables 4.1 and 4.2)**

This approach of looking at levels of knowledge was different to the one taken in 1995 and the different methods used in 1995 and 1996 are discussed in the Annex to this chapter. It is not possible, therefore, to make direct comparisons between the two years.

4.3 What informants look for when shopping for food

> HEA suggested health promotion indicator: The proportion of people who buy food who look for the following nutrition information on the label: total fat, sugar

People may be aware of what a healthy diet should be but to achieve a healthy diet they need to know what is contained in the food they eat. By law, most pre-packed food should contain a list of ingredients in descending order of weight and many now give nutritional information such as the amount of calories contained in the product, the amount of protein, carbohydrates and fat. Manufacturers may also choose to give information about saturated fat, sugars, sodium and fibre.

Interviewers asked respondents if they looked at the list of ingredients or the nutritional information when they went shopping. As in 1995, the question was asked as an open one and interviewers coded the answers according to a pre-coded list. Two new categories were added to the list in 1996: 'suitable for vegetarians' and 'fibre content'.

Almost two thirds (65%) of men and over one third (36%) of women never shopped or never looked at the ingredients. Charles and Kerr in 1988[5] reported that women still have most of the responsibility for food provision, although they said gender differences were less marked in the middle classes. HEMS found that although only 54% of men in Social Classes I and II said that they never shopped or looked at ingredients, compared with 71% of men in Social Classes IV and V, the gender differences existed

Figure 4.2 Percentage who examine ingredients when they shop, and what they look for by sex: adults aged 16–74

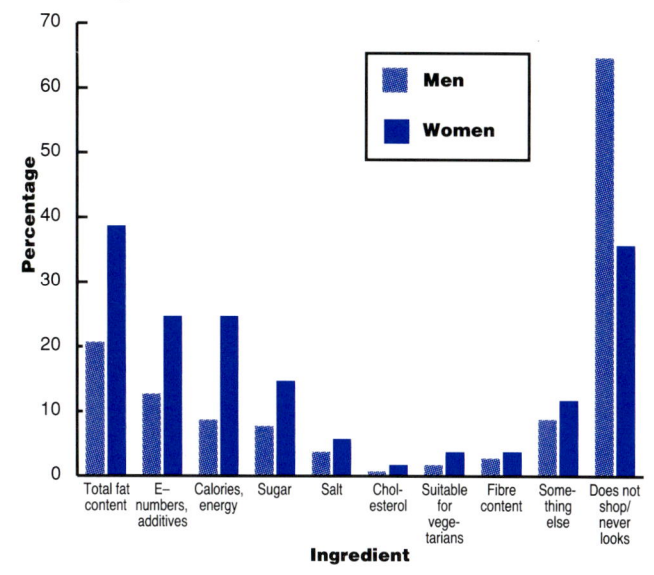

Base numbers are given in Table 4.3
Respondents could mention more than one ingredient

in all social classes. Respondents qualified at 'A' level or above were more likely to look at the ingredients and at the nutritional content than people who were less highly qualified. These findings were not significantly different from 1995.
(Tables 4.3–4.5)

Respondents were most likely to look at fat content; 30% did so, compared with 11% who looked at the sugar content. Nineteen per cent looked at E-numbers and additives, and 17% at the calories or energy content. Three per cent of adults looked at whether food was suitable for vegetarians and 4% looked at the fibre content. **(Figure 4.2)**

Table 4.3 shows that there were differences between men and women in what they looked for; 39% of women looked at the total fat content compared with 21% of men, and 15% of women looked at the sugar content compared with only 8% of men. Women were much more likely than men to look at E-numbers and additives (25% compared with 13%) and at calories (25% and 9% respectively). Of course, these differences are related to the fact that women are more likely than men to do the shopping. The HEA suggested health promotion indicator refers to the proportions of those who actually shop for food. Among those who did shop for food, there were some differences between men and women in what they looked for; 40% of women looked at the fat content compared with 24% of men and 16% of women but only 9% of men looked at the sugar content. **(Table 4.6)**

Respondents in Social Classes I and II and those qualified at 'A' level or above were more likely than people in other groups to look at total fat content, E-numbers and additives, calories and sugar. Respondents with a greater knowledge of a healthy diet were more likely than other respondents to look at the total fat content, the sugar content, the salt content and the fibre content of the food they bought. Over half (55%) of women who correctly mentioned four ways of achieving a healthy diet looked at the total fat content and more than a third (35%) looked at the sugar content, compared with just over a third (36%) and under a sixth (14%) of women who mentioned fewer than three ways.
(Table 4.7)

Health in England 1996 : What people know, what people think, what people do   35

4.4 Eating habits

Increased knowledge about healthy eating does not necessarily result in a change in eating behaviour. Stockley[3] argues that information is interpreted and evaluated in a way that makes sense to a person. People can be influenced in their choice of food by many factors for example price, accessibility of shops, time, advertising, cultural factors such as religion, social factors are important and habit and familiarity may also influence eating habits.

Respondents were asked about their consumption of different types of food. This can only be used to give a broad indication of types of food people were eating and does not provide a detailed analysis of diet. New questions were added in 1996 asking about the consumption of confectionery, such as sweets or chocolate, and about consumption of biscuits and cakes.

4.4.1 Consumption of foods containing starch and fibre

The main dietary change recommended for reduction of heart disease is to reduce the proportion of calories from fat in the diet and substitute some fatty foods with starchy carbohydrates such as bread, cereals, potatoes, rice and pasta, and fruit and vegetables[3].

Eighty three per cent of respondents reported eating bread or rolls at least once a day and 21% wholemeal bread daily. Women were more likely than men to say they ate wholemeal bread; 25% did so, compared with 17% of men. Over half (55%) of respondents reported eating potatoes, pasta or rice daily. **(Table 4.8)**

Fruit and vegetables contain soluble fibre which may help to reduce the amount of cholesterol in the blood[2]; they may also be important in reducing the risk of heart disease. Two thirds of respondents said they ate fruit, vegetables or salad daily; again there was a difference between men and women with 72% of women reporting that they ate fruit, vegetables or salad daily compared with only 59% of men.

The data on consumption of carbohydrates were combined to measure the proportion of respondents who reported eating bread, fruit, vegetables or salad and potatoes, rice or pasta daily[6], 38% did so.

Although the same proportion of respondents reported eating bread daily as in 1995, there has been a slight reduction in the proportion of men and women who report eating wholemeal bread; 21% did so in 1996 compared with 24% in 1995. It was not possible in the survey to compare the proportions of people reporting eating starchy carbohydrates or eating fruit, vegetables or pasta between 1995 and 1996 because of changes in the question wording between the two years[7].

As reported in 1995 and in other surveys[8] the likelihood of eating foods containing starch and fibre every day increased with age, suggesting that in this respect older people tend to have healthier diets (although, of course, in other respects they may have less healthy diets). This is an example of where knowledge is not necessarily related to diet as although younger people were more likely than older people to cite starchy carbohydrates as being important in a healthy diet, it was the older people who were more likely to actually include them in their diets. **(Figure 4.3)**

Figure 4.3 Percentage eating bread; fruit, vegetables or salad; potatoes, pasta or rice daily, by age and sex: adults aged 16–74

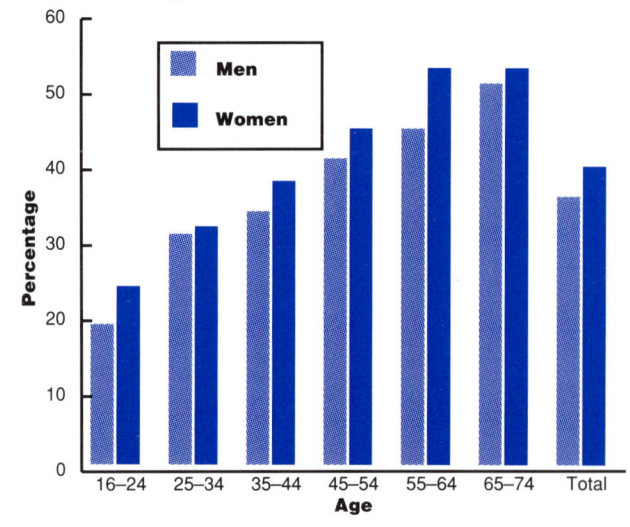

Base numbers are given in Table 4.8

Women in Social Classes I and II or those qualified at 'A' level or above were more likely than other respondents to report eating wholemeal bread and to say they ate fruit, vegetables and salad daily. **(Table 4.9–4.10)**

Respondents living in East Anglia reported eating foods containing starchy carbohydrates more frequently than those living in other regions; 52% of women and 45% of men said that they ate bread, fruit, vegetables or salad and potatoes, rice or pasta daily. Men in the North were the least likely to eat these types of foods daily (21%). Gregory[9] has reported that people in the North eat less fruit, vegetables and salad than other people and HEMS found this was the case for men (50%), but not for women (72%). **(Table 4.11)**

Respondents showing a high level of knowledge about the foods which constitute a healthy diet were more likely to eat a healthy diet; 64% of women who correctly stated the four main ways of achieving a healthy diet said they ate wholemeal bread and vegetables, fruit or salad and potatoes, rice or pasta daily compared with only 38% of women who could only state up to two ways. **(Table 4.12)**

4.4.2 Consumption of foods containing fat

There are three main types of fat: saturates, monounsaturates and polyunsaturates. Saturates can increase the level of cholesterol in the blood and are found in milk and dairy foods, meat and meat products, some cooking and spreading fats, cakes, biscuits and pastry. It is recommended that people cut down on the total amount of fat they consume and choose low-fat varieties of food such as skimmed or semi-skimmed milk rather than full-fat milk. When fats are used it is better to choose unsaturated fats such as vegetable oils wherever possible[2].

Respondents were asked about the type of milk they usually used in tea, coffee and on cereals, how often they ate chips, what kind of fat or oil they used for frying food, and what kind of spread they used on bread.

The majority of respondents (71%) reported using skimmed or semi-skimmed milk; women (74%) were more likely than men (67%) to do so. Women were also much more likely than men to

Figure 4.4 Percentage drinking semi-skimmed or skimmed milk; using no fat, or low- or reduced-fat spread; using oil for cooking and eating chips less than once a week, by age and sex: adults aged 16–74

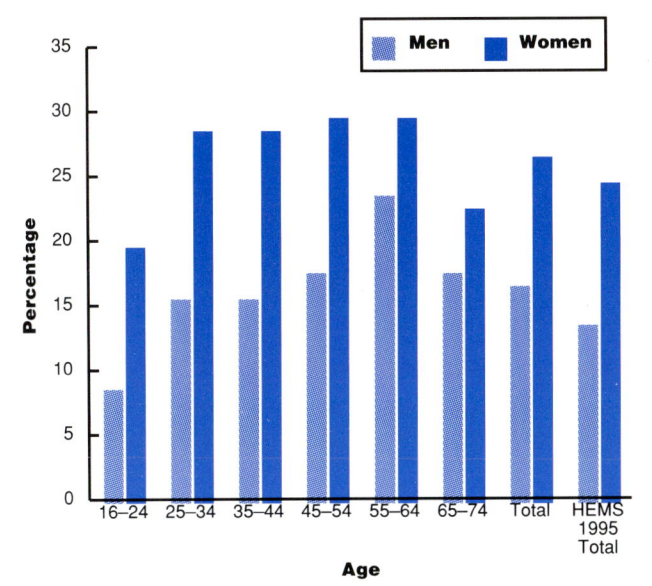

Base numbers are given in Table 4.13

say they ate chips less than once a week (53% did so compared with 35% of men). A large majority of people (90%) reported using oil for cooking and there was no difference between men and women. Just over half (54%) of the respondents said they used no fat, low- or reduced-fat spread; women being slightly more likely than men to do so (56% compared with 52%). **(Table 4.13)**

The information from these questions was combined to show that 22% of respondents used semi-skimmed or skimmed milk, no fat, low- or reduced-fat spread and ate chips less often than once a week. Women were more likely than men to do these things (27% compared with 17%).

It is not possible make comparisons between 1995 and 1996 of the proportion of men and women eating chips less than once a week because of changes in the question wording[10].

The relationship between age and consumption of fats was not clear cut; while older people were more likely than younger people to say they ate chips less than once a week, younger people were more likely to report using oil for cooking. **(Figure 4.4)**

Women in Social Classes I and II and those with 'A' levels or higher qualifications were more likely than other respondents to say that they used low-fat varieties of milk, cooking fat and spread low in saturated fat and that they ate chips less than once a week. **(Tables 4.14–4.16)**

4.4.3 Consumption of confectionery and biscuits or cakes

Confectionery, biscuits and cakes are high in sugar and cakes, biscuits and some confectionery can also be high in fat. The fats in cakes, chocolate and biscuits are sometimes called 'hidden fats' as it is not always obvious to people how much fat they do contain. Fat is particularly dense in calories and sugar contains only calories and no other nutrients; excess calories in the diet can cause obesity if not balanced by physical activity. Health promotion advice is to cut down on confectionery, biscuits and cakes[2].

A third (33%) of respondents said they ate confectionery less than once a week; there was no significant difference between men and women. This finding was also reported for the 1993 Health Survey[8] although Gregory[9] reported in 1990 that women were more likely than men to eat chocolate or sugar confectionery. Just over a quarter (26%) of adults said they ate biscuits or cakes less than once a week; women (28%) were more likely than men (24%) to give this answer.

People aged 55–64 ate confectionery less frequently than younger people; 44% of those aged 65–74 reported eating confectionery less than once a week compared with only 16% of those aged 16–24. Older men, however, reported eating biscuits and cakes more frequently than those in the younger age groups; 14% of men aged 65–74 said they only ate biscuits and cakes once a week compared with at least 22% of other men. **(Figures 4.5–4.6 and Table 4.17)**

Figure 4.5 Percentage eating confectionery less than once a week by age and sex: adults aged 16–74

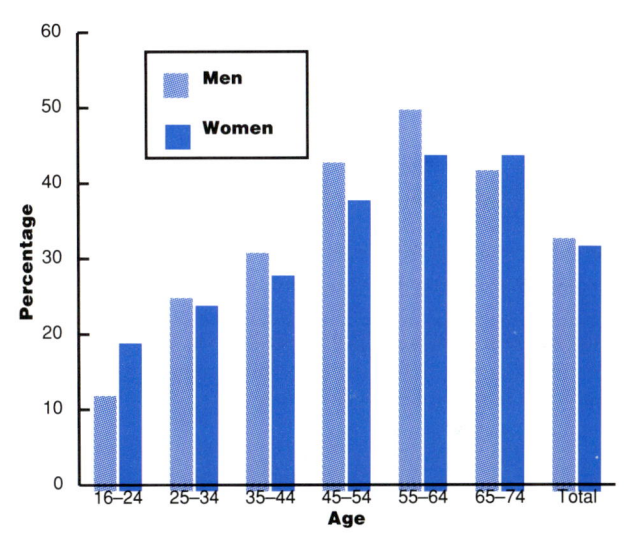

Base numbers are given in Table 4.17

Figure 4.6 Percentage eating biscuits or cakes less than once a week by age and sex: adults aged 16–74

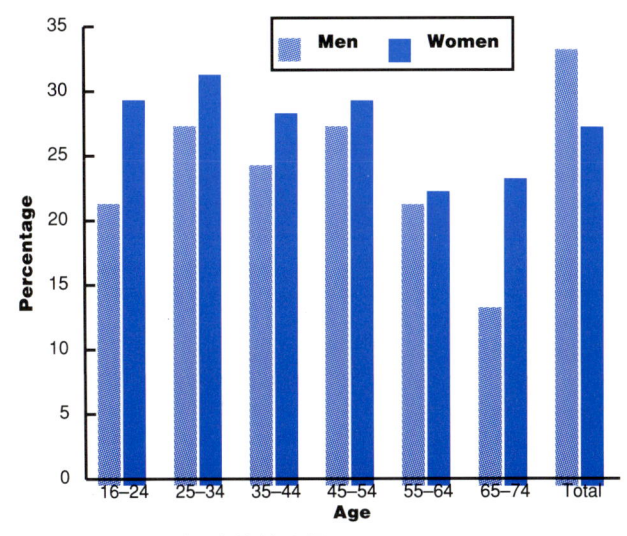

Base numbers are given in Table 4.17

Figure 4.7 Percentage who thought their diet was as healthy as it could be by age and sex: adults aged 16–74

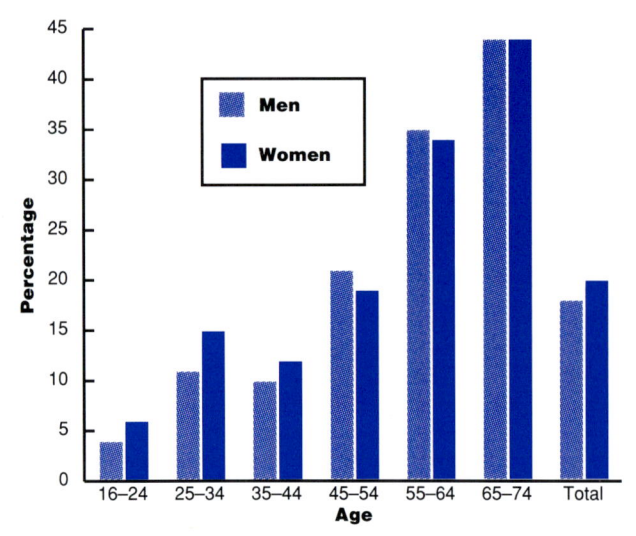

Base numbers are given in Table 4.21

The consumption of confectionery and biscuits or cakes did not seem to be clearly related to social class or level of qualification. Men with no qualifications were the most likely to report eating confectionery less than once a week (46%). **(Tables 4.18–4.20)**

4.4.4 Intentions to change eating habits

Respondents were asked if they thought their diet was as healthy as it could be or whether it could be improved. Almost a fifth (19%) thought their diet was a healthy one, almost three quarters (73%) thought it was quite good but could improve, and the rest either thought their diet was not very healthy (7%) or didn't know (1%). There was no significant difference in the answers given by men and women. The proportion of people who described their diet as healthy increased with age; only 5% of people aged 16–24 gave this answer compared with 44% of those aged 65–74. **(Figure 4.7 and Table 4.21)**

People who ate bread, fruit, vegetables or salad and potatoes, rice or pasta daily were more likely than other respondents to say their diet was healthy (26% compared with 15%). A quarter (25%) of those who reported eating low fat foods said their diet was as healthy as it could be compared with just under a fifth (17%) of other respondents. **(Tables 4.22–4.23)**

Respondents who thought their diet was not as healthy as it could be were asked about their intentions to change: 36% did not want to change, 30% wanted to change but did not think it was likely; 11% intended to change in the next month; 15% in the next six months; and 7% in the next year. Men (40%) were more likely than women (31%) to say they did not want to change and women were more likely to say they intended to change in the next month (15% compared with 8%). Older people were more likely than younger people to say they did not want to change (53% of people aged 65–74 did not want to change, compared with 31% of those aged 16–24). **(Table 4.24–4.25)**

4.5 Attitudes towards diet

Ajzen[11] argues that attitudes towards a behaviour, as well as intentions, are important in influencing whether or not behaviour will change. Respondents were asked about their attitudes towards healthy eating.

> HEA suggested health promotion indicator: The proportion of the population who are confused about what constitutes a healthy diet

> HEA suggested health promotion indicator: The proportion of the population who agree that 'experts never agree about what foods are good for you'

> HEA suggested health promotion indicator: The proportion of the population who believe that: 'eating healthy food is expensive', 'healthy foods are enjoyable' and 'the tastiest foods are the ones that are bad for you'

Almost a third (32%) of respondents agreed with the statement 'I get confused over what's supposed to be healthy and what isn't'. Men (34%) were more likely than women (30%) to say they got confused and men in the older age-groups were the most likely to be confused; 43% of men aged 65–74 said they were. **(Figure 4.8 and Table 4.26)**

Respondents in manual social classes were more likely than those in non-manual social classes to say they got confused about a healthy diet; for example, 42% of respondents in Social Classes IV and V did so, compared with only 25% of those in Social Classes I and II. **(Table 4.27)**

Figure 4.8 Percentage agreeing 'I get confused over what's supposed to be healthy and what isn't' by age and sex: adults aged 16–74

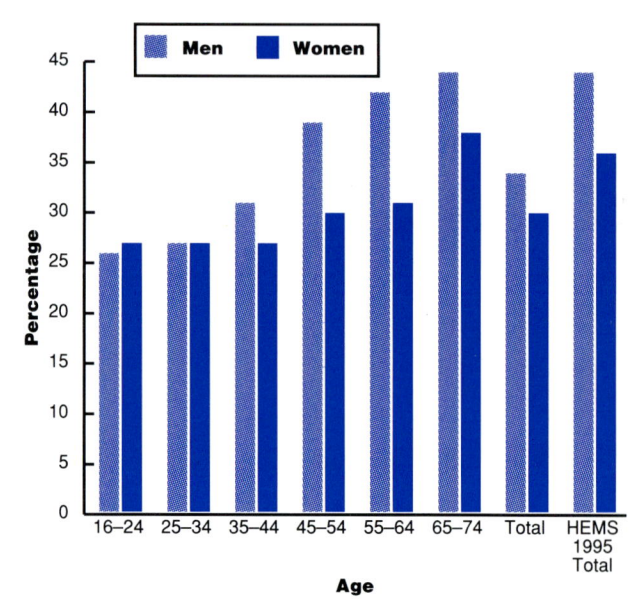

Base numbers are given in Table 4.26

---

38 Health in England 1996 : What people know, what people think, what people do

Figure 4.9 Percentage agreeing that 'experts never agree what foods are good for you' by age: adults aged 16–74

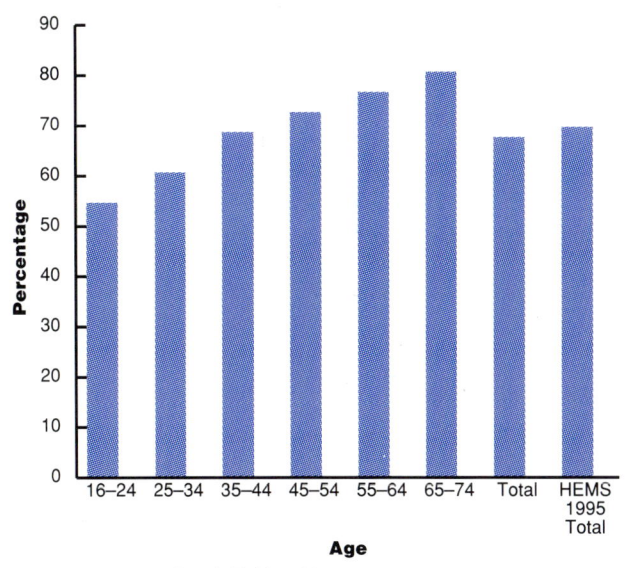

Base numbers are given in Table 4.29

It was reported earlier in the chapter that older people and those in manual social classes did not report such high levels of knowledge as other respondents and Table 4.28 shows that there is a relationship between level of knowledge and whether people felt confused about a healthy diet. While a third (33%) of those who were only able to mention correctly fewer than three ways of achieving a healthy diet agreed that they got confused, under a quarter (22%) of those who could mention three ways described themselves in this way. **(Table 4.28)**

Stockley reported that although there is actually a lot of consensus among experts as to what constitutes a healthy diet the public do not always perceive this[3]. If the public thinks that 'experts never agree' they may be less likely to follow the changes suggested by the experts so this perceived idea may act as a barrier towards following health promotion advice. Sixty eight per cent of HEMS respondents agreed with the statement 'experts never agree about what foods are good for you.' The proportion agreeing increased with age from 55% of those aged 16–24 to 81% of those aged 65–74. **(Figure 4.9 and Table 4.29)**

People are more likely to change their eating behaviour if they perceive it as being easy to do so; the 1986 British Social Attitudes Survey[12] reported that cost was one of the barriers to healthy eating. Thirty seven per cent of HEMS respondents agreed with the statement 'eating healthy food is expensive'. People aged 65–74 were more likely than younger respondents (42% compared with 30% of those aged 16–24) and those in Social Classes IV and V were most likely (49%), and those in Social Classes I and II least likely (29%) to agree with the statement. Not surprisingly there was also a relationship between income and whether or not a person agreed with the statement; just over half (51%) of those with a total household income of less than £5,000 a year agreed that eating healthy food was expensive compared with 29% of those with a household income of £20,000 or more. **(Table 4.30)**

Three quarters of respondents, however, agreed with the statement 'healthy foods are enjoyable'; women were more likely than men to say so, 79% compared with 70%. Older people were more likely than younger people to agree with the statement; 81% of those aged 65–74 did so compared with 70% of those aged 16–24. **(Table 4.31–4.32)**

Although the majority of respondents thought that healthy foods were enjoyable, 38% agreed with the statement 'the tastiest foods are the ones that are bad for you'. **(Table 4.33)**

The wording of these attitude statements changed between the 1995 and 1996. In 1995 the third response option was 'don't know' but in 1996 this was changed to 'neither agree nor disagree' for all the questions; a higher proportion of respondents chose this option. This meant that proportionally fewer chose the other answers. Although the proportions saying they agreed or disagreed with the statements was different between the two years, the pattern of responses was otherwise similar.

Notes and references

1. Department of Health. *The Health of the Nation: a strategy for health in England.* HMSO (London 1992).

2. Health Education Authority. *Enjoy healthy eating: the balance of good health.* Health Education Authority (London 1995).

3. Stockley L. *The promotion of healthier eating: a basis for action.* Health Education Authority (London 1993).

4. Sheiham A et al. Food values, health and diet. In Jowell R et al. *British Social Attitudes: The 1987 report.* Gower (Aldershot 1987).

5. Charles N and Kerr N. *Women, food and families.* Manchester University Press (Manchester 1988) cited in Stockley L. *The promotion of healthier eating: a basis for action.* Health Education Authority (London 1993).

6. The type of carbohydrate in fruit and vegetables is different to that found in bread, potatoes, rice and pasta so nutritionists would not look at consumption of these foods in combination as has been done in this chapter.

7. In the 1995 survey the questions asked were:
    'How often do you eat fruit, vegetables or salad?'
    and
    'How often do you eat potatoes, rice or pasta?'
    whereas in 1996 the questions were changed slightly to say
    'How often do you eat fruit or vegetables or salad?'
    and
    'How often do you eat potatoes or rice or pasta?'
    It is possible that some respondents may have misunderstood the questions in 1995 and thought that they were being asked how often they ate all three items in the question; adding 'or' to the question made it clear they were being asked how often they ate any of the items. There was also a difference in the question order; in 1996 the question on frequency of eating potatoes, rice or pasta was asked before the question about eating chips. In 1995 respondents may have under-reported their consumption of potatoes because they may not have included chips as potatoes; in 1996 interviewers were instructed to tell respondents to include chips in their answers to both the question on chips and the question on potatoes, rice or pasta.

8. Bennett N et al. *Health Survey for England 1993.* HMSO (London 1995).

9. Gregory J et al. *The dietary and nutritional survey of British adults.* HMSO (London 1990).

10. In 1996 the question was 'How often do you eat chips and other fried foods; please do not include oven chips'. In 1995 the instruction not to include oven chips was only an instruction to the interviewer and would not have been read out to all respondents. Oven chips may have been included by some respondents in their answer to this question in 1995 but not in 1996. The question order was also changed; in 1995 this question was asked before the question on consumption of potatoes, rice or pasta whereas in 1996 it was asked afterwards.

11. Azjen I. The theory of planned behaviour. *Organisational Behaviour and Human Decision Processes*, vol. 50, 1991, pp. 179-211.

12. Jowell R et al. *British Social Attitudes: The 1987 report.* Gower (Aldershot 1987).

Annex to Chapter 4

Methodological notes

HEA suggested health promotion indicator: The proportion of the population who are able to state correctly three of the following ways of achieving a healthier diet - eat less fat; eat more fruit, vegetables and salad; eat more starchy carbohydrates (potatoes, pasta or rice); eat more fibre.

Different methods were used in 1995 and 1996 to look at this indicator. In 1995 interviewers read out a list of foods, and for each food respondents were asked whether it was best to:

- eat plenty
- cut down
- neither
- don't know

The types of food asked about were:

- sugar
- salt
- fibre/roughage
- starchy carbohydrates such as potatoes or pasta
- fat
- fresh fruit and vegetables

Asking the questions in this way provided a prompt for the respondent. What it did not show was whether respondents would spontaneously mention these foods if they were asked to.

In 1996 respondents were asked an open question:

'In a few words, how would you describe a healthy diet?'

Interviewers were briefed not to prompt respondents in any way and to record their answers verbatim. If the respondent said 'eat a balanced diet' or 'eat everything in moderation' the interviewer was instructed to ask what was meant by this and to probe fully. The interviewers entered the answers into a coding frame during the interview; any answers which could not be coded in the interview were coded later in the office.

The results show that, although a very high proportion were able to state correctly whether we should eat more or cut down on certain foods, a much smaller proportion said spontaneously that we should do this when asked to define a healthy diet.

Annex Table 1
Knowledge of what constitutes a healthy diet: 1995 and 1996

Healthy diet	1995	1996
	%	%
Cut down on sugar	97	12
Cut down on salt	95	3
Eat plenty of fibre	94	27
Eat plenty of starchy carbohydrates	62	20
Cut down on fat	98	45
Eat plenty of fresh fruit and vegetables	99	67
Identified at least three of 'eat less fat'; 'eat more fruit'; 'eat more starch'; 'eat more fibre'	96	16
Base = 100%	4664	4582

5 Drug use

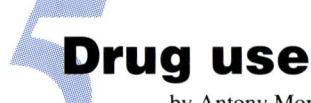

by Antony Morgan, Mary Hickman, Christine Callum, Paige Sinkler
and Hilary Whent – *Health Education Authority*

Summary of main findings

- Thirty two per cent of respondents aged 16–54 had ever used at least one of the drugs asked about, 14% had done so in the past year and 9% in the past month. (Section 5.2.1).

- Twenty eight per cent had ever taken cannabis, 13% had ever taken amphetamines and 9% had ever taken amyl nitrates. (Section 5.2.1).

- A higher proportion of men than of women had ever taken drugs, for example 34% of men had taken cannabis compared with 22% of women. (Section 5.2.1).

- Drug use was less prevalent among older than among the younger age-group. For example, 42% of respondents aged 16–29 had ever taken cannabis, compared with 21% of those aged 30–54 .(Section 5.2.1).

- Drug use was most likely to be reported by the 19–21 age-group: 74% of men and 50% of women in this group had ever tried a drug. (Section 5.2.3).

- Among those who had ever used a drug, 56% of those aged 19–21 had used a drug in the past month, compared with 16% of those aged 30–54. (Section 5.2.4).

- Those aged 16–19 were most likely to know someone who had used drugs (85% did so compared with 26% of 45–54 year-olds). (Section 5.3).

- One in ten of those who had used drugs in the past month did not see the need ever to stop using drugs. (Section 5.4).

- Only a small proportion of respondents had taken two or more drugs in the past year; among this group about half (49%) had taken two or more drugs in combination. (Section 5.6).

- Seventy per cent of respondents agreed that 'all use of drugs is wrong unless with a doctor's prescription or bought from a chemist'. (Section 5.7).

5.1 Introduction and background

Although there were no specific targets for reducing drug use in the *Health of the Nation* White Paper[1], this health topic has since been addressed by the Government in the White Paper 'Tackling Drugs Together'[2]. This presents the government's strategy for tackling drug use and focuses on three main areas: crime, young people and public health. As well as emphasising the need for accessible treatment for drug users the paper also commits the Department of Health to producing guidance for purchasers of drug use services, in time to inform the 1997–8 purchasing round[3].

One recent government report by the Parliamentary Office of Science and Technology has brought together a variety of sources on drug use. It presented a picture of increasing drug-taking, especially amongst young people, mainly those in their late teens and early twenties. As well as looking at the prevalence of drug-taking, the report described the health and psychological effects of taking drugs[4].

Reports on non-prescribed drug use have relied largely on information collected in an ad hoc fashion by both regional and national surveys because reliable on-going surveys, such as the General Household Survey, have never collected data on the prevalence of drug use. It has also been recognised that as the prevalence of the use of some drugs is very low, a large sample would be needed for any survey designed to establish patterns of use[5].

In order to address the problem of scarcity of information about the prevalence of drug use a number of national surveys have recently investigated the topic. The Home Office commissioned the British Crime Survey (BCS) in 1992, 1994, and 1996; data from the 1994 survey have recently been published. Of its three self-completion sections, one was devoted to the prevalence of drug use. No detailed comparisons have been made with the BCS, however, because 1996 data were not available at the time of writing[6].

As part of 'Tackling Drugs Together' the Department of Health commissioned the HEA to manage a drug awareness publicity campaign. Work on this project included a household survey of 11–35 year-olds. This survey, entitled 'Drug Use in England' was carried out in 1995 to measure awareness of drugs and knowledge of health risks associated with drug use (defined as non-medical use/misuse/abuse). The survey also included questions on attitudes towards drugs[7]. Data from this survey were used to develop health promotion indicators on drug use. However, these were finalised after the fieldwork for HEMS 1996 began.

To supplement the data collected on the 1995 National Drugs Campaign Survey, questions about knowledge and use of non-prescribed drugs were asked of all HEMS respondents aged 16–54 years. Respondents were asked to complete this section themselves; the interviewer handed the laptop computer over to the respondent, who keyed in his or her own answers. Ninety eight per cent of those eligible for this part of the interview agreed to take part. A small proportion asked the interviewer to record the answers for them[8].

The questions were designed to measure prevalence rather than frequency of use or amounts taken and asked about all drugs used that had not been prescribed by a doctor. As well as the normal designations, drugs were given their 'street names' to increase the likelihood that respondents understood the questions. The drugs asked about were:

- Amphetamines
- Cannabis
- Cocaine
- Crack
- Ecstasy
- Heroin
- LSD
- Magic mushrooms
- Methadone
- Amyl nitrate
- Glues and solvents
- Anabolic steroids
- Tranquillisers.

Non-prescription use was stressed for the final two drugs. To test for false claiming, respondents were asked, as in similar surveys, about 'Semeron' use. This bogus drug was included as a check on the reliability of the data. However, no one claimed to have taken it.

Respondents were asked if they had ever taken any of the drugs; those who had will be referred to as 'ever users'. Respondents who had ever taken a drug were asked if they had taken it in the past twelve months and finally, where appropriate, in the past month. As with the BCS, *current users have been defined as those who had taken any drug in the past month*. Similar age categories to those used in the BCS report have been used in this chapter. However no detailed comparisons have been made because 1996 BCS data were not available at the time of writing[9].

Respondents were also asked about the methods they had used to take drugs and, if they had injected drugs, whether they had shared needles. Those who had used cannabis in the past month were asked if they had smoked it mixed with tobacco. Informants who had used two or more drugs in the past twelve months were asked if, during one session, they had ever taken two or more drugs in combination or one or more drug in combination with alcohol. Finally, all respondents were asked a number of questions about their attitudes towards drugs, and current users were asked their future intentions with regard to using drugs.

5.2 Prevalence of drug use

5.2.1 Overall prevalence

Nearly one third (32%) of respondents aged 16–54 had ever used at least one of the drugs listed above. However, there were a large number of drugs listed in the survey, and while ever use of drugs such as cannabis, amphetamines and amyl nitrates was not uncommon, prevalence of the use of other drugs such as heroin was very low. Overall, just over one quarter (28%) of the sample had ever used cannabis, slightly more than one in ten (13%) had used amphetamines, less than one in ten (9%) amyl nitrates and a very small percentage heroin (1%).

Within the twelve months preceding the interview just over one in eight (14%) respondents had used at least one drug. Again the most commonly used drug was cannabis (13%), whilst less than one per cent of those interviewed had used heroin in that period.

Health in England 1996 : What people know, what people think, what people do

Figure 5.1 Percentage who had used specific drugs ever, in the past year or in the past month: adults aged 16–54

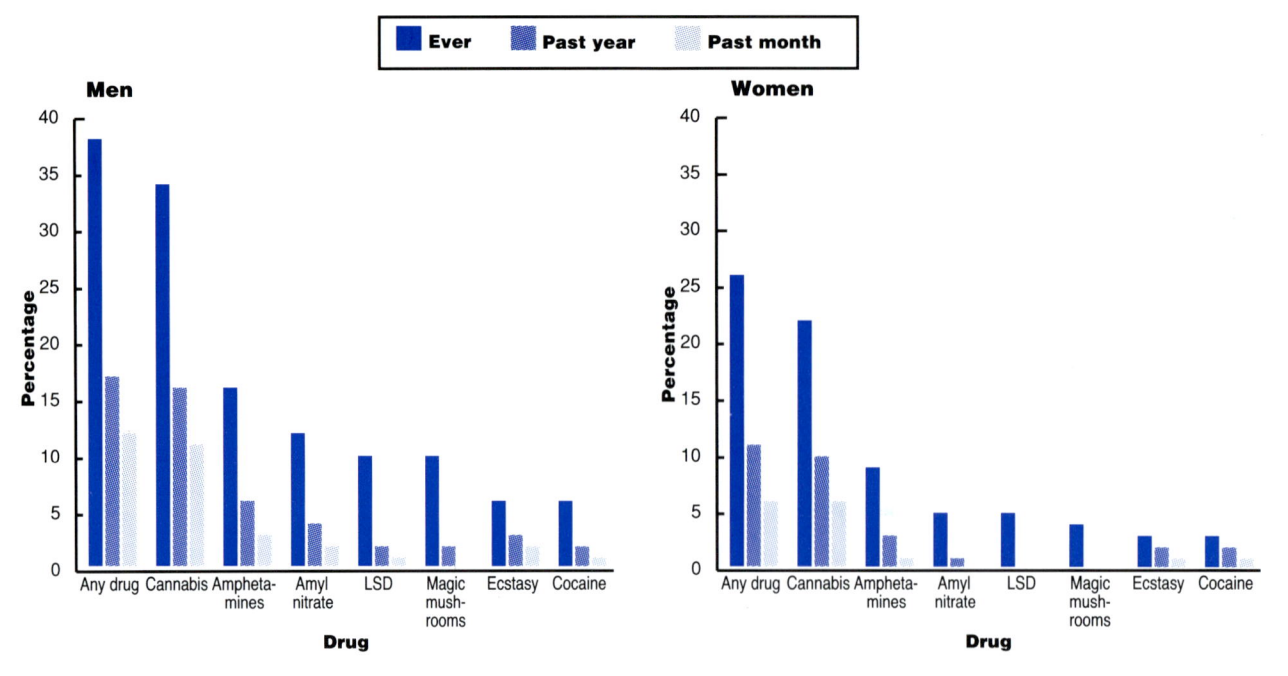

Base numbers are given in Table 5.1

Just under one in ten (9%) respondents had used at least one drug in the past month. Almost all current users had used cannabis (8%). Many of the drugs, for example LSD and magic mushrooms, had been used by less than one per cent of respondents during that period. **(Table 5.1 and Figure 5.1)**

Drug use was analysed by age and sex and was found to be strongly associated with both[10]. Men were more likely than women to have ever used any drug. For example, over one third (34%) of men had ever used cannabis, compared with over one in five (22%) women. Drug use was less likely to be reported by the older than by the younger age-group; two fifths (42%) of respondents aged 16–29 had ever used cannabis, compared with one in five (21%) of those aged 30–54.

In both age-groups, women were less likely than men to report drug use. Whilst nearly half (49%) of men aged 16–29 had ever used cannabis, just over one third (36%) of women in this age-group had done so. This pattern was repeated in the older age-group, but at a lower level of prevalence. Just over one quarter (26%) of men aged 30–54 had ever used cannabis, compared with one in seven (15%) women. **(Table 5.2 and Figure 5.2)**

5.2.2 Drug groupings

As has been seen above, some drugs on the list had only been used by a very small percentage of respondents. Because of this, some surveys have grouped these drugs into categories, so that more detailed analysis is possible. The groups used in this report are the same as those used in the 1994 BCS report on drug use. Whilst, as the BCS authors suggested, these categories are open to argument because they are based on social attributes rather than pharmacological definitions[6], it was felt that using similar categories for reporting the HEMS data would enable comparison. Thus, as in the BCS report, drugs were divided into four groups:

- Cannabis
- Hallucinants (amphetamines, amyl nitrates, magic mushrooms, LSD, Ecstasy)
- Opiates (heroin, methadone, cocaine, crack)
- Other drugs (tranquillisers, glues and solvents, steroids, anything else)

Within the sample there were a small number of respondents who did not want to answer questions on current or past drug use. Unless otherwise indicated in tables, these have been included in the 'not taken' category.

Nearly one third (32%) of respondents had ever used a drug. Of these over a quarter (28%) had used cannabis and nearly one in five (18%) had used hallucinants. One in twenty had used either opiates or drugs from the 'other' category (5% and 6% respectively).

Fourteen per cent of respondents had used a drug in the past year. Thirteen per cent had used cannabis, 6% hallucinants, 2% opiates and 1% drugs from the 'other' category.

Nearly one in ten (9%) respondents were current users. For current use, both age and sex were important differentiators. One in five (21%) men and one in eight (12%) women aged 16–29 were current users of cannabis and one in ten (9%) men and one in twenty (5%) women in that age-group were current users of hallucinants. One in twenty (5%) men and a small proprotion of women (2%) aged 30–54 had used cannabis in the past month. The prevalence of current use of hallucinants was very low for this age-group (1% of men and less than 1% of women). **(Table 5.3)**

Figure 5.2 Percentage who had ever used specific drugs by age: adults aged 16–54

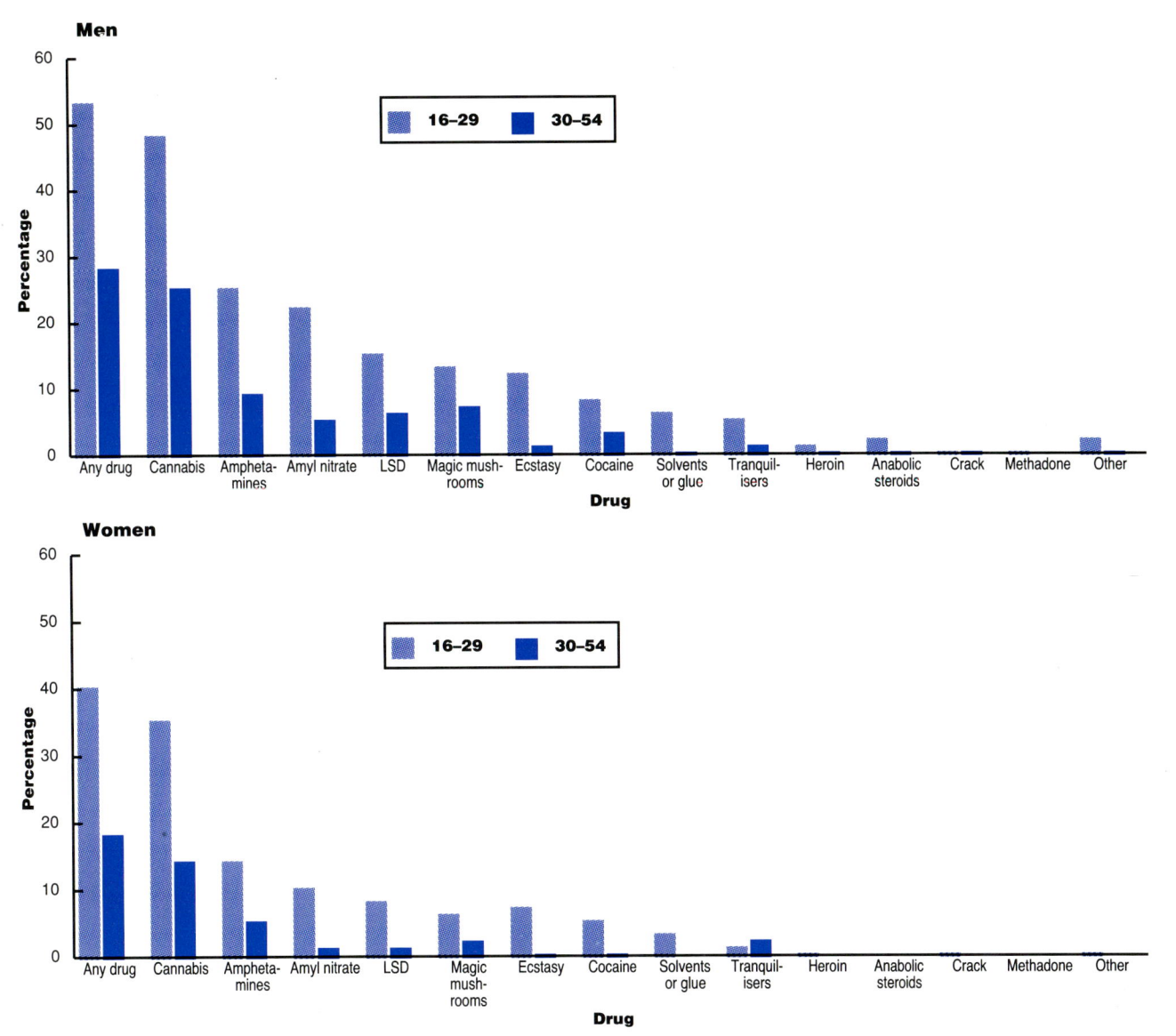

Base numbers are given in Table 5.2

5.2.3 Drug use amongst younger people

In order to get a clearer picture of the strong relationship between drug use and age, the data were broken down into seven age-groups, as was done in the 1994 BCS report.

Prevalence in the ever use of any drug was highest among those aged 20–24; over half (57%) of this age-group had ever used a drug. The next highest prevalence of ever use was among those aged 16–19 and 25–29 (44% and 41% respectively). After the age of 30 prevalence decreased as age increased. However, one quarter (25%) of those aged 40–44 had used a drug at some time.

The pattern of high prevalence in the 20–24 age-group was especially strong for men. Seven in ten (70%) men in that age-group had ever used a drug, compared with two in five (42%) men aged 16–19 and half (50%) of men aged 25–29. However, the pattern was less clear for women; nearly half (47%) of women aged 16–19 and 20–24 (46%) had ever tried a drug, compared with one third (32%) of women aged 25–29. **(Table 5.4 and Figure 5.3)**

Figure 5.3 Ever use of any drug by age and sex: adults aged 16–54

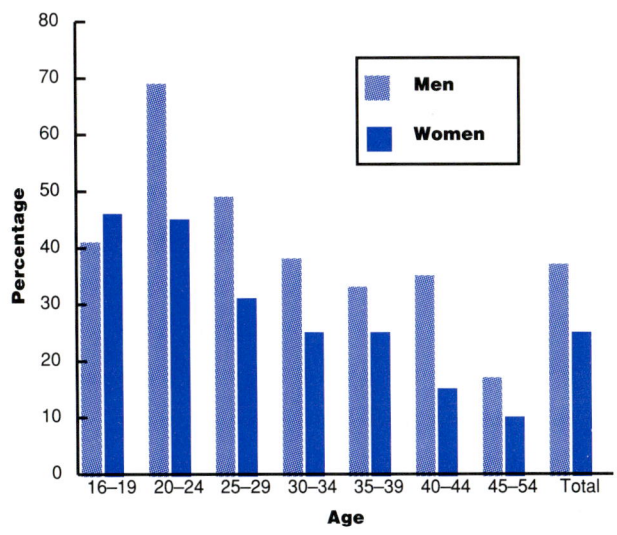

Base numbers are given in Table 5.4

Health in England 1996 : What people know, what people think, what people do   **45**

The relationship between age and current use was slightly different. Current use was very similar for those in the 16–19 and the 20–24 year age-group (26% and 25% respectively). Thereafter, prevalence decreased sharply, with one in ten (10%) of those aged 25–29 being current users. Whilst the pattern of current use was similar for both men and women, prevalence of drug use was higher among men than women for all drugs in all age-groups. The exception was hallucinant use among those aged 16–19 but the difference was not statistically significant. **(Table 5.6)**

Even the age categories discussed above still mask the concentration of drug use amongst the younger age-groups. Therefore the data were further divided to investigate this pattern. The 16–24 age-group was divided into three, rather than two groups (16–18, 19–21 and 22–24), to try to determine the peak age of drug use. Because of the lower levels of prevalence among the older age-groups, respondents aged 30 and over have been grouped into one category for this analysis. When looking at these data it must be remembered that the number of respondents in each age category is fairly small, so that large differences between groups would be needed to make those differences statistically significant.

Prevalence of drug use was highest among those aged 19–21. Three in five (61%) of them had ever used a drug, over half (57%) had ever used cannabis and over one third (37%) hallucinants. This compares with nearly two fifths (39%) of respondents aged 16–18 who had ever used cannabis and nearly one third (29%) who had ever used hallucinants. Sex differences also show clearly here; nearly three quarters (74%) of men and half (50%) of women aged 19–21 had ever used a drug. However, these differences were reversed in the 16–18 age-group where women were slightly more likely than men to have ever used a drug. Nearly half (47%) of women in this age-group had ever used a drug, compared to just under two in five (39%) men. **(Table 5.7)**

Nearly one quarter (24%) of those aged 16–18 were current drug users. This compared to over one third (34%) of those aged 19–21 and one in five (20%) of those aged 22–24. Current drug use was again most prevalent among men aged 19–21; half (50%) of men in this age group had used a drug in the past month, compared to one in five (20%) women.

Nearly half (46%) of men aged 19–21 had used cannabis in the past month and over one quarter (27%) had used hallucinants, compared with one in five (20%) women in this age-group who had used cannabis and less than one in ten (7%) who had used hallucinants. However, only a small percentage of men aged 19–21 had used opiates (4%) or a drug from the 'other' category (5%) in the past month. The likelihood of use of these drugs by women aged 19–21 was very low (2% and less than 1% respectively).

Cannabis was the most commonly used drug by current users in all other age-groups. It had been used by one in five men and women aged 16–18 years (21% and 22% respectively) and by just under a quarter (24%) of men and one in eight (12%) women aged 22–24 in the past month. The prevalence of current drug use was higher for men than for women in all age-groups, except the youngest, where it was similar for both men and women, but these results are not statistically significant. For both men and women the prevalence of use in the past month decreased quite sharply as age increased; one in eight (12%) men and one in twelve (7%) women aged 25–29 and a small percentage of men (6%) and women (2%) aged 30–54 had taken any drug in the past month. **(Tables 5.9 and Figures 5.4–5.5)**

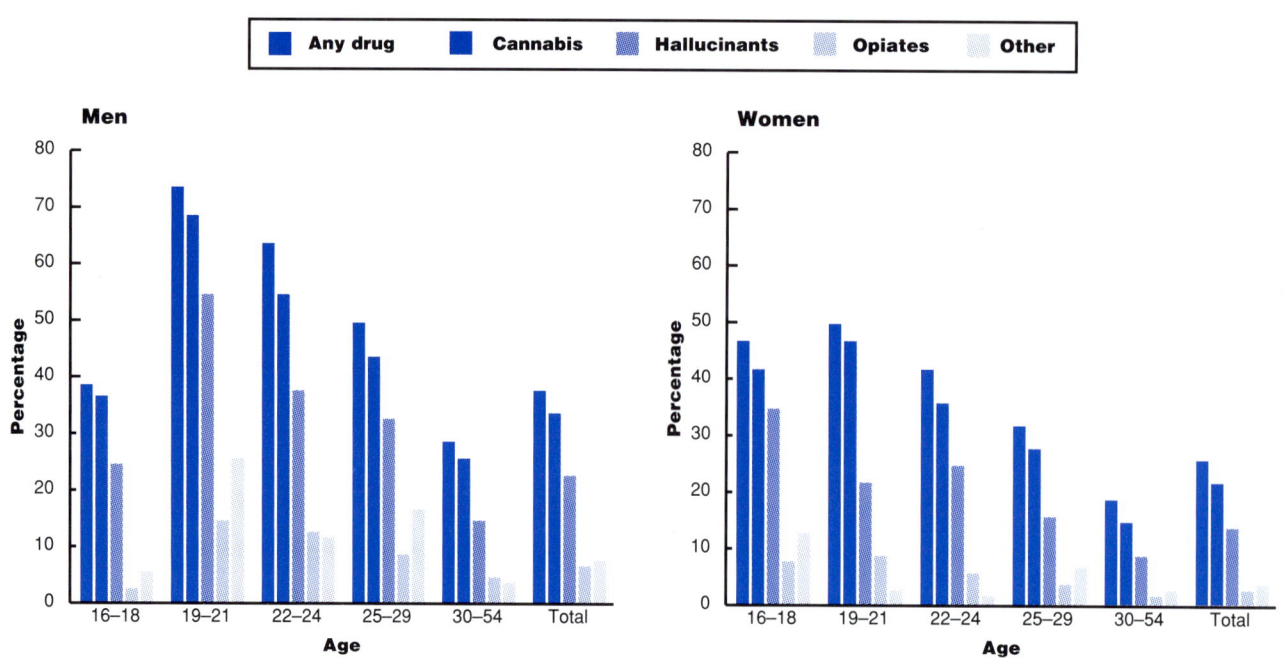

Figure 5.4 Percentage reporting having ever used drugs by drug category and age: adults aged 16–54

Base numbers are given in Table 5.7

Figure 5.5 Percentage who had used drugs in the past month by drug category and age: adults aged 16–54

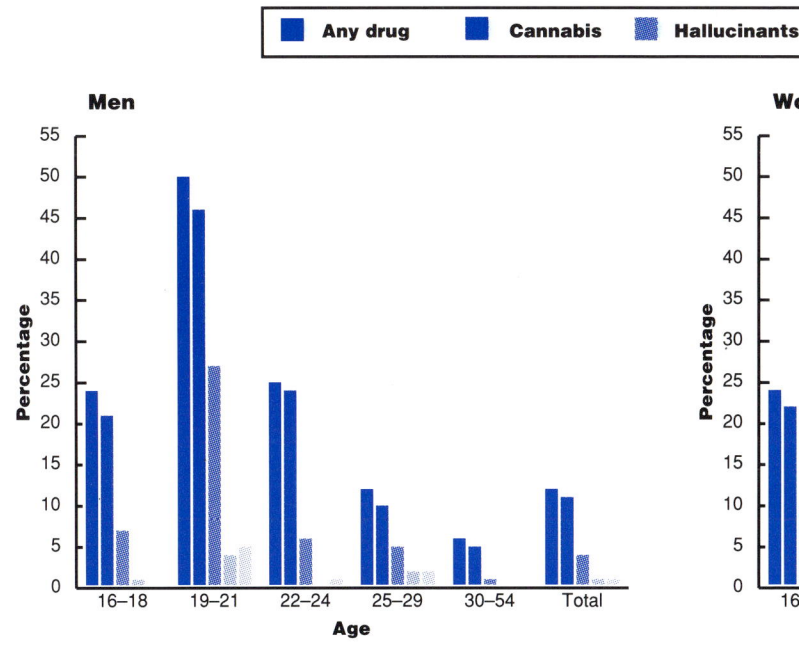

[Legend: Any drug, Cannabis, Hallucinants, Opiates, Other]

[Bar chart: Men — by age group 16–18, 19–21, 22–24, 25–29, 30–54, Total]

[Bar chart: Women — by age group 16–18, 19–21, 22–24, 25–29, 30–54, Total]

Base numbers are given in Table 5.9

5.2.4 Current use as a proportion of ever use

Ever use of a drug gives an overall picture of drug use, and use in the past month shows current use. However, studies such as the 1994 BCS[6] have shown that many people have tried a drug only once or twice and that the high proportions of ever use reported provide a rather simplified picture of drug use. The HEMS data were therefore further analysed to provide more information on this aspect of drug use. Those who had ever used a drug were used as the base figure for current use and use in the past twelve months.

This analysis, although based on small numbers, further highlights the strong relationship between age and drug use; for the older age-groups use in the past month was much lower as a percentage of ever use than for the younger age-groups. Thus, of those aged 19–21 who had ever used drugs, seven in ten (70%) had done so in the past year and over half (56%) in the past month. Current use was highest for those aged 16–21 (among whom, 56% of those who had ever taken a drug had done so in the past month) and declined quite sharply after that. Thus, in the 30–54 age-group, less than one quarter (24%) had ever used drugs; of these just over one quarter (27%) had done so in the past year and one in eight (16%) had done so in the past month. The relationship between age and current use was true for both men and women. **(Table 5.10 and Figure 5.6)**

5.2.5 Number of drugs taken

This section will look at the number of different drugs taken, both including and excluding cannabis. Overall, nearly half (46%) of ever users had used only one type of drug, one in five (20%) had used two drugs, one in ten (10%) had used three drugs and one in four (25%) had used four or more drugs. A higher proportion of women than men had only ever taken one drug, 51% and 43% respectively. However, men were more likely than women to have taken six or more drugs (14% and 6% respectively).

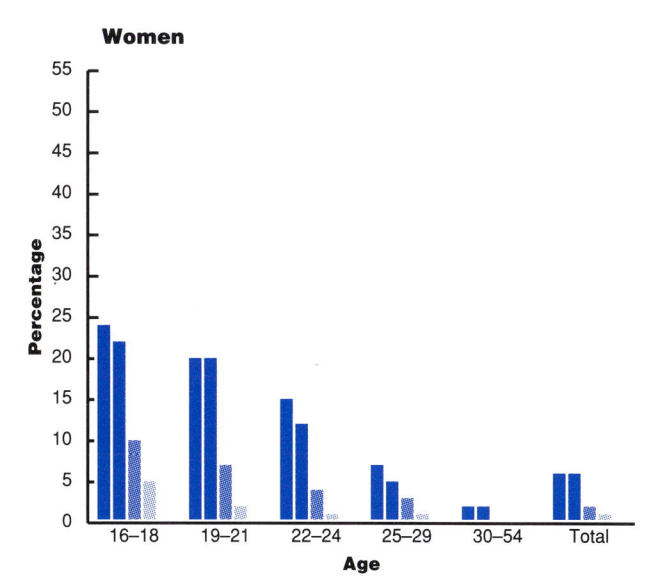

Seven in ten (72%) current users had used one drug, one in eight (12%) had used two drugs and one in twelve (8%) had used three drugs. Again women were more likely to have used only one type of drug; three quarters (77%) of current users had taken only one type of drug, compared to seven in ten (69%) men. Only a small proportion of women had taken more than two different drugs; 4% had taken three in the past month, compared to one in ten (11%) men. **(Table 5.12 and Figure 5.7)**

As has been seen in earlier tables the most common drug used was cannabis. However, other drugs had been used, either with or without cannabis[11]. One third (36%) of respondents who had ever used drugs had used cannabis only, one in five (18%) had used cannabis and one other drug and one third (33%) had used

Figure 5.6 Percentage who had used any drug in the past month, as a proportion of ever users by age and sex: adults aged 16–54 who had ever used any drug

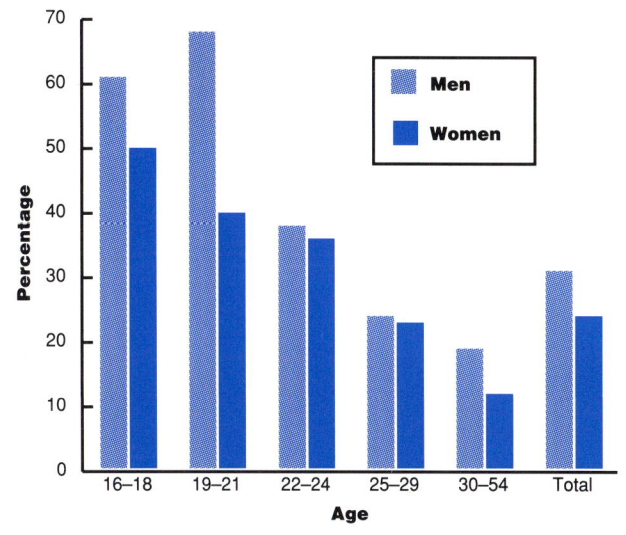

[Bar chart showing Men and Women by age group 16–18, 19–21, 22–24, 25–29, 30–54, Total]

Base numbers are given in Table 5.10

Health in England 1996 : What people know, what people think, what people do

Figure 5.7 Number of different drugs ever used by recency of use and sex: adults aged 16–54 who had ever used any drug

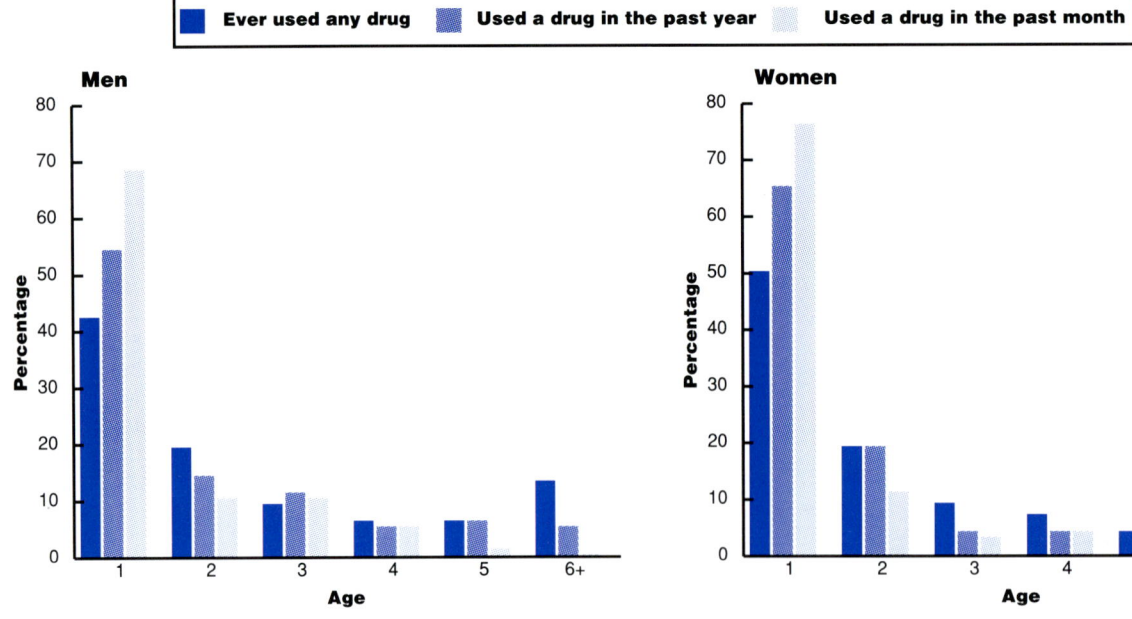

Legend: Ever used any drug | Used a drug in the past year | Used a drug in the past month

Men / Women (bar charts by number of drugs: 1, 2, 3, 4, 5, 6+)

Base numbers are given in Table 5.12

cannabis and two other drugs. One in ten (10%) ever users had used one drug, not cannabis, 2% had used two drugs but not cannabis and 1% had used three or more drugs but not cannabis. There were no sex differences.

Three in five (64%) current drug users had used cannabis only, whilst one in ten (9%) had used cannabis and one other drug and one in six (16%) had used cannabis and two or more other drugs. Less than one in ten (7%) current drug users had used one drug only, but not cannabis, in the past month, 2% had used two drugs other than cannabis and 1% had used three or more drugs but not cannabis. (**Table 5.13 and Figure 5.8**)

5.3 Knowing people who use drugs

All respondents aged 16–54 were asked whether they knew people who used drugs; half (50%) did. Men (55%) were more likely than women (45%) to know drug users. As might have been expected, respondents in the younger age-groups were more likely to know people who used drugs. In fact there was a significant age gradient in these data, ranging from over four in five (85%) 16–19 year-olds to just over a quarter (26%) of 45–54 year-olds who knew someone who used drugs. Such large percentages of young people knowing others who used drugs is reflective of the high percentage of young people in our survey who had ever taken drugs. (**Table 5.14 and Figure 5.9**)

Figure 5.8 Percentage of respondents who used cannabis and/or other drugs by recency of use: adults aged 16–54 who had ever used drugs

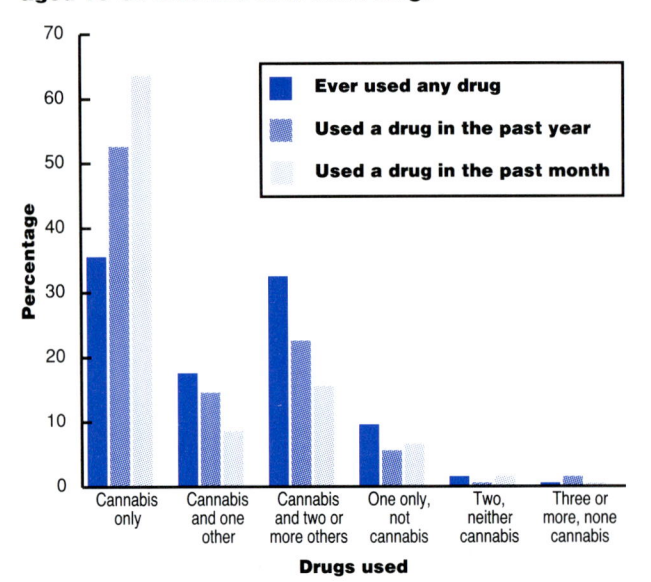

Categories: Cannabis only | Cannabis and one other | Cannabis and two or more others | One only, not cannabis | Two, neither cannabis | Three or more, none cannabis

Base numbers are given in Table 5.13

Figure 5.9 Percentage who know people who use drugs by sex and age: adults aged 16–54

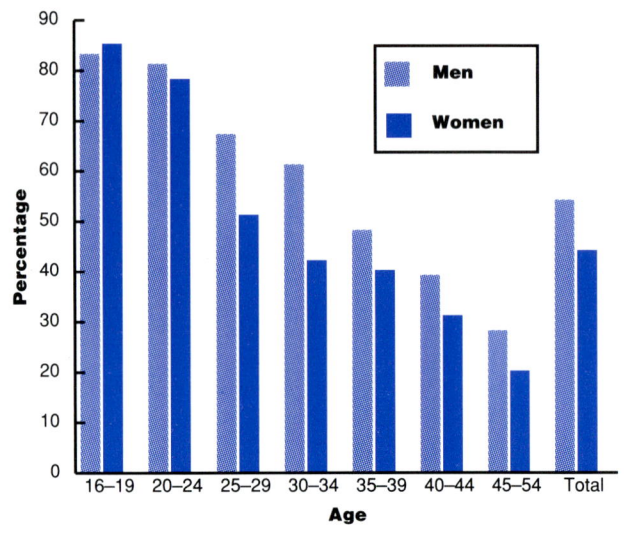

Age groups: 16–19, 20–24, 25–29, 30–34, 35–39, 40–44, 45–54, Total

Base numbers are given in Table 5.14

48 Health in England 1996 : What people know, what people think, what people do

Those respondents who had used drugs were more likely than non-users to know other people who had used drugs. Seven in ten (71%) ever users who had not used drugs in the past year, almost all of those who had used drugs in the past year (95%) and 97% of current users reported knowing people who had used drugs. However, only one third (35%) of those who had never used a drug knew people who used drugs. (**Table 5.15**)

5.4 Intentions to stop using drugs

All current users were asked about their future intentions with regard to drug use. They were asked to select from the following statements the one that fitted most closely with their intentions: 'I'd like to stop using drugs altogether'; 'I see no need to stop using drugs at the moment'; or 'I don't see the need to ever stop using drugs'.

Almost a third (31%) of current users said that they would like to give up using drugs altogether. A higher proportion of men than of women wanted to give up (32% and 27% respectively). Over half (59%) saw no need to give up at the moment and one in ten (10%) did not see the need to ever stop using drugs.

Women were more likely than men to say that they did not see the need to stop using drugs at the moment (64% and 57% respectively). Because of the small numbers involved it was not possible to look at intentions broken down by any but the two main age-groups, 16–29 and 30–54. However, no significant differences between the two groups in intentions to give up were found. (**Table 5.16**)

If respondents said either that they would like to give up using drugs altogether or they saw no need to stop using drugs at the moment, they were then asked to choose from a selection of statements and identify which best described them:

- I intend to stop using drugs within the next month
- I intend to stop using drugs within the next 6 months
- I intend to stop using drugs within the next year
- I intend to stop using drugs but not within the next year
- I am unlikely to ever stop using drugs

The order of the items was different depending on whether the respondent had said that they would like to stop using drugs altogether or they saw no need to stop using drugs at the moment.

Over one third (37%) of current users said that they intended to stop using drugs at some point but not in the next year. Just under one-fifth (18%) said they would be unlikely ever to stop, whilst a similar proportion (18%) said that they intended to stop in the next month. One in ten (10%) saw no need to ever stop, whilst slightly fewer said they intended to stop using drugs within the next six months or within the next year, (9% and 8% respectively). (**Table 5.17 and Figure 5.10**)

5.5 Methods of taking drugs

All respondents who had ever taken drugs were asked by which method they had taken them. Over four fifths (84%) of this group had smoked drugs. This is perhaps not surprising when the most common drug taken was cannabis, which is often smoked. Men who had ever used drugs were more likely than women to have smoked

Figure 5.10 Intentions to stop taking drugs by sex: adults aged 16–54 who had taken drugs in the past month

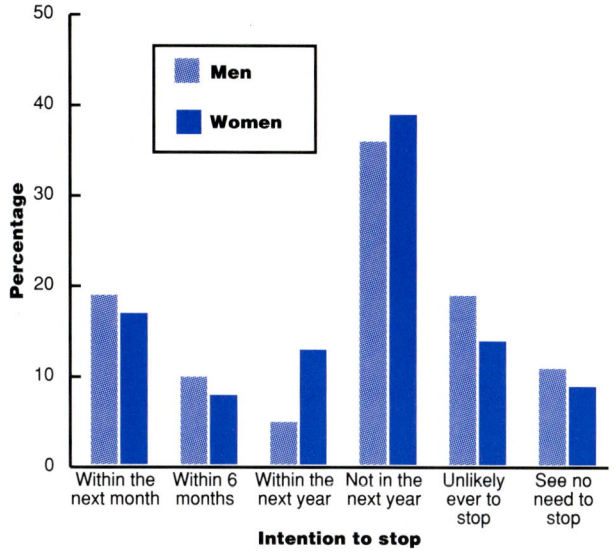

Base numbers are given in Table 5.17

them (87% and 78% respectively). Men aged 30–34 who had ever taken drugs were most likely, and men aged 45–54 least likely, to have smoked drugs (93% and 80% respectively).

Just over one third (34%) of ever users had swallowed drugs. There were no significant differences in either age or sex. One fifth (20%) of ever users had sniffed drugs, and those in the younger age-groups were more likely than those in the older age-groups to have taken drugs by this method. For example, over one quarter (29%) of ever users aged 20–24 had sniffed a drug at some time, compared to fewer than one in ten (7%) of ever users aged 45–54. Just over one in ten (11%) respondents who had ever used drugs had inhaled them. There were no significant age or sex differences here.

Only one per cent of those who had ever used drugs had injected them, so no further analysis was possible on these data. (**Table 5.18**)

5.6 Taking drugs in combination

Respondents who had used two or more drugs in the past twelve months were asked if they had used two or more in combination in one session. The numbers who had used two or more drugs in the past year were very small. These small numbers must be taken into account when looking at these data. Of this group, nearly half (49%) had used two or more in combination. Men were more likely to have done so than women (55% and 36% respectively) but these differences were not significant. (**Table 5.19**)

Respondents who had used one or more drugs in the past twelve months were asked if they had used one or more drugs in combination with alcohol; over half (58%) had done so. Men were more likely than women to have used a drug in combination with alcohol (65% and 47% respectively). Although numbers were too small to report the findings by small age-groups, those in the 16–29 age group were more likely than those in the 30–54 age-group to have used at least one drug in combination with alcohol (64% and 46% respectively). (**Table 5.20**)

Health in England 1996 : What people know, what people think, what people do 49

Figure 5.11 Whether agrees that 'All use of drugs is wrong unless with a doctor's prescription or bought from a chemist': adults aged 16–54

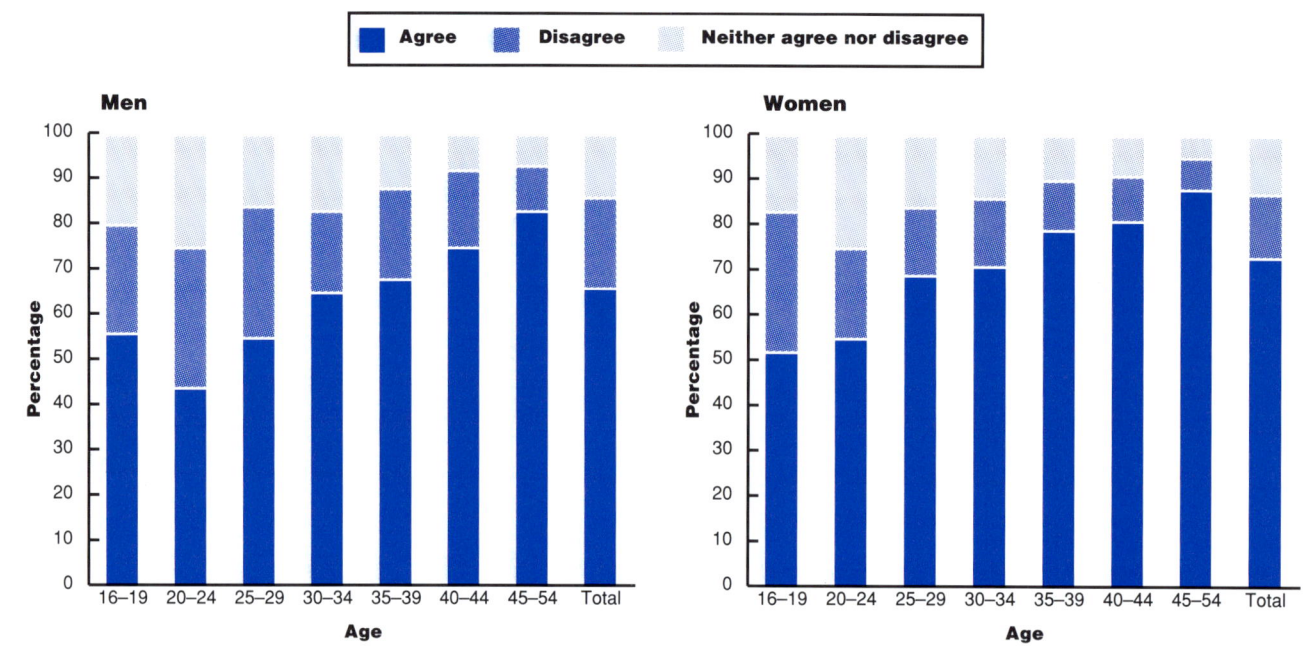

■ Agree   ▨ Disagree   ░ Neither agree nor disagree

Men

Women

Base numbers are given in Table 5.21

5.7 Attitudes to drugs

To explore the climate of opinion and public attitudes towards drug use, respondents were asked whether they agreed or disagreed with two statements:

- All use of drugs is wrong unless with a doctor's prescription or bought from a chemist
- I don't mind other people using drugs

They were also asked about their perceptions of the safety of drug use. For the purposes of interpretation it was assumed that people understood 'drugs' to be the list of substances asked about prior to these attitudinal statements.

Seven in ten (70%) respondents agreed that 'all use of drugs is wrong unless with a doctor's prescription or bought from a chemist'. Women were more likely to agree than men (74% and 66% respectively). Older people were more likely to agree than those in younger age-groups; so that, for example, half (50%) of those aged 20–24 agreed with the statement, compared with over eight in ten (85%) of those aged 45–54. **(Table 5.21 and Figure 5.11)**

Those who had ever taken drugs were less likely to agree with the statement than those who had not. For example, less than one in five (17%) of current drug users agreed with the statement compared with nearly nine in ten (86%) of those who had never used a drug. This low level of agreement amongst users compared to non-users was true for both men and women. **(Table 5.22 and Figure 5.12)**

Just over half (55%) of respondents disagreed with the statement, 'I don't mind other people using drugs', about one fifth (21%) agreed and a quarter (24%) neither agreed nor disagreed. Older people were less likely to agree than younger people; nearly two in five (37%) of those aged 16–19 agreed that they did not mind others using drugs, compared to one in eight (12%) of those aged 45–54. **(Table 5.23)**

There was an association between drug use and agreement with the statement. Whilst over half (52%) of current users did not mind others using drugs, only one in eight (13%) of those who had never used a drug agreed that they did not mind. **(Table 5.24)**

Figure 5.12 Whether agrees that 'All use of drugs is wrong unless with a doctor's precription or bought from a chemist' by drug use: adults aged 16–54

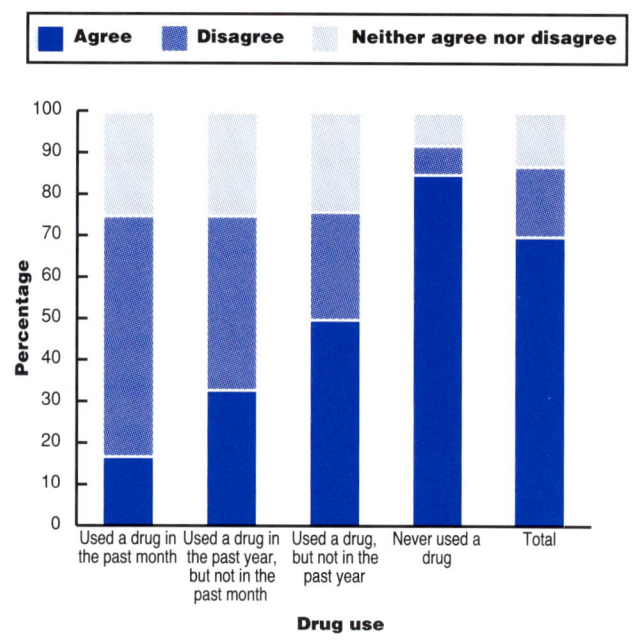

■ Agree   ▨ Disagree   ░ Neither agree nor disagree

Base numbers are given in Table 5.22

Figure 5.13 Whether agrees that drugs are safe to use by sex: adults aged 16–54

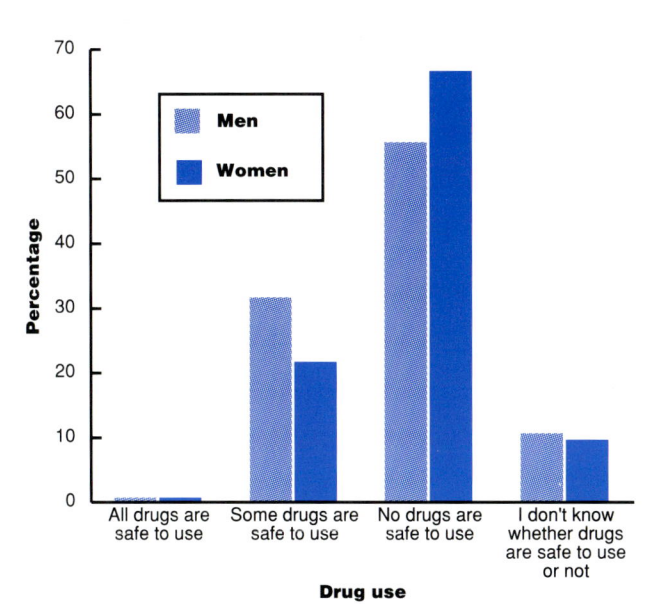

Base numbers are given in Table 5.25

Figure 5.14 Whether agrees that drugs are safe to use by drug use: adults aged 16–54

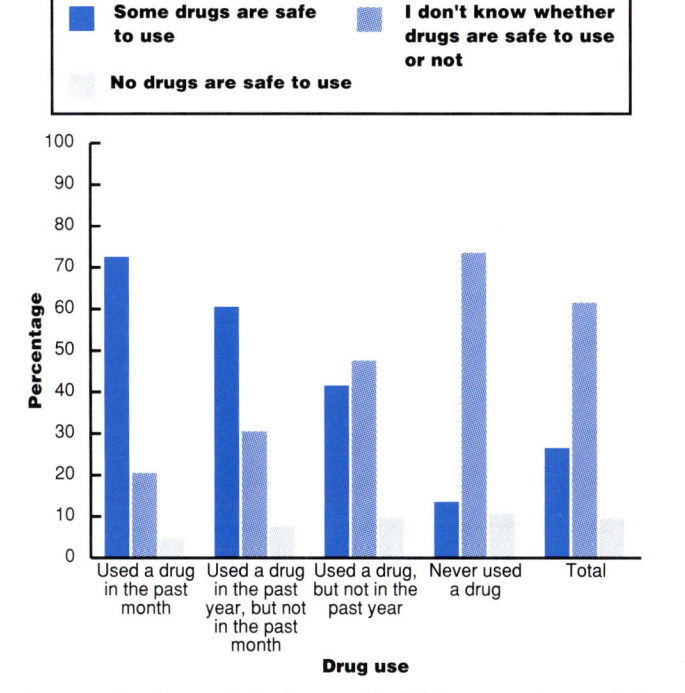

The proportion of respondents who agreed that 'All drugs are safe to use (as long as you know what you are doing)' was too small to show on the chart.

Base numbers are given in Table 5.26

Only a very small proportion of respondents agreed that 'all drugs are safe to use as long as you know what you are doing' (1%); one third (32%) of men and one in five (22%) women, agreed that 'some drugs are safe to use as long as you know what you are doing'. The majority of respondents (61%), agreed that 'no drugs are safe to use', although one in ten (10%) felt that they did not know how safe drugs were. The proportion agreeing that 'some drugs are safe as long as you know what you're doing' declined with age among both men and women. Nearly half (49%) of men and over one third (38%) of women aged 16–19 agreed with this statement, compared to one in five (20%) men and one in eight (12%) women aged 45–54. The proportion of respondents agreeing that 'no drugs are safe' generally increased with age, although men aged 16–19 were more likely to agree with the statement than those aged 20–24. (46% and 38% respectively). **(Table 5.25 and Figure 5.13)**

Only 1% of current drug users agreed with the statement that 'all drugs are safe to use as long as you know what you're doing'. Current drug users were much more likely than those who had never used a drug to agree that 'some drugs are safe to use as long as you know what you're doing' (73% and 14% respectively). Seven in ten (73%) of those who had never used a drug agreed that 'no drugs are safe to use', compared to one in five (21%) current users. **(Table 5.26 and Figure 5.14)**

Notes and references

1. Department of Health. *The Health of the Nation: a strategy for health in England*. HMSO (London 1992).

2. *Tackling Drugs together; a strategy for England 1995-1998*. HMSO (London 1995).

3. Department of Health. *The Task Force to Review Services for Drug Misusers: Report of an Independent Review of Drug Treatment Services in England*. Department of Health (London 1996).

4. Parliamentary Office of Science and Technology. *Common Illegal Drugs and Their Effects*. (London 1996).

5. Institute for the Study of Drug Dependence. *Drug Misuse in Britain 1994*. Institute for the Study of Drug Dependence (London 1994).

6. Ramsey M and Percy A. *Drug misuse declared: results of the 1994 British Crime Survey*. Home Office (London 1996).

7. Health Education Authority. *Drug Use in England: results of the 1995 National Drugs Campaign Survey*. To be published by the HEA in 1997.

8. Appendix A gives more detailed information on response to the self-completion section of the interview.

9. Comparisons with 1994 data were not possible because the published data were not in a comparable format.

10. Three summary tables showing the associations betweeen drug use and other characteristics are included at the end of the chapter. See Tables 5.27–5.29.

11. This section only looks at the number of drugs used, drugs taken in combination are looked at in Section 5.6.

6 Sexual Health

Summary of main findings

- Sixteen per cent of men and 10% of women aged 16–54 reported two or more sexual partners in the 12 months before interview. (Section 6.2).

- Thirty per cent of men and 31% of women thought they had 'no risk' of being infected with HIV, while 33% of men and 34% of women made the same assessment of their risk of contracting another sexually transmitted disease (STD). Older respondents were less likely than younger ones to see themselves as at risk. (Section 6.3).

- Only a minority (18%) of respondents thought it would be 'difficult to raise the subject of using a condom with a new partner'. (Section 6.4.1).

- More than two thirds of women (67%), and almost three fifths of men (58%) said they would always use a condom 'if in the near future they did have sex with a new partner', while 17% of women and 31% of men said it would depend. Only 1% of respondents stated that they would never use a condom. (Section 6.4.2).

- Among those who reported a new partner in the last year, 60% of men and 63% of women used a condom the first time they had intercourse with their most recent partner. (Section 6.4.3).

6.1 Introduction and background

The *Health of the Nation* White Paper[1] argues that good personal and sexual relationships can actively promote health and well-being; they can therefore contribute to the overall goal of 'adding life to years'. On the other hand, sexual activity can sometimes result in unwanted pregnancies, ill-health or disease. HIV/AIDS and sexual health were included in the White Paper as a Key Area because AIDS/HIV 'is perhaps the greatest new threat to public health this century'. AIDS/HIV was not included as a target in the HEA's Targets Project because of surveillance difficulties (including a long latent period between infection with HIV and the appearance of symptoms associated with AIDS).

Estimates from the United Nations AIDS programme, published in November 1996, are that 29.4 million people world-wide have been infected with HIV, with 8.4 million AIDS cases and 6.4 million deaths[2]. The rate of increase in HIV infection, including in the UK, is greatest among those infected through heterosexual intercourse[3]. In England, 24,134 cases of HIV infection were notified to the Communicable Disease Surveillance Centre between 1985 and June 1996, with 11,961 AIDS cases[4]. In England and Wales, 517 men and 57 women were certified as dying from HIV in 1994, compared with 458 men and 48 women in 1993[5].

In the 1995 HEMS, all respondents aged 16–54 were asked to do a self-completion module on sexual health. The module included questions on age at first intercourse, number of sexual partners in the last year, attitudes towards and use of condoms, and knowledge of safer sex. Many of the questions were taken from the *National Survey of Sexual Attitudes and Lifestyles*[6] to allow comparisons to be made between the two sets of data. In 1996, the module was shortened considerably, as the main focus of the self-completion section of the interview was on drug use, reported on in Chapter 5. A few questions on sexual health were retained in the self-completion module to enable two risk behaviours, drug use and unprotected intercourse, to be examined together. This chapter therefore presents a broad, rather than a detailed, picture of sexual health.

Ninety eight per cent of those eligible for this part of the interview agreed to take part. Respondents were asked to complete this section themselves; the interviewer handed the laptop computer over to the respondent, who keyed in his or her own answers. A small proportion asked the interviewer to record their answers for them[7].

6.2 Number of sexual partners in the last year

The likelihood of HIV infection increases with the number of partners with whom one has unprotected intercourse; unprotected intercourse with more than one partner can therefore be seen as a risk behaviour, in the sense that it increases the probability of infection by the HIV virus. Those respondents who had ever had sexual intercourse were asked how many partners they had had in the 12 months before interview[8]. Apart from those who reported a new partner in the last year, however, respondents were not asked about their use of condoms; those who did report a new partner were only asked if they had used a condom when they first had intercourse with their most recent partner. Although HEMS data show the number of partners in the last year, they therefore do not provide information on what proportion of respondents were having *unprotected* intercourse.

Figure 6.1 Percentage reporting two or more sexual partners in the last 12 months by age and sex: adults aged 16-54

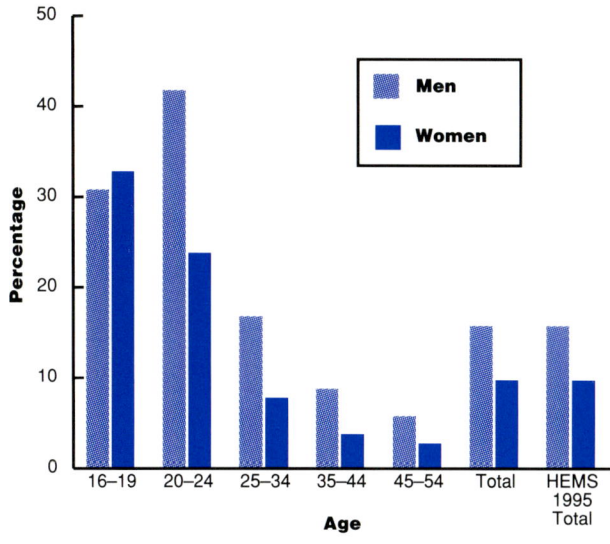

Base numbers are given in Table 6.1

Not surprisingly, the youngest respondents (those aged 16–19) were most likely to say they had not had a partner in the last year and they are therefore shown separately in Table 6.1[9]. Almost half (47%) of men and over a quarter (27%) of women in this age-group reported no partner, compared with 14% or fewer of older men and 17% or fewer of older women. As in 1995[10], the majority of respondents (69% of men and 78% of women) reported only one partner in the last year[11]. With the exception of those aged 16–19, men were more likely than women in the same age-group to say they had had more than one partner, but the differences were not always significant. These proportions are very similar to those reported in the 1992 *Health and Lifestyles Survey*[12] (68% of men and 79% of women in that survey said they had had only one partner in the last year) and the *National Survey of Sexual Attitudes* (73% of men and 79% of women reported one [opposite sex] partner), except that the latter survey had a statistically slightly higher proportion of men reporting only one partner. Sixteen per cent of men and 10% of women in the HEMS sample had had more than one partner in the last year, not significantly different from 1995. A very small proportion (1% of men and less than 1% of women) reported ten or more partners. (**Figure 6.1 and Table 6.1**)

The likelihood of reporting two or more sexual partners in the last year was highest among those aged under 25, but dropped markedly after this. More than a third of men and more than a quarter of women aged 16–24 had had more than one partner, compared with only 6% of men and 3% of women in the 45–54 age-group. Wellings et al note that the youngest age-groups are starting on their sexual careers and may explore a series of relationships before (in the future) adopting a long-term relationship with a monogamous lifestyle. Knox et al[13] believe, however, that there is a cohort effect; when the total number of lifetime partners reported by respondents in their study was analysed, some of the youngest age-groups, who might be thought to have the least complete sexual careers, had already had more partners than some of the oldest age-groups.

Among HEMS respondents, there was no clear association between social class and the likelihood of reporting two or more partners in the last year. There was no significant difference in the proportion of women in different social classes reporting more than one partner; among men, those in Social Class III (Non-Manual) were most likely, and those in Social Classes I and II least likely, to say they had had two or more partners in the last year, but this relationship did not hold for all age-groups. Because of the strong association between sexual behaviour and age, it is important to take age into account when investigating the relationship between the number of sexual partners and other social characteristics such as social class; this can be done by calculating age-standardised ratios[14]. A ratio of more than 100 indicates a greater likelihood of reporting two or more sexual partners than would be expected in that group on the basis of age distribution alone. Conversely, a ratio of less than 100 indicates that the members of the group are less likely to report this many partners than would be expected from the age composition of the group. The lack of a clear relationship between the number of sexual partners and social class was supported by age-standardised ratios; none of the ratios differed signficantly from 100. (**Tables 6.2–6.3**)

Several studies, including the *National Survey of Sexual Attitudes and Lifestyles* and the 1995 HEMS, have demonstrated that, in addition to sex and age, marital status is most strongly associated with the number of partners; the likelihood of reporting two or more sexual partners in the last year being highest among the widowed, divorced and separated group. In 1996, although HEMS respondents who were single were most likely to say they had had more than one partner, the difference between this group and the widowed, divorced and separated group was not significant. Married respondents were least likely to report two or more partners. These relationships held for both sexes in all age-groups. Age-standardised ratios show that, with the exception of cohabiting men, the ratios of men and women of all marital statuses differed significantly from 100; when age was taken into account, widowed, divorced and separated respondents, followed by single people, had higher than expected ratios, while married respondents and cohabiting women had lower than expected ratios; supporting the findings of the 1995 HEMS and the *National Survey of Sexual Attitudes and Lifestyles*. (**Tables 6.4–6.5**)

Tables 6.1–6.5 show sex, age, social class and marital status separately. They do not show how much these attributes interact with each other and with other characteristics such as economic activity status. As noted in Chapter 2, it is possible to look at how different factors interrelate by using logistic regression (see Appendix D.1), a multivariate statistical technique which can be used to predict the odds of a behaviour (in this case, reporting two or more sexual partners in the last year or not) occurring for people with different combinations of the characteristics under consideration (odds refers to the ratio of the probability that the event will occur to the probability that the event will not occur).

Data from the 1995 and 1996 surveys were combined and a logistic regression model was run to look at the odds of reporting more than one sexual partner in the 12 months before interview. The independent variables used in the model were:

- sex
- age
- marital status
- highest qualification level
- economic activity status
- social class
- tenure
- income
- whether the respondent had any children aged under 16 in the household

Practitioners engaged in health promotion at local level are likely to have information about the socio-demographic profile of their area; showing whether these characteristics increase or decrease the likelihood of a particular behaviour occurring may help them to target campaigns at key groups. The results of the logistic regression are shown in Figure 6.2. The figures in the columns headed 'Multiplying factors' can be thought of as 'weights'; they represent the factor by which the odds of a respondent reporting two or more partners increase with the attribute shown compared to a reference category. For each characteristic shown, the reference category (shown with a value of 1.00) was taken to be the group of respondents least likely to report two or more sexual partners in the last year. The characteristics are listed in order of importance.

The most important characteristic influencing the odds of reporting more than one partner was marital status, followed by sex, age, economic activity status and tenure status. The other variables were eliminated by the model. The logistic regression supported the results of the age-standardisation in that the widowed, divorced and separated group had the highest odds; their odds were increased 13-fold, while those of single people were increased by a factor of almost nine, compared with those of married respondents. Men had twice the odds of women, and the youngest age-group almost three and a half times the odds of those aged 45–54. (**Figure 6.2**)

6.3 Perceptions of risk

Respondents were asked two questions designed to measure their assessment of the risk of being infected with HIV or of contracting another sexually transmitted disease; they were asked whether the risk of 'someone like me getting HIV (the AIDS virus)' or 'another sexually transmitted disease' was 'very high', 'quite high', 'low', or 'is there no risk at all?'

The pattern of responses to the two questions was very similar; 30% of men and 31% of women thought there was 'no risk' of them being infected with HIV, while 33% of men and 34% of women made the same assessment of their risk of contracting another sexually transmitted disease (STD). These proportions are slightly higher than in 1995. Older respondents were less likely to see themselves as at risk; 43% of men and 44% of women aged 45–54 thought they had 'no risk' of contracting HIV, while 42% and 51% respectively said the same about other STDs. Among those aged 16–24, 15% of men and 14% of women thought there was no risk of HIV infection and 16% of men and women said there was no risk of contracting another STD. Younger respondents in the 1992 *Health and Lifestyles Survey* were less likely than older respondents to agree with the statement; 'I don't think I'll ever get HIV'.

Three per cent of respondents thought their risk of getting HIV (the AIDS virus) was 'very high', while 2% assessed their risk of getting another sexually transmitted disease (STD) in this way; 6% thought their risk of either was 'quite high'. Statistically, the probability of contracting another STD is higher than that of contracting HIV, so it is interesting that respondents' assessments of risk were so similar for the two questions. Research on risk has

Figure 6.2 Odds of an individual reporting two or more sexual partners in the last year
Adults aged 16–74 (HEMS 1995 and HEMS 1996)

Characteristics	Multiplying factors	95% confidence intervals
Marital status		
Married	1.00	
Cohabiting	1.81	1.23–2.68
Single	8.62*	6.64–11.19
Widowed/divorced/separated	13.39*	10.07–17.80
Sex		
Male	2.12*	1.78–2.53
Female	1.00	
Age		
16–24	3.41*	2.48–4.69
25–34	2.47*	1.86–3.28
35–44	1.35*	1.01–1.81
45–54	1.00	
Economic activity status		
Working	1.63*	1.25–2.12
Unemployed	2.05*	1.40–2.99
Economically inactive	1.00	
Tenure		
Owner occupied	1.00	
Rented from Local Authority or Housing Association	0.86	0.66–1.11
Privately rented	1.27*	1.02–1.59
Number of cases in the model	5839	
Baseline odds	0.008	

shown that perceptions of risk are often at odds with the actual probability[15] of an event happening, and that people often overestimate the likelihood of a rare event happening, and underestimate the likelihood of a common risk[16].

As noted above, just under one in ten respondents thought that someone like them had a 'very high' or 'quite high' risk of infection by HIV or another STD. There were no significant differences between the assessments made by men and women. The likelihood of respondents seeing themselves as at risk declined with age; about one in five of the 16–24 age-group thought their risk of contracting either type of disease was 'very' or 'quite' high, compared with about one in 20 or fewer of those aged 45–54. **(Figures 6.3–6.4 and Tables 6.6–6.7)**

There was also an association between assessments of risk and marital status. Single respondents were most likely and married people least likely to see themselves as being at risk of contracting either type of disease; this was true for both sexes. For example, about one in twenty five married respondents thought they had a very or quite high chance of getting HIV (the AIDS) virus, compared with one in five or fewer single respondents. **(Tables 6.8–6.9)**

Figure 6.3 Percentage who thought there was no risk of 'someone like me getting HIV/the AIDS virus' by age and sex: adults aged 16–54

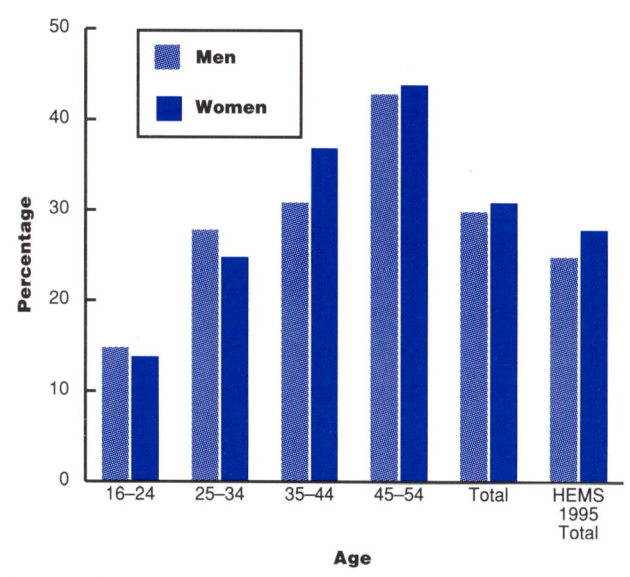

Base numbers are given in Table 6.6

Figure 6.4 Percentage who thought there was no risk of 'someone like me getting another sexually transmitted disease' by age and sex: adults aged 16–54

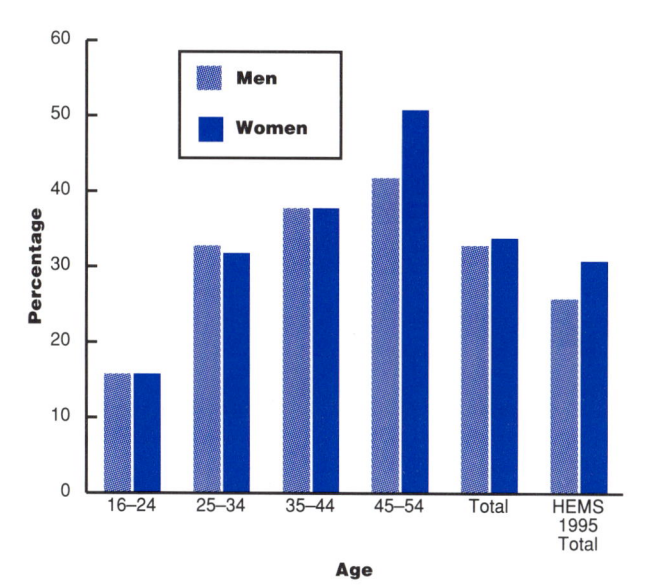

Base numbers are given in Table 6.7

It was noted earlier in the chapter that single people were most likely and married people least likely to report two or more partners in the last 12 months, so the responses to these two questions were analysed by the number of sexual partners. Those who reported two or more partners during the last year were most likely to perceive themselves as at risk; 11% of men and 10% of women thought there was no risk of being infected with HIV, while only 10% of this group thought they were not at risk of contracting another STD. About a quarter of men and a fifth of women reporting more than one partner thought they had a very or quite high chance of contracting HIV, while about a quarter gave the same estimate of their chance of getting another STD. In contrast, less than a tenth of those reporting no or one partner in the last year thought the likelihood of them contracting HIV was very or quite high, while fewer than one in twenty saw themselves as at this level

Health in England 1996 : What people know, what people think, what people do

of risk for another STD. Respondents who had never had sexual intercourse, objectively the group least at risk, were more likely than those reporting no or one partner in the 12 months before interview to see themselves as at risk, although the differences were not always significant. Seventeen per cent of men and 10% of women who said they had never had intercourse, for example, assessed their risk of contracting another STD as very or quite high, compared with 4% of those who reported one partner in the last year. When age was taken into account, however, this pattern was no longer apparent; age-standardised ratios showed that those who reported two or more partners in the last year were most likely to see themselves as at risk. (**Tables 6.10–6.13**)

6.4 Use of condoms with a new partner

Two of the main routes for the transmission of HIV are unprotected sexual intercourse (anal or vaginal) and shared needles, hypodermic syringes and any other injecting equipment.[17] Unprotected intercourse also increases the risk of contracting other sexually transmitted diseases (STDs), themselves a significant cause of ill-health. The White Paper therefore developed targets relating to sexually transmitted diseases and injecting drug users[18]. In order to reduce the risk of infection with HIV (or with any other STD) health promotion campaigns advise people to use a condom with a new partner. As noted in Chapter 1, Prochaska[19] argues that people who are not considering changing their behaviour, in this case using condoms, are in a 'pre-contemplation' stage. Those who wish to change pass through 'contemplation' and 'preparation' stages before taking action to change their behaviour. As outlined in Chapter 3, the Theory of Reasoned Action[20], and the later Theory of Planned Behaviour[21] argue that intentions and behaviour are predicted by two pathways; the 'attitudinal component' comprises individual beliefs and attitudes, while the 'normative component' is concerned with the beliefs of significant others and the extent to which people wish to comply with such beliefs. The interview therefore included a number of questions to measure respondents' attitudes, intentions and behaviour in relation to condom use with new partners.

6.4.1 Discussing the use of condoms with a new partner

HEA suggested health promotion indicator: The proportion of young people who say they would find it difficult to raise the subject of using a condom with a new partner

Whether or not to use a condom can be a delicate matter to raise with a new partner; it may be embarrassing or seem unspontaneous and unromantic. As a way of assessing attitudes to this issue, respondents were asked whether they would find it difficult to raise the subject of using a condom with a new partner. As in 1995, only a minority (18%) said they would. Women were slightly more likely than men to say they would find it difficult, and the proportion saying this increased with age, although the age difference was only significant among women. The relationship between the potential difficulty of raising the subject and other characteristics was very similar to that found in 1995; those belonging to the manual social classes, the widowed, divorced and separated, respondents with no qualifications, and those who had never had a sexual partner or who reported no partner in the last year were most likely to believe that they would find it difficult to discuss using a condom with a new partner. (**Figure 6.5 and Tables 6.14–6.15**)

Figure 6.5 Percentage who would find it difficult to raise the subject of using a condom with a new partner by age and sex: adults aged 16–54

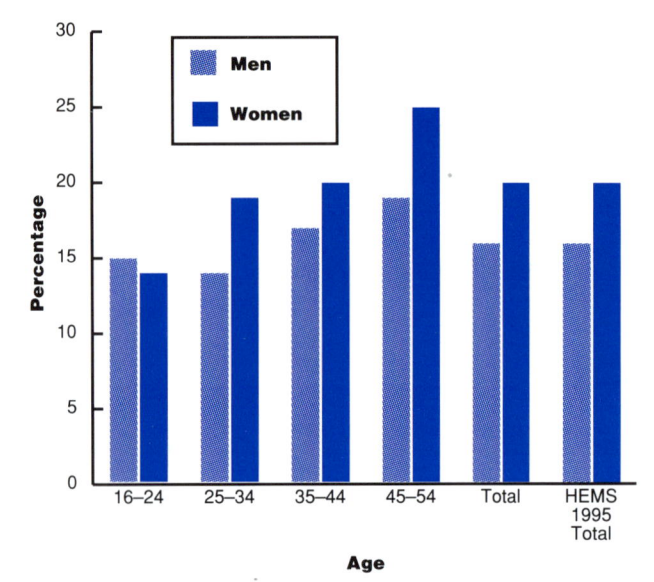

Base numbers are given in Table 6.14

6.4.2 Intention to use condoms with a new partner

HEA suggested health promotion indicator: The proportion of people who claim that if in the near future they did have sex with a new partner they would use a condom

Whether or not someone would find it difficult to raise the subject of using a condom does not tell us whether they intend to use a condom in the event of starting a new sexual relationship. Respondents were therefore asked whether 'if, in the near future, you did have sex with a new partner, would you use a condom?'. More than two thirds of women (67%), and almost three fifths of men (58%) thought they would always use one, while 17% of women and 31% of men said it would depend. Only 1% of respondents stated that they would never use a condom. These proportions do not differ significantly from those recorded in 1995. This suggests that the majority of respondents were at the 'contemplation' stage, and had at least considered how they would behave when first having intercourse with a new partner. The proportion who said they would always use a condom declined with age, from 65% of men and 75% of women aged 16–24 to 51% of men and 56% of women in the 45–54 age-group. This was largely because older respondents were more likely than younger ones to say they were not contemplating having sex with someone new. (**Figure 6.6 and Table 6.16**)

The risk of HIV infection increases with the number of partners with whom people have unprotected intercourse; among women, the proportion saying they would always use a condom did not differ significantly by the number of partners in the last year. Among men, however, almost three quarters of those who had never had intercourse said they would always use a condom, compared with fewer than three fifths of other men. It may be that this group is being unduly optimistic about how they would behave in a situation which they have probably not yet experienced. (**Table 6.17**)

Figure 6.6 Percentage who would always use a condom with a new partner by age and sex: adults aged 16-54

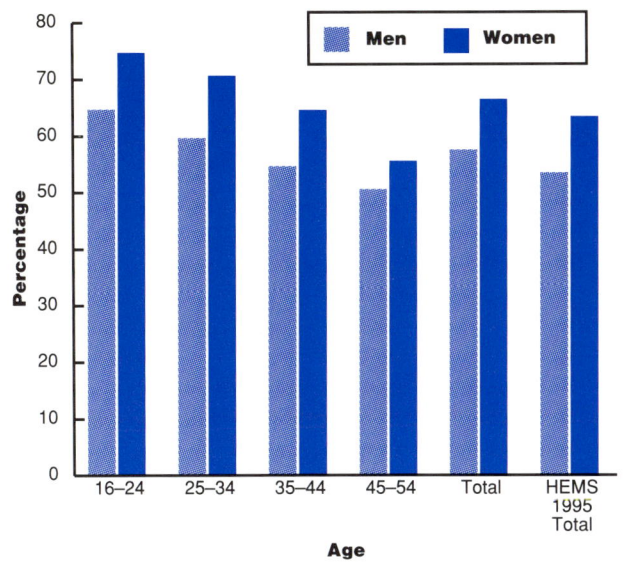

Base numbers are given in Table 6.16

Figure 6.7 Percentage using a condom with a new partner by age and sex: adults aged 16–54 who reported a new partner in the last 12 months

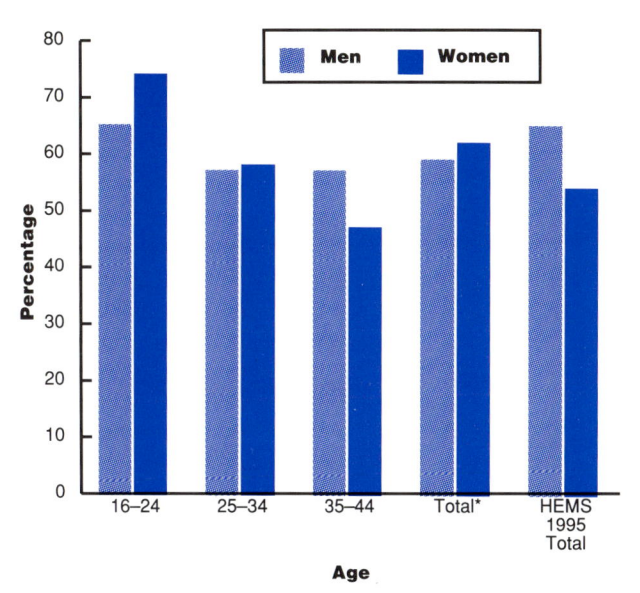

* Includes a small number of respondents aged 45–54

Base numbers are given in Table 6.19

Respondents who thought it would not be difficult to discuss using a condom with a new partner were most likely to say they would always use one; 64% of men and 74% of women in this group gave this answer. The group least likely to say they would always use a condom were those who neither agreed nor disagreed that they would find it difficult to raise the subject. **(Table 6.18)**

6.4.3 Use of condoms with a new partner

> HEA suggested health promotion indicator: The proportion of the population (aged 16–54) who used a condom when they last had sex with a new partner.

As Prochaska and DiClemente's[22] model of behaviour change suggests, not all intentions are translated into action; respondents who reported having at least one new partner during the 12 months prior to interview were therefore asked whether they had used a condom when they first had intercourse with their most recent partner. The number of respondents in this group was small, so it was possible to carry out only limited analysis. Sixty per cent of men and 63% of women in this group said they had used a condom, not significantly different from 1995. The youngest age-group, respondents in Social Class III (Non-Manual), single people, those who said they would always use a condom and those who said they would not find it difficult to raise the subject of using a condom were most likely actually to have used one. This means, however, that 21% of those who said they would always use a condom had not done so when they first had intercourse with their most recent partner, suggesting that a proportion had not moved from the 'contemplation' to the 'action' stage of behaviour change. **(Figure 6.7 and Table 6.19)**

Health in England 1996 : What people know, what people think, what people do

Notes and references

1. Department of Health. *The Health of the Nation: a strategy for health in England.* HMSO (London 1992).

2. Figures released in November 1996 by the United Nations AIDS programme to mark World AIDS Day on December 1, 1996. Cited in *The Guardian*, 29 November 1996.

3. Figures quoted by Peter Piot, Executive Director of the United Nations AIDS programme, on Radio 4's *Today* programme, 28 November 1996.

4. PHLS AIDS Centre – Communicable Disease Surveillance Centre, and Scottish Centre for Infection and Environmental Health. *Unpublished Quarterly Surveillance Tables, No. 32,* June 1996. Tables 3 and 5. These data were kindly supplied by the Communicable Disease Surveillance Centre. The number of people infected through heterosexual intercourse in the UK is small.

5. *Mortality statistics: review of the Registrar General on deaths by cause, sex and age, England and Wales 1993 (revised) and 1994.* HMSO (London 1996). These figures are almost certainly an underestimate; a comparison of data from death registrations with the number of AIDS or HIV-related deaths among cases reported to the Communicable Diseases Surveillance Centre shows that for a high proportion HIV or AIDS is not stated as a cause of death. A study of trends in the number of deaths stated to be due to causes which may have been associated with HIV infection, assuming that any increase was HIV-related, suggests that between 1984 and 1991 there were 2,540 deaths from this cause, only 61% of which were assigned to HIV or AIDS as the cause. (See McCormick A. The impact of human immunodeficiency virus on the population of England and Wales. *Population Trends*, vol. 76, 1994, pp. 40–45.)

6. Wellings K et al. *Sexual behaviour in Britain: the national survey of sexual attitudes and lifestyles.* Penguin (Harmondsworth 1994).

7. Appendix A gives more detailed information on response to the self-completion section of the interview.

8. No information is available on the gender of respondents' partners.

9. Tables in this chapter present grouped number of partners, medians and 95th percentiles. The skewed nature of the distribution of number of partners makes the mean an unreliable measure.

10. As outlined in Chapter 8 of the 1995 HEMS report, a proportion of 1995 HEMS respondents who were married, cohabiting, widowed, separated or divorced reported that they had never had a sexual partner. When this group was excluded from analysis, the distribution of HEMS respondents was closer to that found in the National Survey of Sexual Attitudes and Lifestyles and the 1992 Health and Lifestyles Survey. The proportions shown for 1995 in Table 6.1 exclude this group, and therefore differ from the proportions shown in the 1995 published report.

11. Both Knox et al and Wellings et al reported a discrepancy in the number of partners reported by men and women and offered several explanations for this. Wellings et al argue that men may include relationships which involve sexual contact, but not intercourse, in their count of partners. Knox et al suggest that men may exaggerate and women under-estimate the number of partners. Alternatively, there may be a bias in the sample.

12. Health Education Authority. *Health and Lifestyles: a survey of the UK population.* (London 1995)

13. Knox E G MacArthur C and Simons K J. *Sexual behaviour and AIDS in Britain.* HMSO (London 1993).

14. See Appendix D.2 for a full explanation of age standardisation.

15. The Royal Society defines objective risk as 'the probability that a particular adverse event occurs during a stated period of time, or results from a particular challenge'. Cited in Adams J. *Risk.* University College Press (London 1995).

16. British Medical Association. *The BMA guide to living with risk.* Penguin (Harmondsworth 1990).

17. Apart from unprotected intercourse and sharing injecting equipment, the main routes of transmission for HIV are by blood, either through infected blood factor or blood/tissue transfer; and from an infected mother to her infant during pregnancy, birth or via breastfeeding. Health Education Authority. *Health Update 4: Sexual Health.* (London 1994).

18. The White Paper also developed a target relating to teenage pregnancies. This was discussed in the 1995 HEMS report, but the relevant questions were not included in the 1996 survey. See Bridgwood A et al. *Health in England 1995: what people know, what people think, what people do.* HMSO (London 1996).

19. Prochaska J O. Strong and weak principles for progressing from precontemplation to action on the basis of twelve problem behaviours. *Health Psychology*, vol. 13, 1994, pp. 46–51.

20. Fishbein M and Ajzen I. *Belief, attitudes, intentions and behaviour: an introduction to theory and research.* Addison-Wesley (Boston 1975).

21. Ajzen I. The theory of planned behaviour. *Organisational Behaviour and Human Decision Processes*, vol. 50, 1991, pp. 179–211.

22. Prochaska J O and DiClemente C C. Towards a comprehensive model of change. In Miller W R and Heather N (eds). *Treating addictive behaviours.* Plenum Press (New York 1986).

7 Behaviour in the sun

Summary of main findings

- Just over a quarter of respondents had been sunburnt in the last 12 months; men (29%) were more likely than women (23%) to have been sunburnt. (Section 7.2.1).

- The proportion of people saying they had been sunburnt decreased with age from 41% of those aged 16–24 to only 8% of those aged 65–74. (Section 7.2.1).

- Over two thirds (68%) of adults used a suncream; women were more likely than men to have done so (74% compared with 61%). (Section 7.2.2).

- Suncreams were most commonly used when sunbathing either abroad or in this country. (Section 7.2.2).

- Women were more likely than men to think that having a suntan was important; 31% said it was, compared with 20% of men. (Section 7.3).

- Forty five per cent of respondents agreed that having a suntan made them feel healthier and 45% thought that a suntan made them look more attractive. Women were more likely than men to agree with each of these statements. (Section 7.3).

7.1 Introduction and background

Skin cancer is one of four types of cancer which are focused on in the *Health of the Nation* White Paper and is the second most common cancer in this country. There are two types of skin cancer; non-melanotic and malignant melanoma. Non-melanotic skin cancer is seldom life-threatening if detected in time; it tends to occur in older people who have had a lot of exposure to the sun throughout their lifetime. Malignant melanoma is much more dangerous as it can result in secondary tumours in other parts of the body[1]; it tends to occur in younger people who have had intermittent but intense exposure to the sun[2].

The *Health of the Nation* White Paper states that the number of cases of skin cancer has been increasing in recent years. The incidence of malignant melanoma is increasing more rapidly than the number of cases of non-melanotic skin cancer. The most recent figures available for cancer registrations in England show that 3,703 cases of malignant melanoma were registered in 1991[3]. The number of cases of non-melanotic skin cancer is much higher; there were 31,495 cases in England and Wales in 1989[4]. There were 1,375 deaths from malignant melanoma in 1994 and 436 from non-melanotic skin cancer[5]. Behaviour in the sun is the main risk factor which accounts for this increase[6].

Most cases of skin cancer are avoidable; the British Association of Dermatologists estimated that four out of five cases could be avoided[7]. The most effective way to do this is to avoid exposure to the sun, as even minimal exposure can cause damage to the skin.

One of the *Health of the Nation* targets is to stop the year-on-year increase in the incidence of skin cancer but it is difficult to monitor success in this because of the long time period between initial cell damage and the clinical manifestation of skin cancer. The HEA has developed interim indicators to look at the knowledge of and attitudes towards exposure to the sun, and behaviour in the sun; this chapter looks at behaviour in the sun and then goes on to examine attitudes towards having a suntan[8].

7.2 Behaviour in the sun

7.2.1 Prevalence and frequency of sunburn

> HEA suggested health promotion indicator: The proportion of people who reported having sunburn in the last 12 months causing redness and soreness of the skin lasting for at least 1–2 days

When people expose themselves to the sun they are also exposing themselves to ultra-violet (UV) radiation. Ultraviolet B radiation (UVB) is the main cause of skin cancer[9] but it is now known that ultraviolet A radiation (UVA) can also contribute to skin cancer[10]. As sunburn is an indication that people have had excessive exposure to the sun, interviewers asked respondents if they had had sunburn causing redness and soreness of the skin which lasted for at least 1–2 days in the last 12 months; just over a quarter (26%) said they had. Men were more likely than women to have been sunburnt (29% compared with 23%). The proportion of people saying they had been sunburnt decreased with age from 41% of those aged 16–24 to only 8% of those aged 65–74. Most people reporting sunburn had only been burnt on one occasion in the last 12 months and only 2% of respondents had been sunburnt four or more times. Younger people were more likely than those in the older age-groups to have been sunburnt more than once. Men in Social Class III (Non-Manual) were more likely than men in other social classes to have been sunburnt: 36% had been compared with 26% of those in Social Classes I and II. Among women, those in Social Class III (Manual) were the least likely to have been sunburnt: 16% had been. The proportion of people reporting sunburn increased slightly from 24% in 1995 to 26% in 1996 but this difference was only just significant. **(Figure 7.1 and Table 7.1– 7.2)**

People most at risk of damage from ultraviolet radiation are those with fair or freckled skin which never tans and always burns, while those less at risk have skin that always tans and rarely burns[1]. Respondents were asked to describe what happened to their skin when they went out in the sun without protection. Men were less likely than women to say that their skin 'always burns and never tans' (8% compared with 14%) but more likely to say that it 'rarely burns and tans easily' (29% compared with 23%). It is unlikely that the proportion of men whose skin actually burns easily is different from the proportion of women with skin that burns easily; the answers to this question, therefore, suggest that men see themselves as being less at risk of sunburn than women which may explain why they are more likely than women to get sunburnt and less likely to use a suncream (see section 7.22). **(Table 7.3)**

Not surprisingly respondents who said their skin 'never burns and always tans' were the least likely to report having been sunburnt in the last 12 months; only 2% did so. At least a third of those who said their skin 'always burns and never tans', 'burns at first and tans with difficulty' or 'burns at first then tans easily' had been sunburnt in the last year. Women who said their skin 'always burns and never tans' were less likely than men who described their skin in the same way to have been sunburnt; 26% had been compared with 48% of men, which suggests that women with this type of skin take more care in the sun than men do. **(Table 7.4)**

Figure 7.1 Percentage who reported being sunburnt in the 12 months prior to interview by age and sex: adults aged 16–74

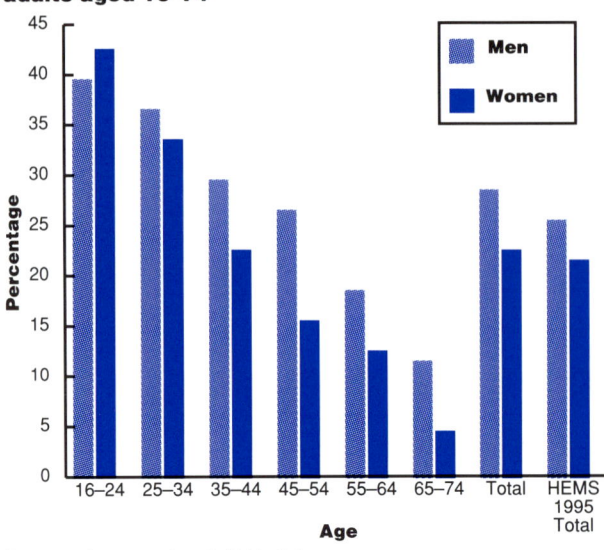

Base numbers are given in Table 7.1

7.2.2 Use of suncream

Although the most effective way of avoiding sunburn is to minimise exposure to the sun; using a suncream is another way of reducing the chances of sunburn. The majority (68%) of adults aged 16–74 said that they did use a sunscreen although women (74%) were more likely than men (61%) to do so. Below the age of 55, around 70% of respondents used a suncream but people aged 55 or above were less likely to do so; 60% of those aged 55–64 used a suncream and only 44% of people in the 65–74 age-group did so. Respondents were asked when they used a suncream and the answers most commonly given were sunbathing abroad, mentioned by 44% of respondents, followed by sunbathing in this country, mentioned by 41%. Women in the younger age-groups were the most likely to give these answers. **(Figure 7.2 and Table 7.5)**

Figure 7.2 Percentage using a suncream by age and sex: adults aged 16–74

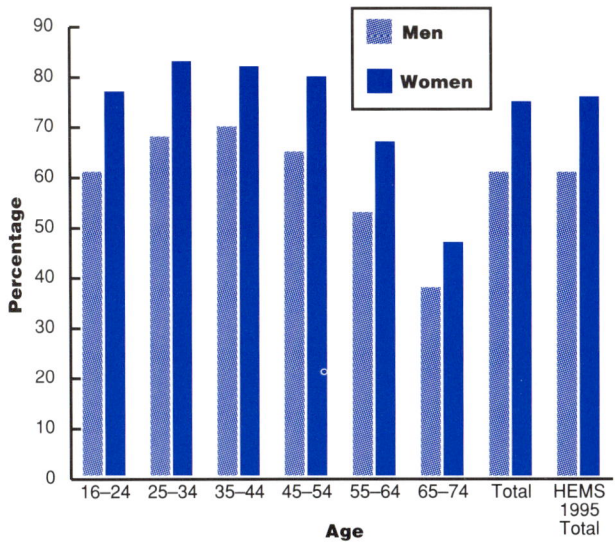

Base numbers are given in Table 7.5

Respondents in the non-manual social classes were more likely than those in the manual social classes to use a suncream; for example, 77% of those in Social Classes I and II did so compared with only 58% of those in Social Classes IV and V. Those in the non-manual social classes were most likely to say they used a suncream when sunbathing abroad. **(Table 7.6)**

The proportion of people saying that they use a suncream when sunbathing in this country increased from 34% in 1995 to 41% in 1996, while the proportion of people saying they use a suncream when outdoors abroad but not sunbathing decreased from 36% in 1995 to 31% in 1996[11].

The Sun Protection Factor (SPF) of suncreams tells people how much longer they can stay out in the sun before getting burnt; for example, if a person burns after 10 minutes in the sun a suncream with an SPF of two would double the amount of time they could spend in the sun before burning. It is recommended that people use a sunscreen with an SPF of 15 or more[12]. Nine per cent of respondents used a cream with the highest factor (SPF of 17 or more), 17% used one with an SPF of 11–16, 24% used one with an SPF of 6–10 and 10% used one with an SPF 2–5. Seven per cent did not know what factor level they used. As stated earlier, women were more likely than men to use a suncream; and they were also more likely to use one with a higher factor level; 20% of women used one with an SPF of 11–16 compared with 14% of men. When people who didn't use a suncream were excluded there were no significant differences in the proportions of men and women who used a cream with an SPF of 2–5, 6–10 or 17 or over. Women were more likely than men to say they used a suncream with an SPF of 11–16; a higher proportion of men than of women, however, said they did not know what factor level they used (14% compared with 7%) which may account for at least some of the difference. **(Tables 7.7–7.8)**

Respondents with skin that 'always burns and never tans' were the most likely to use a suncream with an SPF of 17 or more; 19% did so compared with 13% or fewer of respondents with other skin types. Those who said their skin tanned easily were more likely to use a suncream with a lower factor. **(Table 7.9)**

Although suncreams protect against UVB radiation and allow people to stay in the sun for a longer length of time before they get burnt they do not actually prevent burning if people stay out in the sun for too long. In addition, in a recent article in the *British Medical Journal,* McGregor and Young argued that although suncreams protect against sunburn, they may be less effective at protecting against skin cancer. While there is evidence that suncreams reduce the incidence of non-melanotic skin cancer, there have been reports of an increased risk of malignant melanoma in sunscreen users because some suncreams may fail to protect against UVA, although most British suncreams do now contain effective UVA blocking agents[9]. Table 7.10 shows that a higher proportion of people who used a suncream actually reported sunburn in the last 12 months; 30% compared with 17%. This may be because people using a suncream feel more protected and therefore may stay out in the sun longer than is safe. **(Table 7.10)**

7.3 Attitudes towards a suntan

> HEA suggested health promotion indicator: The proportion of people to whom having a suntan is very important or fairly important

In order to change people's behaviour in the sun attitudes towards having a suntan need to change. Respondents were asked whether it was important to them to have a suntan; a quarter said it was. Women were more likely than men to think a suntan was important; 31% said it was compared with 20% of men. The importance of having a suntan decreased with age; 44% of women and 24% of men aged 16–24 said that it was important compared with 12% of women and 14% of men aged 65–74. The proportion of people who thought a suntan was important has decreased slightly since 1995 from 28% to 25%. **(Figure 7.3 and Table 7.11)**

Two new questions were added to the questionnaire in 1996 asking respondents whether they agreed or disagreed with the following statements:

- Having a suntan makes me feel healthier
- Having a suntan makes me look more attractive

The pattern of response to these two questions was similar; 45% of respondents agreed with both statements. Women were more likely than men to agree with each statement; 49% of women

Figure 7.3 Percentage who thought it was important to have a suntan by age and sex: adults aged 16–74

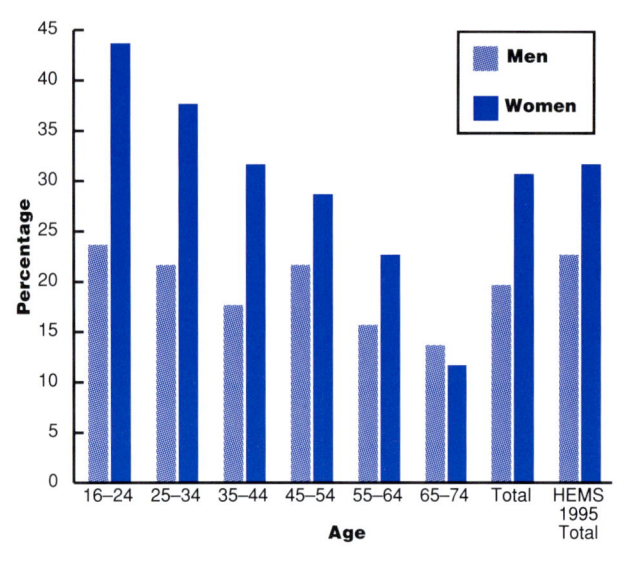

Base numbers are given in Table 7.11

Figure 7.4 Percentage agreeing that 'having a suntan makes me look more attractive' by age and sex: adults aged 16–74

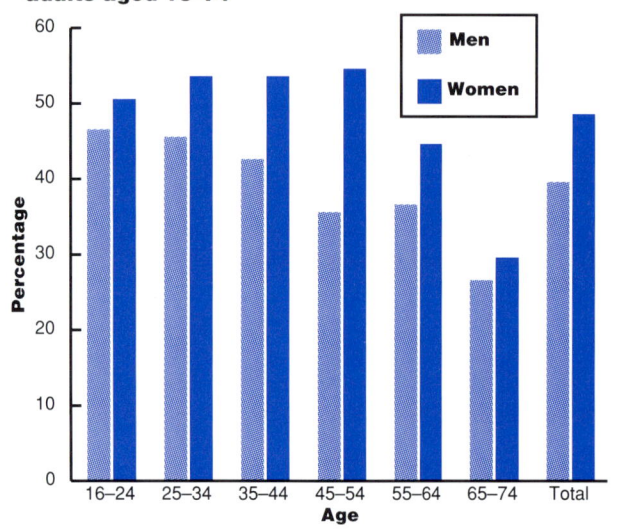

Base numbers are given in Table 7.14

agreed with both while 41% of men said that having a suntan made them feel healthier and 40% that it made them look more attractive. Respondents aged 65–74 were least likely to agree with either statement; only 28% did so. **(Figure 7.4 and Table 7.12 and 7.14)**

People in the manual social classes were less likely to agree that having a suntan made them feel healthier; only 39% of those in Social Classes IV and V did so, compared with 47% of those in Social Classes I and II. The pattern was similar for the statement 'having a suntan makes me look more attractive; only 38% of people in Social Classes IV and V agreed, compared with 48% of those in Social Classes I and II. **(Tables 7.13 and 7.15)**

People whose skin 'always burns and never tans' were least likely to agree that having a suntan made them more attractive, possibly because they felt they were unlikely to get a tan. Women whose 'skin burns at first and then tans easily' were the most likely to think that having a tan made them look more attractive; 60% said it did. **(Table 7.16)**

Notes and references

1. Skinner E. *Skin cancer: A brief review of incidence and causes*. Health Education Authority (London).

2. Blackmore R and Reddish A. *Global environmental issues*. Hodder & Stoughton (1996).

3. *ONS Monitor: Population and Health Registrations of cancer diagnosed in 1991, England and Wales*. Series MB1, 19 September 1996.

4. OPCS *Cancer Statistics Registration; England and Wales 1989*. Series MB1, Number 22, HMSO (London 1994).

5. *OPCS Monitor: Deaths in 1994 by cause, and by area of residence*. DH2/95/1 (18/7/95).

6. Department of Health. *The Health of the Nation: a strategy for health in England*. HMSO (London 1992).

7. Melia J and Bulman A. Sunburn and tanning in a UK population. *Journal of Public Health Medicine*, vol. 17, no. 2, 1995, pp 223-229.

8. Questions on knowledge about exposure to the sun were included in the 1995 survey but were not asked in 1996.

9. McGregor J M and Young A R. Sunscreens, suntans and skin cancer. *British Medical Journal*, vol. 312, 1996, pp1621-1622.

10. Health Education Authority. *Ultraviolet radiation: Sun know how factsheet 3* (1996).

11. In 1996 respondents were shown a card with the answer codes on and this may account for some of the difference between 1995 and 1996.

12. Health Education Authority. *Sun protection and sunscreens. Sun know how factsheet 2* (1996).

General health and doctor consultations

Summary of main findings

- Eighty per cent of men and 78% of women said that their general health was 'very good' or 'good'. (Section 8.2).

- Women were slightly more likely than men to report a long-standing illness or disability, 37% did so, compared with 35% of men. (Section 8.3).

- Sixty nine per cent of women and 62% of men said they had experienced a 'moderate' or 'large' amount of stress in the 12 months prior to interview. More than two fifths of men and more than half of women had experienced stress which they felt was harmful to their physical or mental health. (Section 8.4).

- When asked to choose which, if any, of a list of factors were currently good for their health, respondents were most likely to cite relationships and family (mentioned by 59%); what they ate (56%); and exercise (47%). Pollution, lack of exercise and 'my weight' were most often seen by respondents as currently bad for their health; 29%, 27% and 27% respectively mentioned these. (Section 8.6).

- When asked for their general opinions about health, 88% of respondents agreed that to have good health is the most important thing in life and 67% that it is sensible to do exactly what the doctors say. Only 25% agreed with the statement that generally health is a matter of luck. (Section 2.8).

- Almost three quarters (73%) of women and three fifths (60%) of men had talked to a GP at his or her surgery in the last year. An additional 3% of men and 4% of women had spoken to another health professional, such as a nurse or health visitor, at the surgery or health centre. (Section 8.8).

- Thirty per cent of male and 36% of female current and ex-smokers who had given up smoking in the last year had discussed smoking with a GP or other health professional; 13% of male and 6% of female current and ex-drinkers had discussed drinking. (Section 8.8).

8.1 Introduction and background

This chapter reports on respondents' general health and well-being, their attitudes to health, and doctor consultations about some of the health behaviours discussed in previous chapters. The first part of the chapter considers four self-reported measures of health and well-being; general health, long-standing illness or disability, stress, and whether respondents felt they were leading a healthy life. These topics were reported on in detail in the 1995 HEMS report[1]; in 1996, a question asking respondents about the effect of stress on their health was added to the questionnaire.

Although the four measures are based on respondents' perceptions and are therefore subjective, there is widespread evidence of the validity of subjective assessments of health. Health is an abstract and multi-dimensional concept which is difficult to define. Blaxter[2] argues that much of modern medicine is based on a biomedical model, which defines disease as 'deviations of measurable biological variables from the norm, or the presence of defined and categorised forms of pathology'. The World Health Organisation (WHO) offers a much wider definition of health as a 'state of complete physical, social and mental well-being and not merely the absence of disease or infirmity'[3].

Neither objective nor subjective accounts of health are sufficient on their own. On the one hand, individuals may misinterpret, be misinformed or unaware of their biomedical condition; on the other, they have information about their symptoms and feeling states which only they can give. Subjective assessments of health have also been shown to be related to objective measures such as standardised mortality ratios, doctor diagnoses and use of services.

8.2 Self-reported general health

Self-reported general health has been shown to be a strong predictor of mortality; it is also associated with the use of health services[4]. HEMS respondents were asked to rate their health as 'very good', 'good', 'fair', 'bad' or 'very bad'[5]. Eighty per cent of men and 78% of women said their health was 'very good' or 'good'. Four fifths or more of those aged under 55 reported good health; this fell to just under two thirds of the 65–74 age-group. There was no significant difference in the proportions reporting good health in 1995 and 1996. (**Figure 8.1 and Table 8.1**)

Respondents in non-manual social classes were more likely than those in manual classes to report good health; this was true for both men and women and for all age-groups. Thus, for example, 80% of men and women aged 45–64 in Social Classes I and II reported good health, compared with 68% of men and 64% of women of the same age in Social Classes IV and V. (**Table 8.2**)

Because of the strong association between health and age, it is important to take age into account when investigating the relationship between health and other social characteristics such as social class. Age-standardised ratios (see Appendix D.2) are therefore presented for all four self-reported measures discussed in this part of the chapter[6]. An age-standardised ratio of more than 100 indicates a greater likelihood of reporting good general health than would be expected in that group on the basis of age distribution alone. Conversely, a ratio of less than 100 indicates that the members of the group are less likely to report good health than would be expected from the age composition of the group. The standardised ratios shown in Table 8.3 reinforce the results shown in Table 8.2; among both men and women, those in Social Classes I and II were more likely to report good general health than would be expected on the basis of age alone (ratios of 106 and 107 respectively), while those in Social Classes IV and V were less likely to do so (ratios of 91 for men and 92 for women). (**Table 8.3**)

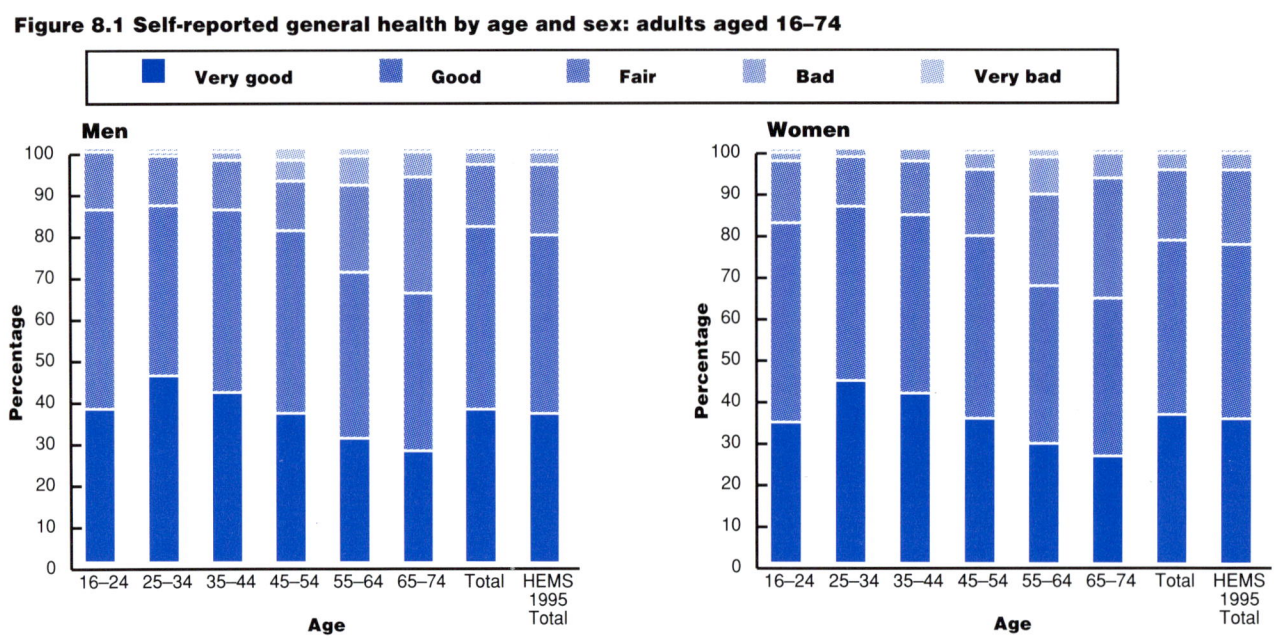

Figure 8.1 Self-reported general health by age and sex: adults aged 16–74

Base numbers are given in Table 8.1

64 Health in England 1996 : What people know, what people think, what people do

8.3 Self-reported morbidity

Questions on self-reported long-standing illness or disability are commonly asked in surveys; they have been included in the General Household Survey (GHS) since its inception in 1971. A question on limiting long-standing illness was included in the Census for the first time in 1991.

Several studies have confirmed the validity of this measure; there is a high level of agreement between prevalence based on self-reporting and on medical examinations[7]. Associations between self-reported illness and standardised mortality ratios have also been demonstrated[8]. Commentators note that discrepancies do not necessarily indicate that data from self-reported sources are inaccurate; informants may not have brought a condition to the attention of a doctor, medical records could be inaccurate[1], doctors may not have informed patients of their diagnosis, and lay descriptions may differ from those given by doctors[9,10].

HEMS respondents were asked if they have any long-standing illness or disability which had troubled them for some time. Those who did were asked whether this illness or disability limited their activities in any way. Over a third of men (35%) and women (37%) reported a long-standing illness or disability, while 18% of men and 21% of women said that their illness limited their activities. These proportions did not differ significantly from those reported in 1995. The likelihood of reporting a chronic illness increased with age; 28% of men and 24% of women aged 16–24 reported a long-standing illness, compared with 53% of men and 57% of women aged 65–74. For limiting long-standing illness, the corresponding proportions were 10% of men and 9% of women aged 16–24 and 31% of men and 36% of women in the 65–74 age-group.

The data may under-estimate prevalence in the oldest age-groups. Evidence from several sources indicates that questions on self-reported long-standing illness underestimate the prevalence of chronic illness and disability among the elderly; among those aged 65 and over, a proportion of those who are assessed as having a disability[11] or who report difficulties with activities of daily living[12,13] nevertheless say they have no chronic illness or disability. Even when there is no reference in the question to 'people of your age', it appears that elderly people regard limitations in their daily activities, particularly difficulties with eyesight and hearing, as a normal part of growing old, not as evidence of illness or disability[14]. This should be less of a problem for HEMS than for other surveys as those aged 75 and over, among whom prevalence of chronic conditions tends to be highest, are excluded from the survey. It should also be remembered that some people are more troubled by a certain kind of symptom than others, and that the need to limit activities will depend on what people usually do[15].

There were no significant differences in the proportions reporting a long-standing condition between HEMS and the 1994 Health Survey for England, with the exception of men aged 65–74. Among this group, Health Survey respondents were more likely to report a chronic illness; 62% did so, compared with 53% of HEMS respondents. HEMS respondents were more likely than 1995 GHS respondents to report a long-standing illness, but the difference was only significant among women. **(Figure 8.2 and Table 8.4)**

Figure 8.2 Percentage reporting a long-standing illness by age and sex: adults aged 16–74

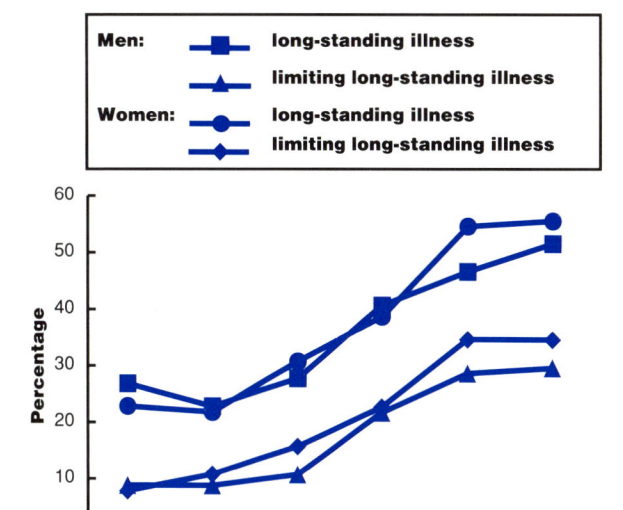

Men: ■ long-standing illness
▲ limiting long-standing illness
Women: ● long-standing illness
◆ limiting long-standing illness

Base numbers are given in Table 8.4

Respondents classified as belonging to Social Classes I and II were least likely to report a chronic condition; 34% did so, compared with 37% or more of other respondents. Although this pattern held for both men and women, the difference was only significant among women. **(Table 8.5)**

The age-standardised ratios showed that, once age was taken into account, there were no significant differences in reported prevalence between different social classes. In an analysis of the 1984–5 Health and Lifestyles Survey data, Blaxter found that those belonging to a non-manual social class were more ready to declare a chronic condition, even if it was not functionally troublesome or accompanied by symptoms. Informants in manual social classes, particularly men, were likely to say they had a named disease only if it was actually troublesome; this was particularly true for mental disorders[1]. Analysis of the level of agreement between self-reporting and doctor diagnosis for specific conditions, as opposed to overall prevalence, has also demonstrated that agreement between the two measures was lower among the manual than among the non-manual social classes[16]. HEMS data, in common with those collected for other surveys, may therefore under-estimate the prevalence of long-standing illness and disability among respondents, particularly men, in the manual social classes. The exclusion of the oldest age-group, those aged 75 and over, may also partly account for the lack of difference between the age-standardised ratios for different social classes. **(Table 8.6)**

8.3.1 Self-reported morbidity and self-reported general health

As in 1995, there was an association between self-reported general health and self-reported morbidity; those reporting no long-standing condition were most likely and those with a limiting long-standing illness least likely to say they had good general health. This was true for both men and women and for all age-groups. Among those aged 45–64, for example, 93% of men and 94% of women with no chronic illness said they had good general health, compared with 34% of men and 36% of women with a limiting condition. **(Table 8.7)**

Figure 8.3 Percentage reporting a large or moderate amount of stress in the last 12 months by age and sex: adults aged 16–74

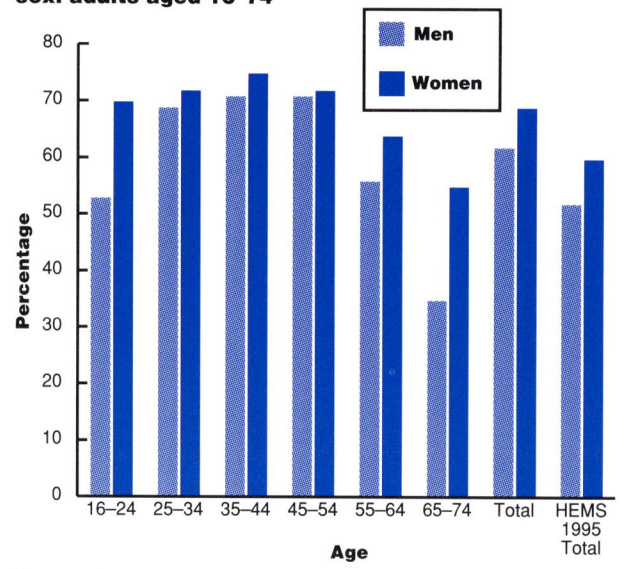

Base numbers are given in Table 8.8

8.4 Self-reported stress

Stress has been identified as a major contributory factor to both mental and physical ill health[17]; more specifically, several studies have shown that psychological factors are implicated in the development of cardiovascular disease[18].

Respondents were shown a card and asked which of the statements on the card best described the amount of stress or pressure they had experienced in the 12 months before interview. Sixty two per cent of men and 69% of women reported a 'moderate' or 'large' amount of stress; an increase on the 52% and 60% respectively reported in 1995. Conversely, 7% of men and 5% of women said they had been completely free of stress, compared with 11% and 7% respectively in 1995.

Although the proportions reporting stress were higher in 1995 than in 1996, the *pattern* of reporting was very similar. In both years, women were more likely than men to say they had experienced a moderate or large amount of stress in the 12 months prior to interview. There was also the same inverted U-shaped relationship between stress and age, with the youngest and oldest age-groups least likely to report stress or pressure. This was less marked among women than among men; levels of stress were not significantly lower among the 16–24 age-group for women than among those aged 25–34. Among men, those aged 35–54 were most likely to say they had experienced moderate or large amounts of stress (71%); among women, stress was most prevalent among the 35–44 age-group, 74% of whom reported this amount of stress. **(Figure 8.3 and Table 8.8)**

As in 1995, reported levels of stress and pressure were highest among respondents in Social Classes I and II and lowest in Social Classes IV and V. This was true for both men and women, but the pattern did not hold for all age-groups. Age-standardised ratios confirmed the relationship with social class; men and women in Social Classes I and II had ratios of 112 and 110 respectively, while the corresponding ratios for men and women in Social Classes IV and V were 87 and 95. **(Tables 8.9–8.10)**

8.4.1 Perceived effects of stress on health

Respondents who reported some stress or pressure in the last 12 months were asked:

> How harmful would you say the amount of stress and pressure you have experienced in the last 12 months has been to your physical and mental health?

In order to show the proportion of the total HEMS sample who felt that stress had been harmful to their health, Tables 8.11–8.12 include respondents who reported no stress in the last 12 months. They show that over two fifths of all men and more than half of all women felt that stress had had a harmful effect on their health; 6% of men and 10% of women said the effect had been 'very harmful', while an additional 35% of men and 43% of women said it was 'quite harmful'. The inverted U-shaped relationship between stress and age was again apparent; among women, it was more marked for this question than for the amount of stress experienced; 51% of men aged 45-54 and 60% of women aged 35–44 said that stress had had a quite or very harmful effect on their health. **(Table 8.11)**

One of the criticisms made of estimates of self-reported general health and morbidity based on only one or two questions is that they tend to measure physical rather than psychosocial health[19]. The data on the perceived effect of stress on health were therefore analysed by self-reported general health and long-standing illness to examine the associations. Respondents whose health was not good and those who reported a long-standing illness were more likely than others to say that stress had had a harmful effect on their health in the last 12 months. Almost three fifths of men and almost three quarters of women who said they did not enjoy good health, and half of men and almost two fifths of women with a chronic condition, said this. However, more than a third of men and almost half of women who reported good health or who said they had no long-standing illness or disability also felt that stress had been harmful to their health. **(Table 8.12)**

These results are not necessarily contradictory; the effects of stress may have been temporary and not affecting the respondent at the time of interview. Even if the effects of stress were longlasting, some respondents may not have classified this as a 'long-standing illness'. In addition, as noted earlier, health is multi-dimensional. Blaxter points out that it can be 'good' in some respects and 'bad' in others. Individuals can have a disease, but assess themselves as in 'good' health; have poor psychosocial health, but good physical health[1]. It is possible that HEMS respondents were thinking of one dimension of health when asked about their 'health in general' and another when asked about the effect of stress on their health. It is also possible that some psychosocial morbidity was not being measured by the questions on self-reported general health and morbidity.

Not surprisingly, the perceived effect of stress on health was related to the amount of stress reported; about one fifth of those who had experienced a small amount of stress said that it was harmful to their health, compared with about half of those reporting a moderate amount and four fifths of those reporting a large amount in the last year. Seventy six per cent of men and 86% of women reporting a large amount of stress felt that it had been harmful to their health. **(Table 8.13)**

8.5 Respondents' assessments of whether they led a healthy life

Respondents were asked whether they led a 'very healthy', 'fairly healthy', 'not very healthy' or 'unhealthy' life. Overall, 91% believed they led a 'very' or 'fairly' healthy life. Only 1% thought they led an unhealthy life. There were no significant differences between men and women. Although the oldest age-group was most likely to say they led a 'very healthy' life (26% of men and 31% of women), the overall proportion who reported leading either a 'very' or 'fairly' healthy life did not differ significantly by age. There were no significant differences between 1995 and 1996. **(Table 8.14)**

There were also no significant differences between the proportion of men and women in different social classes reporting that they led a healthy life. Age-standardised ratios confirmed that this was still the case when age was taken into account. **(Tables 8.15–8.16)**

8.6 Respondents' assessments of which factors are good and bad for their health

Respondents were shown a card listing a number of factors and asked which, if any, they felt were currently good or bad for their health. Similar questions were asked in 1995, but differences in question wording meant that it was not possible to make direct comparisons between the data from the two years. This is discussed in more detail in a methodological Annex to this chapter.

'Relationships and family', 'exercise' and 'what I eat' were most likely to be thought by respondents to be good for their health; these items were chosen by 59%, 47% and 56% respectively. When asked what was currently bad for their health, 29% of respondents chose 'pollution', 27% 'lack of exercise' and 27% 'my weight'.

Women were more likely than men to say that 'relationships and family' (61% compared with 56%) and 'what I eat' (58% and 54%) were currently good for their health, while a higher proportion of men chose 'exercise' (50%, compared with 44% of women). Women were more likely (31%) than men (23%) to say that their weight was currently bad for their health, while a higher proportion of men chose smoking (24% compared with 19% of women), not having a job (11% and 7%) and their alcohol consumption (11% and 6%). **(Figures 8.4–8.5, and Tables 8.17–8.18)**

The relationship between social class and the proportions choosing an item varied; men in Social Classes IV and V were most likely to say both that their work was currently good for their health (27%) and that 'not having a job' was currently bad for their health (16%). Both men (31%) and women (30%) in Social Classes I and II were most likely to report that 'lack of exercise' was currently bad for their health. **(Tables 8.19–8.20)**

8.7 General attitudes towards health

As a way of measuring some general attitudes towards health, interviewers read out six statements and asked respondents to say whether they 'strongly agreed', 'agreed', 'neither agreed nor disagreed', 'disagreed', or 'strongly disagreed' with each of them. The statements were:

- To have good health is the most important thing in life
- It's sensible to do exactly what the doctors say
- Generally health is a matter of luck
- If you think too much about your health you are more likely to be ill

Figure 8.4 Factors which are currently good for respondents' health by sex: adults aged 16–74

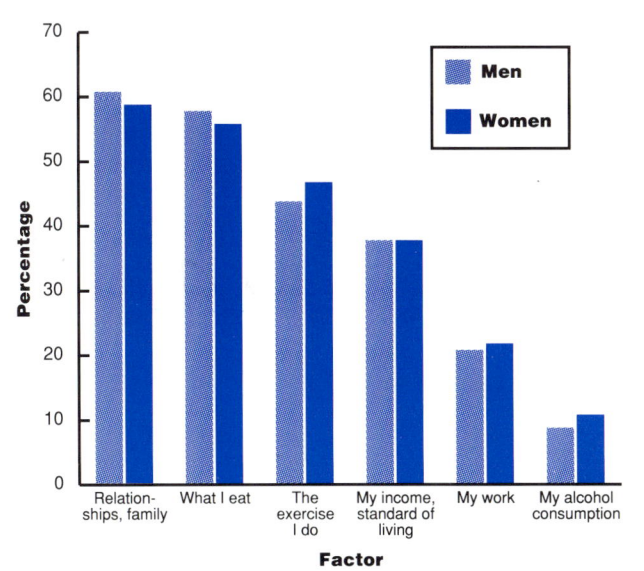

Base numbers are given in Table 8.17

Figure 8.5 Factors which are currently bad for respondents' health by sex: adults aged 16–74

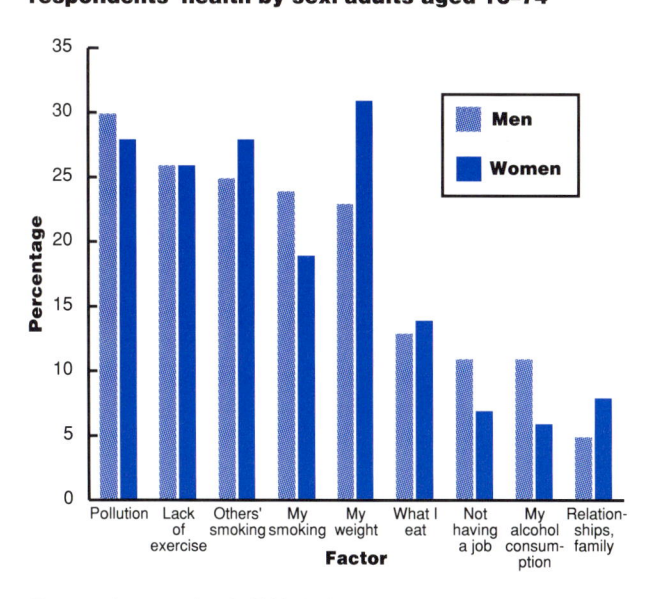

Base numbers are given in Table 8.18

Health in England 1996 : What people know, what people think, what people do

- I have to be very ill before I go to the doctor
- I don't really have time to think about my health

The items were chosen from among those which were developed for the Health and Lifestyles Surveys[20]. For those surveys, the statements were used to develop a 'locus of control' scale, which gave a measure of the extent to which respondents felt in control of their own health. As noted in Chapter 1, Ajzen argues that perceived behavioural control is one of three basic determinants of a person's intention to perform a given behaviour[21]. This is similar to Bandura's concept of 'self-efficacy'[22], the belief that one's own efforts play a critical role in the face of difficult situations, which Prochaska sees as important in the action stage of change[23]. A 'locus of control' scale was not developed for the present survey, as only some of the items used in the scale were included in the questionnaire. The statements were, however, analysed using principal components analysis to see if they were measuring one or more underlying factors[24]. The analysis identified two underlying factors, which differentiated between the first two and the last four statements. The last four statements ('Generally health is a matter of luck', 'If you think too much about your health you are more likely to be ill', 'I have to be very ill before I go to the doctor' and 'I don't really have time to think about my health') were most highly correlated with the first factor, which accounted for 26% of the total variance of the six statements. The first two statements ('To have good health is the most important thing in life' and 'It's sensible to do exactly what the doctors say') were most highly correlated with the second factor, which accounted for 20% of the total variance. If all six statements were contributing equally to the variance, each would account for approximately 17%. Little is gained by combining the statements into two factors. The statements were therefore analysed separately, and the results are shown in **Tables 8.21–8.26**.

A large majority, 88%, strongly agreed or agreed that 'to have good health is the most important thing in life', while 67% thought it sensible 'to do exactly what the doctors say' and 65% said they had to be very ill to go to the doctor. Only 25% agreed that 'generally health is a matter of luck', and 30% that they 'don't really have time to think about my health'.

Women were more likely than men to agree that health is the most important thing in life, that if you think too much about your health, you are more likely to be ill, and that they don't really have time to think about their health. Older respondents were more likely than younger ones to say it is important to do exactly what the doctors say, that health is largely a matter of luck, and that you are more likely to be ill if you think about your health too much.

The third response option 'neither agree nor disagree' was changed from 1995; then, respondents were given a 'don't know' option. For every statement, the change in wording increased the proportions who chose this category; for example, whereas only 8% said they 'did not know' whether they didn't really have time to think about their health in 1995, 19% said they neither agreed nor disagreed with the statement in 1996. With this exception, the pattern of responses was very similar in the two years, with very similar proportions agreeing with each of the six statements. (**Tables 8.21–8.26**)

8.8 Consultations with GPs and other health professionals

The *Health of the Nation* White Paper identified primary health care as a key setting for promoting the health of the population as a means of achieving the targets set out in the White Paper. Thus, for example, GPs' terms of service state that, where appropriate, they should give advice on the use of tobacco and record quantified information on patient smoking habits[25]. All respondents were asked:

> During the past year, apart from any visit to a hospital, have you talked to a GP either in person or by telephone about your health?

Those who had not seen a GP in his or her surgery were asked if they had talked to another health professional, such as a nurse or health visitor, at the surgery or health centre.

Sixty per cent of men and 73% of women had consulted a GP at the surgery or health centre and another 2% had seen the doctor at home; these proportions did not differ significantly from those reported in 1995. An additional 3% of men and 4% of women had spoken to another health professional at the surgery or health centre. Among men, the likelihood of seeing their GP at the surgery increased with age, but this was not true for women. The difference between men and women was greatest among the younger age-groups; 71% of women, but only 48% of men aged 16–24, for example, had talked to the doctor at the surgery. It is likely that some of the consultations sought by younger women were about birth control, pregnancy or in relation to children, which would account for at least some of the difference. (**Figure 8.6 and Table 8.27**)

Figure 8.6 Percentage consulting a GP at the surgery in the last 12 months by age and sex: adults aged 16–74

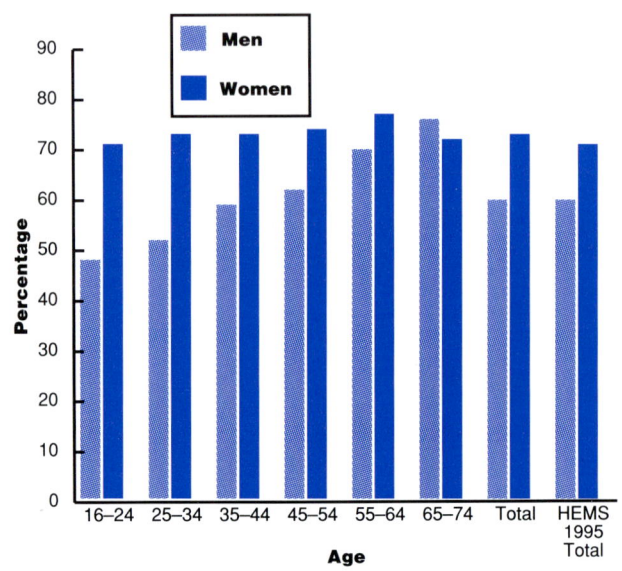

Base numbers are given in Table 8.27

Table 8.28 shows no significant difference in the proportion of respondents in different social classes who had consulted a GP or other health professional during the last year. The age-standardised ratios show, however, that once age was taken into account, men in Social Classes I and II were more likely than other men to have consulted a GP or other health professional. **(Tables 8.28–8.29)**

As noted earlier, self-reported general health and morbidity are associated with use of health services; HEMS data confirmed this. Respondents with good health and those with no long-standing illness or disability were less likely than others to have seen their GP at the surgery in the 12 months prior to interview. Among men, 78% of those whose general health was not good and 79% of those with a chronic illness had seen their GP at the surgery, compared with 55% of men with good health and 49% of men with no long-standing illness or disability. Eighty five per cent of women who did not report good health and 86% of those with a long-standing condition had visited their GP at the surgery, compared with 70% of women reporting good health and 66% of those with no long-standing illness. **(Table 8.30)**

8.8.1 Discussions with GPs and other health professionals about health behaviours

HEA suggested health promotion indicators:

The proportion of smokers and ex-smokers who gave up less than a year ago who have discussed smoking with a member of staff at the surgery in the last 12 months and agree that the discussion was helpful

The proportion of current and ex-drinkers who have discussed sensible drinking with a member of staff at the surgery in the last 12 months and agree that the discussion was helpful

The proportion of the population who have discussed physical activity with a member of staff at the surgery in the last 12 months and agree that the discussion was helpful

The proportion of the population who have discussed diet/healthy food with a member of staff at the surgery in the last 12 months and agree that the discussion was helpful

As part of its Targets Project (see Appendix B), the HEA has developed a set of suggested health promotion indicators relating to the proportion of people who had discussed health behaviours with GPs or other health professionals. HEMS respondents who had talked to a GP or other health professional in the 12 months before interview were therefore asked, in subsequent sections of the interview, whether they had discussed smoking, drinking, physical activity and nutrition. The findings from these questions were discussed separately in the relevant chapters of the 1995 HEMS report; this year, they have been brought together to allow common patterns to be examined. Data relating to the indicators are highlighted in Table 8.31.

Of the four health behaviours, smoking was most likely and drinking least likely to have been discussed during the last year. Among current and ex-smokers who gave up less than a year ago, 27% of men and 33% of women had discussed smoking with their GP and another 2% had discussed it with another health professional. This compares with 11% of male and 5% of female current and ex-drinkers who had discussed drinking with their GP and 1% who had spoken to another health professional.

Discussions on smoking were, however, the least likely to be perceived as helpful; whereas 66% of men and 61% of women who had discussed diet and healthy eating had found the discussions helpful, only 31% of men and 22% of women who had talked about smoking had done so.

In general, GPs and health professionals were more likely than respondents to have initiated discussions. The exception was discussions on physical activity between GPs and women. Smoking was most likely, and physical activity least likely, to have been raised by health professionals. **(Table 8.31)**

The data on discussions with doctors and other health professionals were analysed by health-related behaviour and attitudes. Current smokers smoking 10–19 cigarettes a day were least likely to have spoken to anyone about their smoking, but the likelihood of having a discussion about drinking increased both with level and frequency of alcohol consumption. Nineteen per cent of the heaviest drinkers (men drinking 51 units a week or more and women with a weekly consumption of 36 or more units) had spoken to someone about drinking, compared with only 5% of those drinking less than a unit a week. Similarly, almost a quarter (23%) of those who drank every day reported a discussion. Apart from smoking, respondents who wanted to change their behaviour, for example by taking more exercise, were more likely than those who did not wish to change, to have discussed health behaviours.

As the number of respondents reporting a discussion was small, it was possible to carry out only limited analysis of the data. There was no association between health-related behaviour and whether the respondent or a health professional had initiated the discussion. Those who wanted to give up smoking or to have a healthier diet were more likely to have raised the subject than those who did not. Discussions were most likely to be perceived as helpful by smokers who wanted to give up, and by respondents who had initiated discussions about smoking and drinking. **(Table 8.32)**

Notes and references

1. Bridgwood A et al. *Health in England 1995: what people know, what people think, what people do.* HMSO (London 1996).

2. Blaxter M. *Health and Lifestyles.* Routledge (London 1990).

3. *Second consultation to develop common methods and instruments for health interview surveys: report on a WHO meeting, 18–20 Sep 1990.* World Health Organisation Regional Office for Europe and Netherlands Central Bureau of Statistics (1990).

4. Blaxter M. Self-definition of health status and consulting rates in primary care. *Quarterly Journal of Social Affairs*, 1987, vol 1, pp. 131–171; Bennett N et al. *Health Survey for England 1993.* HMSO (London 1995). See also Section 8.8 of this chapter.

5. This five-fold classification is recommended by the World Health Organisation Regional Office for Europe. It is used by a number of UK surveys, including the Health Survey for England and the ONS Psychiatric Morbidity Surveys. It is used also by a number of other European countries. See reference 3, above.

6. Age-standardised ratios reflect the *average* relationship across all age-groups, but this may vary between different age-groups. They are therefore not a substitute for the detail available in Tables 8.2, 8.5 and so on, which show each age-group separately. In addition, standardised ratios only take account of age differences and do not make adjustments for other characteristics, such as the presence of a long-standing illness, which may help to explain the observed differences. These tables should therefore be treated with caution. See Foster K. The use of standardisation in survey analysis. *Survey Methodology Bulletin*, 1993, vol. 33, pp. 19–27.

7. Blaxter, M. Self-reported health. In *The Health and Lifestyles Survey*. Health Promotion Research Trust (London 1987).

8. *General Household Survey 1972*. HMSO (London 1975).

9. White A et al. *Health Survey for England 1991*. HMSO (London 1993).

10. When respondents are asked for details of their illnesses (HEMS respondents are asked 'what is the matter with you?' only as a courtesy question; interviewers do not probe fully and the answers are not coded); there is a high level of agreement between the answers and doctor diagnoses, although levels of agreement vary for specific conditions and for different social groups. See Blaxter (reference 2, above) and Bennett N et al. *Health Survey for England 1993, Appendix D*. HMSO (London 1995).

11. Martin J et al. *The prevalence of disability among adults: OPCS surveys of disability in Great Britain; Report 1*. HMSO (London 1988).

12. Hunt A. *The Elderly at Home*. HMSO (London 1976).

13. *First results from the quality check element of the 1991 Census Validation Survey*. OPCS Monitor SS94/2, March 1994.

14. Goddard E. Measuring morbidity and some of the factors associated with it, in *Health and Lifestyle surveys: towards a common approach: report of a workshop held on 7 November 1989 organised by the HEA and OPCS*. HEA and OPCS (London 1990).

15. Bennett N et al. *Living in Britain: results from the 1994 General Household Survey*. HMSO (London 1996).

16. Bennett N et al. *Health Survey for England 1993, Appendix D*. HMSO (London 1995).

17. Goldberger EL and Brenitz S (eds). *Handbook of stress*. Free Press (New York 1993).

18. Fredrikson M. Psychophysiological and biochemical indices in 'stress' research: applications and pathophysiology. In Turpin G (ed). *Handbook of clinical psychophysiology*. Wiley and Sons (1989), cited in Colhoun H et al. *Health Survey for England 1994*. HMSO (London 1996).

19. Leavey R and Wilkin D. A comparison of two survey measures of health status. *Social Science Medicine*, 1988, vol. 27, pp. 269–275.

20. Blaxter M. Attitudes to health. In Cox B D et al. *The Health and Lifestyle Survey* Health Promotion Research Trust (London 1987).

21. Ajzen I. The theory of planned behaviour. *Organisational Behaviour and Human Decision Processes*, 1991, vol. 50, pp. 179–211.

22. Bandura A. Self-efficacy mechanism in human agency. *American Psychologist*, 1982, vol. 37, pp. 122–147.

23. Prochaska JO. Strong and weak principles for progressing from precontemplation to action on the basis of twelve problem behaviours. *Health Psychology*, 1994, vol. 13, pp. 46–51.

24. Principal components factor analysis is a technique which analyses the correlations between a set of variables to identify any underlying independent constructs. The first stage is the creation of a correlation matrix, which is then used to generate a factor loading matrix. The values in this matrix range from -1 to +1, and show the strength of the association between each of the items and the derived factors. The larger the factor loading (negative or positive), the greater the degree of association between the variable and the factor.

    Thus, in the present example, the factor loadings were as follows:

Statement	Factor 1	Factor 2
1	0.24	0.69
2	0.14	0.74
3	0.50	0.15
4	0.60	0.03
5	0.65	-0.28
6	0.67	-0.27

    showing that the last four statements were most highly correlated with the first underlying factor and the first two with the second.

    Each 'eigenvalue' of the correlation matrix can be linked to one factor and shows the percentage of the total variance of the set of variables that is accounted for by that factor Factors with eigenvalues of less than one are usually ignored on the grounds that they account for less variance than any one of the original variables. The eigenvalue for the first underlying factor was 1.57 and for the second 1.21, while the two factors explained 26% and 20% respectively of the variance. As each of the original statements would explain approximately 17% of the variance, this does not represent a large increase.

    For further details, see Walsh A. *Statistics for the Social Sciences*. Harper and Row (New York 1990).

25. Department of Health. *The Health of the Nation: a strategy for health in England*. HMSO (London 1992). Practices are required to submit proposals for health promotion activities to local health promotion committees. If the committees approve the plans, GPs are paid a unified fee for health promotion work. See *NHS Executive letter, GP Health Promotion* FHSL(96)35, 9 July 1996.

Annex to Chapter 8

Methodological notes

As noted in Section 8.6, respondents to both the 1995 and 1996 HEMS were shown a card listing a number of factors and asked which, if any, they felt were good or bad for their health. There were a number of methodological differences in the two years, which makes it difficult to make direct comparisons between the results from the two years.

Firstly, there was a change in question wording. In 1995, respondents were asked:

> Thinking of your own health, could you tell me which of these, if any, is good (bad) for **your** health.

The question was designed to assess what respondents thought was good or bad for their health in general, even if a particular factor, such as housing, was not actually affecting their health at the time of interview. In 1996, it was decided that the focus should be on factors which were affecting respondents' health at the time of interview. In addition, interviewers reported that, despite the emphasis in the question on 'your' health, some respondents to the 1995 HEMS were choosing factors which they felt were good or bad for *anyone's* health, not just their own. In 1996, the wording was changed to:

> Which of these, if any, currently have a good (bad) effect on your health?

The second change was in the showcards which were used. In 1995, the same card was used for both questions (see Annex Table 8.1 below). Analysis of the results showed that some items were chosen by only a small proportion of respondents; only 1%, for example, thought that 'others' smoking' was good for their health, while only 4% said 'housing' was bad for their health. These seldom-chosen items were therefore omitted from the card in 1996, and a different card was used for the two questions; one list contained factors which might be good for respondents' health, while the other listed items which might be bad for their health. In addition, in 1995, the second most commonly chosen item was 'stress'; 52% of men and 56% of women said it was bad for their health. In 1996, this item was omitted from the list as respondents had already been asked about the effects of stress on their health.

The third change was in the wording of individual items. Given that separate cards were being used, it was possible to tailor items more appropriately to the 'good' and 'bad' questions. For example, 'exercise' was changed to 'lack of exercise' for the 'bad' card in 1996; the very marked change in the proportion choosing this item can be largely attributed to the change in question wording; in 1995, 3% of respondents said that 'exercise' was bad for their health, while in 1996, 27% said that 'lack of exercise' was bad for their health.

Although the *pattern* of responses is very similar in the two years, the likelihood of an item being chosen appeared to be affected by the change in wording, particularly for the question asking about the factors which might have a bad effect on health. In general, items were less likely to be chosen in 1996 than in 1995, probably indicating the difference between respondents' assessments of the effects on their health in general and at the time of interview.

In both years, 'relationships and family', 'exercise' and 'what I eat' were most likely to be thought by respondents to be good for their health; these items were chosen by 63%, 63% and 61% of respondents in 1995, but by only 59%, 47% and 56% in 1996. 'What I eat', which was the third most commonly chosen factor in 1995, was ranked second in 1996. Similarly, 'pollution', 'others' smoking' and 'my smoking' were chosen by 53%, 54% and 34% of respondents in 1995, but by only 29%, 26% and 21% in 1996.

Respondents were also more likely to choose 'none of these' in 1996 than in 1995; 10%, compared with 4% for the 'good' question, and 21% compared with 4% for the 'bad' question. There are two possible explanations for this. Firstly, the lists were shorter in 1996 than in 1995, thus reducing the likelihood that they would include items relevant to respondents. Secondly, it is less probable that something might affect respondents' health at a particular point in time, than at any time.

Annex Table 1
Factors which are good or bad for health: 1995 and 1996

	1995 %		1996 %
Good for health			
Relationships, family	63	Relationships, family	59
What I eat	61	What I eat	56
Exercise	63	The exercise I do	47
Income, standard of living	47	My income, standard of living	38
Work	36	My work	22
My weight	34		
Housing	26		
My alcohol consumption	7	My alcohol consumption	11
Stress	5		
Not having a job	5		
My smoking	3		
Pollution	1		
Others' smoking	1		
None of these	4	None of these	10
*Base = 100%**	*4661*		*4636*
Bad for health			
Pollution	56	Pollution	29
Stress	54		
Exercise	3	Lack of exercise	27
Others' smoking	53	Others' smoking	26
My smoking	34	My smoking	21
My weight	22	My weight	27
What I eat	12	What I eat	13
Not having a job	22	Not having a job	9
My alcohol consumption	18	My alcohol consumption	8
Work	9		
Relationships, family	5	Relationships, family	6
Income, standard of living	8		
Housing	4		
Exercise	3		
None of these	4	None of these	21
*Base = 100%**	*4663*		*4642*

* Percentages total more than 100% because respondents may have given more than one answer.

9 Conclusion: knowledge, attitudes and behaviour

9.1 Introduction

This chapter presents an overview of the findings reported in Chapters 2 to 7 by looking at the knowledge, attitudes and behaviour of different groups in the population. First the chapter will look at the differences by sex, then at the differences between different age-groups and finally at social class differences.

Figures 9.1 to 9.3 show the overall proportions for knowledge, attitudes and behaviour for the key areas covered by the report. They show which groups had the highest and lowest proportions engaging in the health-related behaviours covered by the survey; which were the most likely and least likely to have different types of knowledge; and which were most and least likely to hold selected attitudes. All the differences shown in the figures are significant at the 95% level.

9.2 Sex

Men were more likely than women to take part in the following behaviours; they were more likely to drink more than 21 units of alcohol per week, to have taken drugs, to have had two or more sexual partners in the last year and to have been sunburnt in the last year. However, similar proportions of men and women were current smokers. As well as being less likely to take part in risk behaviours, women were more likely take part in behaviour which was good for their health; they were more likely to eat low-fat varieties of food, to eat three types of starchy carbohydrates daily and to take more care in the sun. The only area where men were more likely than women to engage in behaviour which was good for their health was physical activity; men were more likely than women to have participated in moderate to vigorous exercise for 30 minutes or more at least five days a week. (**Figure 9.1**)

Differences in behaviour between men and women are reflected in the differences in their types of knowledge. It was reported in Chapter 2 that respondents who drank fairly high levels of alcohol were more likely to know the number of units contained in different drinks and as men were more likely than women to drink fairly high levels of alcohol they were also more likely to know the number of alcohol units contained in a pint of beer, a glass of wine and a pub measure of spirits. Women were more likely than men to be able to identify what constitutes a healthy diet. (**Figure 9.2**)

Although there were a number of differences in the proportion of men and women reporting the behaviours covered by the survey there were not so many differences in attitudes. Similar proportions of men and women said they would like to give up smoking, drink less alcohol, take more exercise or stop using drugs and the proportions who actually intended to do these things were similar as well. Women, however, were more likely than men to say they intended to change their diet in the next year and to say it was important to have a suntan. A higher proportion of women than of men said they would always use a condom with a new partner although women were more likely to say they would find it difficult to raise the subject of using a condom with a new partner. (**Figure 9.3**)

9.3 Age

People in the younger age-groups, particularly the 16–24 age-group, were most likely to engage in high risk behaviours. A higher proportion of people aged 16–24 than of people in older age-groups were current smokers, drank more than 21 units of alcohol per week (men) or more than 14 units per week (women), had used drugs and had had two or more sexual partners in the last year. Younger people were more likely to have been sunburnt and less likely to eat low-fat varieties of food or to eat three types of starchy carbohydrates daily. However, they were more likely to take part in moderate to vigorous exercise for 30 minutes or more at least five days a week. (**Figure 9.1**)

Although young people were more likely to take part in physical activity lasting for 30 minutes or more at least five days a week it was the oldest age-group (65–74) who were most likely to know that this was the recommended level of physical activity. People in the oldest age-group were, however, less likely to know the number of alcohol units contained in different drinks and to know what constitutes a healthy diet; people aged 25–44 were most likely to have both these types of knowledge. (**Figure 9.2**)

There were differences in attitude between the different age-groups. Older people were less likely to say they would like to change their behaviour and that they intended to change their behaviour, for example, they were less likely to say they intended to give up smoking, to drink less or to take more exercise. Among younger respondents, the age-group most wanting to change varied between health behaviours; men aged 35–44 and women aged 25–34 were most likely to say they wanted to give up smoking; those aged 16–24 were most likely to say they would like to drink less and men aged 25–34 and women aged 16–24 were most likely to want to take more exercise. However, when

Health in England 1996 : What people know, what people think, what people do

asked about intentions to change those aged 16–24 were the most likely to say they intended to change their behaviour in the next year. It may be that younger people are more optimistic about being able to change their behaviour as they are less likely than older people to have already tried and failed. Prochaska and DiClemente's model suggests that people may try to change their behaviour and fail several times before finally succeeding. **(Figure 9.3)**

9.4 Social class

People in manual social classes were most likely to take part in risk behaviours; they were more likely than those in non-manual social classes to be smokers and less likely to eat low-fat varieties of food or to eat three types of starchy carbohydrates daily although they were more likely to take part in moderate to vigorous activity lasting 30 minutes or more at least five days times a week. This is not surprising given that activity at work is included in this summary measure of activity. People in manual social classes were less likely to say they would use a condom with a new partner. They were also less likely to use a suncream. **(Figure 9.1)**

People in non-manual social classes were more likely than those in manual social classes to know how many units were contained in different drinks and to be able to identify what constituted a healthy diet. **(Figure 9.2)**

There were differences in attitudes between the social classes; people in manual social classes were more likely than those in non-manual social classes to say they would find it difficult to raise the subject of using a condom with a new partner. People in non-manual social classes were more likely to say they would like to take more exercise and that they intended to take more exercise in the next six months. **(Figure 9.3)**

9.5 Conclusion

The findings in this report and in the 1995 report show that there are differences between different social groups in health-related behaviour, knowledge and attitudes. The findings suggest that men, people in younger age-groups and people in manual social classes are more likely to engage in risk behaviours than people in other social groups; the exception to this is physical activity where these people are the most likely to be physically active.

Below are three profiles showing the health-related behaviour, knowledge and attitudes of three different types of people based on the HEMS findings. These profiles show what proportion of people in the groups reported the given behaviour, knowledge and attitudes. Profiles can be drawn up by health promotion practitioners for other groups using the tables in this report.

Profiles of three types of people based on HEMS findings

Men aged 16–24

- 41% were current smokers
- 42% drank more than 21 units of alcohol per week
- 56% took moderate to vigorous exercise for 30 minutes or more at least 5 days a week
- 31% of those aged 16–19 and 43% of those aged 20–24 had had two or more sexual partners in the last 12 months
- 40% had been sunburnt in the last 12 months
- 36% of those aged 16–19 and 46% of those aged 20–24 had used drugs in the last 12 months

Women aged 65–74

- 79% were non-smokers (24% ex-smokers and 46% never or only occasionally smoked)
- 48% drank less than one unit of alcohol per week
- 53% ate three types of starchy carbohydrates daily (bread; vegetables and salad; potatoes, pasta or rice)
- 44% thought their diet was as healthy as it could be
- 46% were sedentary, that is they engaged less than once a week in moderate-intensity activity lasting 30 minutes
- only 17% intended to take more exercise in the next six months and 11% intended to change their diet in the next year

Women in Social Classes I and II

- 77% looked at ingredients when shopping
- 45% ate three types of starchy carbohydrates daily (bread; vegetables and salad; potatoes, pasta or rice)
- 38% used low-fat varieties of milk, cooking fat and spread and ate chips less than once a week)
- 84% used a suncream
- 23% knew what constitutes a healthy diet (i.e. could identify at least three of 'eat less fat', 'eat more fruit', 'eat more starch', 'eat more fibre')

Figure 9.1 Health-related behaviours
Adults aged 16–74

Type of behaviour	Percentage of respondents engaging in this behaviour	Groups most likely to engage in this behaviour	Groups least likely to engage in this behaviour
Current smoker	30	No sex difference 16–24 Manual social classes	65–74 Non-manual social classes
Has tried to give up smoking[1]	77	No sex difference 35–44 Smokes 10 or more cigarettes a day	16–24 Smokes fewer than 10 cigarettes a day
Drinks more than 21 units of alcohol per week (men) or more than 14 units per week (women)	17–31	Men 16–24	Women Women aged 65–74
Takes moderate to vigorous exercise for 30 minutes or more at least five times a week	36	Men Men 16–24, women 25–34 Manual social classes	Women 65–74 Non-manual social classes
Looks at ingredients when shopping	50	Women 35–44 Non-manual social classes Qualified to 'A' level or above	Men 16–24 Manual social classes No qualifications
Eats three types of starchy carbohydrates daily	38	Women 65–74 Non-manual social classes	Men 16–24 Manual social classes
Eats low-fat varieties of four types of food	22	Women Non-manual social classes Women qualified to 'A' level or above	Men 16–24 Manual social classes Women with no qualifications
Has used drugs in the last month	9	Men 16–29	Women 30–54
Has had two or more sexual partners in the last 12 months[3]	13	Men Men aged 20–24, women aged 16–19 Men aged 16–34 in Social Class III (Non-Manual) Single	Women 45–54 Women in Social Class III (Manual) Married
Uses a condom with a new partner[2]	61	Single 16–24 Non-Manual social classes Women qualified to 'A' level or above Two or more sexual partners in the last year	Married 45–54 Manual social classes No qualifications One sexual partner in the last year
Sunburnt in the last 12 months	26	Men 16–24 Social Class III (Non-Manual)	Women 65–74
Uses a suncream	68	Women 35–44 Non-manual social classes	Men 65–74 Manual social classes

1. Current smokers.
2. Respondents reporting a new partner in the last 12 months.
3. Adults aged 16–54.

Health in England 1996 : What people know, what people think, what people do

Figure 9.2 Characteristics associated with different levels of knowledge
Adults aged 16–74

Type of knowledge	Percentage of respondents with this type of knowledge	Groups most likely to have this type of knowledge	Groups least likely to have this type of knowledge
Knowledge of alcohol units contained in a pint of beer, glass of wine, measure of spirits[1]	Beer 40 Wine 41 Spirits 30	Men Men aged 35–44; women aged 25–34 Social Classes I and II Heavier drinkers	Women 65–74 Social Classes IV and V Abstainers and very low drinkers
Knowledge of recommended levels of physical activity (at least 30 minutes on at least five days a week)	25	No sex difference 65–74 No social class difference	 16–24
Knowledge of what constitutes a healthy diet (i.e. can identify at least three of 'eat less fat', 'eat more fruit', 'eat more starch', 'eat more fibre')	16	Women 25–34 Non-manual social classes	Men 65–74 Manual social classes

1. Adults aged 16–74 who had heard about measuring alcohol in units.

Figure 9.3 Attitudes towards health behaviours
Adults aged 16–74

Attitude	Percentage of respondents reporting this attitude	Groups most likely to report this attitude	Groups least likely to report this attitude
Diet is as healthy as it could be	19	No sex difference 65–74 Eats three types of starchy carbohydrates daily Has a diet low in saturated fats	16–24
Some drugs are safe to use[1]	27	Men 16–24 Currently using drugs	Women 45–54 Never used drugs
Would find it difficult to raise the subject of using a condom with a new partner[1]	18	Women Women aged 45–54 Manual social classes Widowed, divorced or separated women No qualifications No sexual partner in the last year	Men 16–24 Non-manual social class Qualified to 'A' level or above Two or more sexual partners in the last year
Important to have suntan	25	Women 16–24	Men 65–74
WISH TO CHANGE BEHAVIOUR			
Would like to give up smoking[2]	65	No sex difference Men aged 35–44, women aged 25–34 Smokes 10 or more cigarettes a day	65–74 Smokes fewer than 10 cigarettes a day
Would like to drink less[3]	17	No sex difference 16–24 Heavy drinkers	55–74 Light drinkers
Would like to take more exercise	68	No sex differences Men aged 25–34, women aged 16–24 Social Class I and II	65–74 Social Class IV and V
Would like to stop taking drugs[4]	31	No sex differences	
INTENTION TO CHANGE BEHAVIOUR			
Intends to give up smoking within the next year[2]	32	No sex difference 16–24 Smokes fewer than 20 cigarettes a day	65–74 Smokes 20 or more cigarettes a day
Intends to cut down on drinking within the next year[5]	44	No sex difference Women aged 35–44 No social class difference	Women aged 25–34 Men aged 45–74

Health in England 1996 : What people know, what people think, what people do

Intends to take more exercise in the next 6 months[6]	45	No sex difference 16–24 Non-manual social classes Participates in moderate-intensity activity for 30 minutes or more 3–4 days a week	65–74 Manual social class Sedentary (participates in moderate intensity activity less than one day a week)
Intends to change diet within the next year[7]	33	Women 16–24	Men 65–74
Would always use a condom with a new partner[1]	62	Women 16–24 No sexual partner in the last year	Men 45–54 Two or more sexual partners in the last year
Intends to give up using drugs within the next year[8]	35	No sex differences	

1. Adults aged 16–54.
2. Current smokers.
3. Respondents who drink at least once or twice a week.
4. Adults aged 16–54 who have used one or more drugs in the past month.
5. Respondents who drink at least once or twice a week and would like to cut down on their drinking.
6. Respondents who would like to take more exercise.
7. Respondents who say their diet is not as healthy as it could be.
8. Adults aged 16–54 who have used one or more drugs in the past month and would like to stop using drugs.

Part B - Reference Section

Table 1.1 Characteristics of the sample by sex
Adults aged 16–74

Characteristic	Men %	Women %	All %
Age			
16–24	16	15	15
25–34	22	21	22
35–44	20	21	20
45–54	18	16	17
55–64	13	13	13
65–74	11	13	12
Base = 100%	*2044*	*2601*	*4645*
Marital status			
Single	26	20	23
Married, cohabiting	67	65	66
Widowed, divorced or separated	7	15	11
Base = 100%	*2044*	*2601*	*4645*
Highest qualification level			
'A' level or above	38	28	33
GCSE Grade A–G or equivalent	38	41	40
No qualifications	24	31	27
Base = 100%	*2037*	*2595*	*4632*
Social class*			
I & II	36	25	31
III (NM)	10	34	22
III (M)	27	9	18
IV & V	18	25	22
Base = 100%	*2043*	*2599*	*4642*
Economic activity status			
Working	70	58	64
Unemployed	6	3	5
Economically inactive	23	39	31
Base = 100%	*2043*	*2601*	*4644*
Tenure status			
Owner occupied	72	70	71
Rented from Local Authority or Housing Association	14	16	15
Rented privately	14	13	13
Base = 100%	*2040*	*2597*	*4637*
Gross annual household income			
Under £5,000	6	11	8
£5,000–£9,999	15	18	17
£10,000–£14,999	16	15	15
£15,000–£19,999	15	15	15
£20,000–£29,999	20	18	19
£30,000 or more	23	18	21
Don't know	4	4	4
Refused	2	2	2
Base = 100%	*2043*	*2598*	*4641*
Standard region			
North	6	7	6
Yorkshire and Humberside	11	11	11
North West	13	13	13
East Midlands	9	9	9
West Midlands	10	11	10
East Anglia	4	4	4
Greater London	13	13	13
Outer Metropolitan and Outer South East	24	24	24
South West	10	9	10
Base = 100%	*2044*	*2601*	*4645*

* Members of the Armed Forces, persons in inadequately described occupations and persons who have never worked are not shown as separate categories but are included in the figures for all persons.

Health in England 1996 : What people know, what people think, what people do

Table 2.1 Cigarette smoking status by age and sex
Adults aged 16–74

Age	16–24	25–34	35–44	45–54	55–64	65–74	Total	HEMS 1995 Total
Smoking status	%	%	%	%	%	%	%	%
Men								
Current cigarette smokers	41	34	29	29	29	20	31	31
Ex-regular cigarette smokers	6	13	25	37	46	56	28	28
Never or only occasionally smoked cigarettes	53	53	46	34	25	23	41	42
Cessation rate *	0.13	0.28	0.46	0.56	0.61	0.74	0.47	0.47
Base = 100%	224	436	396	367	309	310	2042	2117
Women								
Current cigarette smokers	38	32	30	22	26	21	29	28
Ex-regular cigarette smokers	9	15	19	23	26	30	20	19
Never or only occasionally smoked cigarettes	52	54	50	55	48	49	52	53
Cessation rate *	0.19	0.32	0.39	0.51	0.50	0.59	0.41	0.40
Base = 100%	266	586	533	392	362	461	2600	2548
All								
Current cigarette smokers	40	33	30	26	27	21	30	29
Ex-regular cigarette smokers	8	14	22	30	36	42	24	23
Never or only occasionally smoked cigarettes	53	53	48	44	37	37	46	47
Cessation rate *	0.17	0.30	0.42	0.54	0.57	0.67	0.44	0.44
Base = 100%	490	1022	929	759	671	771	4642	4665

* Cessation rate = % ex-regular smokers / % ever smoked.

Table 2.2 Cigarette smoking status by standard region of residence and sex
Adults aged 16–74

Region	North	Yorkshire & Humberside	North West	East Midlands	West Midlands	East Anglia	Greater London	Outer Metropolitan & SE	South West	England	HEMS 1995 England
Smoking status	%	%	%	%	%	%	%	%	%	%	%
Men											
Current cigarette smokers:											
less than 10 a day	5	8	11	8	7	8	8	8	5	8	8
10, less than 20 a day	13	12	8	18	12	8	11	10	16	12	11
20 or more per day	15	7	14	9	14	12	14	9	11	11	11
Total current cigarette smokers *	33	27	34	35	33	28	33	28	32	31	31
Ex-regular cigarette smokers	26	29	24	22	28	33	27	29	32	28	28
Never or only occasionally smoked cigarettes	41	45	42	42	39	39	40	43	36	41	42
Base = 100%	123	220	272	188	218	84	269	455	213	2042	211
Women											
Current cigarette smokers:											
less than 10 a day	9	10	11	5	9	9	10	9	11	9	9
10, less than 20 a day	17	15	13	10	11	14	11	12	11	12	11
20 or more per day	10	9	9	9	6	5	8	5	5	7	8
Total current cigarette smokers *	36	34	33	24	26	28	29	25	27	29	27
Ex-regular cigarette smokers	19	20	18	19	17	19	19	22	22	20	19
Never or only occasionally smoked cigarettes	45	46	49	57	56	52	52	53	52	52	53
Base = 100%	180	308	361	235	285	118	318	544	251	2600	2548
All											
Current cigarette smokers:											
less than 10 a day	7	9	11	6	8	9	9	9	8	9	9
10, less than 20 a day	15	13	11	14	11	11	11	11	13	12	11
20 or more per day	12	8	12	9	10	8	11	7	8	9	9
Total current cigarette smokers *	34	31	34	30	29	28	31	27	30	30	29
Ex-regular cigarette smokers	22	24	21	21	23	26	23	25	27	24	23
Never or only occasionally smoked cigarettes	43	45	45	49	48	46	46	48	43	46	47
Base = 100%	303	528	633	423	503	202	587	999	464	4642	4665

* Includes those for whom number of cigarettes was not known.

Health in England 1996 : What people know, what people think, what people do

Table 2.3 Cigarette smoking status by social class based on own current or last job and sex
Adults aged 16–74

Social class Smoking status	I & II %	III(NM) %	III(M) %	IV & V %	Total† %
Men					
Current cigarette smokers:					
less than 10 a day	7	11	8	9	8
10, less than 20 a day	7	11	14	17	12
20 or more per day	8	8	15	9	11
Total current cigarette smokers *	22	30	36	39	31
Ex-regular cigarette smokers	30	22	32	26	28
Never or only occasionally smoked cigarettes	48	48	32	35	41
Base = 100%	783	195	561	366	2041
Women					
Current cigarette smokers:					
less than 10 a day	8	11	9	9	9
10, less than 20 a day	7	11	19	15	12
20 or more per day	5	5	8	10	7
Total current cigarette smokers *	20	28	35	34	29
Ex-regular cigarette smokers	22	20	17	21	20
Never or only occasionally smoked cigarettes	58	52	47	45	52
Base = 100%	677	862	224	680	2598
All					
Current cigarette smokers:					
less than 10 a day	7	11	8	9	9
10, less than 20 a day	7	11	15	16	12
20 or more per day	7	6	13	12	9
Total current cigarette smokers *	21	28	36	36	30
Ex-regular cigarette smokers	27	20	29	23	24
Never or only occasionally smoked cigarettes	52	51	35	41	46
Base = 100%	1460	1057	785	1046	4639

* Includes those for whom number of cigarettes was not known.
† Members of the Armed Forces, persons in inadequately described occupations and persons who have never worked are not shown as separate categories but are included in the figures for all persons.

Table 2.4 Mean and median cigarette consumption per smoker by age and sex
Current cigarette smokers aged 16–74

Age	16–24	25–34	35–44	45–54	55–64	65–74	Total	HEMS 1995 Total
				Mean and median consumption per smoker				
Men								
Daily cigarette consumption								
- mean	12.0	15.4	17.0	16.6	17.2	14.5	15.3	15.5
- standard deviation	7.1	7.5	9.2	9.7	9.6	11.0	8.9	10.1
- median	10.0	15.0	17.1	17.1	17.9	12.9	15.0	15.0
Weekly cigarette consumption								
- mean	84.1	107.7	118.8	116.1	120.6	101.7	107.3	108.6
- standard deviation	49.9	52.6	64.4	68.1	67.3	76.8	62.4	70.6
- median	70.0	105.0	120.0	120.0	125.0	90.0	105.0	105.0
Base = 100%	96	153	118	114	89	66	636	651
Women								
Daily cigarette consumption								
- mean	10.2	12.4	14.0	15.9	14.3	11.9	12.9	13.8
- standard deviation	7.1	8.1	7.8	9.6	7.5	6.3	8.0	
- median	10.0	11.4	15.0	15.0	15.0	10.0	11.4	12.1
Weekly cigarette consumption								
- mean	71.5	86.8	98.1	111.2	100.0	83.1	90.5	
- standard deviation	49.5	56.9	54.8	67.1	52.7	44.1	56.1	
- median	70.0	80.0	105.0	105.0	105.0	70.0	80.0	85.0
Base = 100%	107	198	171	98	98	89	761	748
All								
Daily cigarette consumption								
- mean	11.2	14.0	15.4	16.3	15.8	13.1	14.2	14.7
- standard deviation	7.2	7.9	8.6	9.7	8.8	8.8	8.6	9.9
- median	10.0	14.1	16.4	16.4	15.0	10.0	13.6	14.0
Weekly cigarette consumption								
- mean	78.2	97.7	107.8	114.1	110.6	91.5	99.1	103.0
- standard deviation	50.1	55.6	60.4	67.7	61.4	61.5	60.0	69.3
- median	70.0	99.0	115.0	115.0	105.0	70.0	95.0	98.0
Base = 100%	203	351	289	212	187	155	1397	1399

Health in England 1996 : What people know, what people think, what people do

Table 2.5 Daily cigarette consumption by current regular cigarette smokers and ex-regular cigarette smokers by sex
Current and ex-smokers aged 16–74

Number of cigarettes smoked per day	Current smokers %	Ex-smokers %
Men		
0–9	26	9
10–19	37	29
20 or more	37	61
Base = 100%	*636*	*598*
Women		
0–9	33	25
10–19	42	37
20 or more	25	38
Base = 100%	*761*	*535*
All		
0–9	29	16
10–19	40	33
20 or more	31	52
Base = 100%	*1397*	*1133*

Table 2.6 Whether current smokers would like to give up smoking altogether by age and sex
Current cigarette smokers aged 16–74

Age	16–24 %	25–34 %	35–44 %	45–54 %	55–64 %	65–74 %	Total %	HEMS 1995 Total %
Men								
Yes	66	72	74	69	60	38	67	68
No	24	23	23	30	36	62	29	25
Don't know	10	5	2	1	4	1	4	7
Base = 100%	*96*	*155*	*120*	*114*	*91*	*66*	*642*	*658*
Women								
Yes	54	74	69	66	60	52	64	68
No	38	23	25	29	36	45	31	24
Don't know	8	3	5	5	4	3	5	8
Base = 100%	*107*	*199*	*171*	*98*	*98*	*89*	*762*	*749*
All								
Yes	60	73	72	68	60	46	65	68
No	30	23	24	30	36	52	30	25
Don't know	9	4	4	3	4	2	5	7
Base = 100%	*203*	*354*	*291*	*212*	*189*	*155*	*1404*	*1407*

Table 2.7 Proportion of current smokers who would like to give up smoking altogether by how easy they would find it to go without smoking and whether they have ever tried to give up
Current cigarette smokers aged 16–74

	Men	Women	All	Men	Women	All
	Proportion of current smokers who would like to give up smoking altogether			Base = 100%		
Ease or difficulty of not smoking for a day						
Very easy	47	53	50	115	123	238
Fairly easy	70	64	67	159	187	346
Fairly difficult	77	63	71	182	173	355
Very difficult	64	71	68	176	272	448
Whether smoker has ever tried to give up						
Yes	72	72	72	505	578	1083
No	48	42	45	137	182	319
Total	67	64	65	636	760	1396

Table 2.8 Proportion of current smokers who would like to give up smoking altogether by age and number of cigarettes smoked per day
Current cigarette smokers aged 16–74

Age	16–24	25–34	35–44	45–54	55–64	65–74	Total
Number of cigarettes smoked per day	Proportion of current smokers who would like to give up smoking altogether						
0–9	61	62	49	60	56	42	57
10–19	59	77	80	76	64	48	70
20 or more	62	77	78	66	59	48	69
All smokers *	60	73	72	68	60	46	65
Bases = 100%							
0–9	81	93	74	54	42	56	400
10–19	82	157	109	69	76	58	551
20 or more	40	101	106	88	69	41	445
All smokers *	203	351	289	211	187	155	1396

* Includes a few smokers who did not say how many cigarettes a day they smoked.

Health in England 1996 : What people know, what people think, what people do

Table 2.9 How easy or difficult smokers would find it to go without smoking for a whole day by age and sex
Current cigarette smokers aged 16–74

Age Ease or difficulty of not smoking for a day	16–24 %	25–34 %	35–44 %	45–54 %	55–64 %	65–74 %	Total %	HEMS 1995 Total %
Men								
Very easy	20	16	14	21	12	23	17	16
Fairly easy	42	24	17	24	31	21	27	28
Fairly difficult	21	32	43	28	18	21	29	30
Very difficult	14	26	26	26	39	32	25	24
Don't know	3	1	–	–	1	4	1	2
Base = 100%	*96*	*155*	*120*	*114*	*91*	*65*	*641*	*658*
Women								
Very easy	31	19	14	9	13	12	18	16
Fairly easy	25	24	25	21	19	27	24	22
Fairly difficult	29	25	20	25	20	25	24	25
Very difficult	15	30	40	44	49	34	34	35
Don't know	–	1	1	1	–	2	1	2
Base = 100%	*107*	*199*	*171*	*99*	*98*	*88*	*762*	*749*
All								
Very easy	25	17	14	16	12	17	17	16
Fairly easy	34	24	21	23	25	24	25	25
Fairly difficult	25	29	31	27	19	23	26	28
Very difficult	14	28	34	34	44	33	30	30
Don't know	2	1	0	0	0	3	1	2
Base = 100%	*203*	*354*	*291*	*213*	*189*	*153*	*1403*	*1407*

Table 2.10 How easy or difficult smokers would find it to go without smoking for a whole day by number of cigarettes smoked per day and sex
Current cigarette smokers aged 16–74

Number of cigarettes per day	0–9	10–19	20 or more	All*
Ease or difficulty of not smoking for a day	%	%	%	%
Men				
Very easy	47	11	3	17
Fairly easy	34	29	21	27
Fairly difficult	14	35	33	29
Very difficult	5	23	42	25
Don't know	1	2	0	1
Base = 100%	160	226	249	635
Women				
Very easy	43	6	3	18
Fairly easy	32	26	8	23
Fairly difficult	17	33	20	24
Very difficult	7	34	70	34
Don't know	1	1	-	1
Base = 100%	239	326	195	760
All				
Very easy	45	9	3	17
Fairly easy	33	27	16	25
Fairly difficult	15	34	28	27
Very difficult	6	29	53	30
Don't know	1	2	0	1
Base = 100%	399	552	444	1395

* Includes a few smokers who did not say how many cigarettes a day they smoked.

Table 2.11 Percentage of smokers who have tried to give up smoking by age, the number of cigarettes smoked per day and sex
Current cigarette smokers aged 16–74

	Men	Women	All	Men	Women	All
	\multicolumn{3}{c}{Percentage of smokers who have tried to give up smoking}	\multicolumn{3}{c}{Base = 100%}
Characteristic						
Age						
16–24	66	66	66	96	107	203
25–34	79	81	80	155	198	353
35–44	82	86	84	120	171	291
45–54	88	73	82	114	99	213
55–64	85	69	77	91	97	188
65–74	73	67	69	66	89	155
Total	79	75	77	642	761	1403
HEMS 1995 Total	76	77	77	658	749	1407
Number of cigarettes per day						
0–9	69	70	69	160	238	398
10–19	81	79	80	226	326	552
20 or more	83	77	80	250	195	445
Total*	79	75	77	636	759	1395

* Includes a few smokers who did not say how many cigarettes a day they smoked.

Table 2.12 Length of time smokers gave up for by age and sex
Current cigarette smokers aged 16-74 who had previously tried to give up

Age	16-24	25-34	35-44	45-54	55-64	65-74	Total
Length of time smokers gave up for	%	%	%	%	%	%	%
Men							
Less than a day	11	7	3	8	9	5	7
A day, less than a week	29	17	28	15	20	25	22
A week, less than a month	23	23	17	21	17	8	20
A month, less than three months	13	15	13	5	9	17	12
Three months, less than six months	8	12	9	13	12	11	11
Six months, less than a year	9	9	9	8	15	8	10
One year or more	8	18	23	30	18	25	20
Base = 100%	64	124	97	97	75	47	504
Women							
Less than a day	10	6	7	6	11	5	7
A day, less than a week	24	20	20	9	22	11	19
A week, less than a month	21	23	20	20	21	28	22
A month, less than three months	12	11	8	11	12	14	11
Three months, less than six months	13	7	12	10	12	16	11
Six months, less than a year	6	11	10	8	4	7	9
One year or more	13	22	23	36	19	19	22
Base = 100%	72	165	146	73	64	58	578
All							
Less than a day	11	7	5	7	10	5	7
A day, less than a week	27	18	23	13	21	18	20
A week, less than a month	22	23	19	21	19	19	21
A month, less than three months	13	13	10	7	10	15	11
Three months, less than six months	10	10	10	12	12	14	11
Six months, less than a year	8	10	10	8	10	8	9
One year or more	10	19	23	32	19	22	21
Base = 100%	136	289	243	170	139	105	1082

Table 2.13 Length of time smokers gave up for by number of cigarettes smoked per day and sex
Current cigarette smokers aged 16–74 who had previously tried to give up

Number of cigarettes per day	0–9	10–19	20 or more	All *
Length of time smokers gave up for	%	%	%	%
Men				
Less than a day	4	6	10	7
A day, less than a week	14	24	24	22
A week, less than a month	11	21	23	19
A month, less than three months	15	10	11	11
Three months, less than six months	13	13	7	11
Six months, less than a year	10	11	8	10
One year or more	32	16	17	20
Base = 100%	*109*	*182*	*209*	*500*
Women				
Less than a day	0	6	18	7
A day, less than a week	9	23	22	19
A week, less than a month	19	22	25	22
A month, less than three months	11	13	7	11
Three months, less than six months	15	9	10	11
Six months, less than a year	10	10	5	9
One year or more	35	17	13	22
Base = 100%	*167*	*261*	*149*	*577*
All				
Less than a day	2	6	13	7
A day, less than a week	12	24	23	20
A week, less than a month	16	21	24	21
A month, less than three months	12	11	10	11
Three months, less than six months	15	11	8	11
Six months, less than a year	10	10	7	9
One year or more	34	17	15	21
Base = 100%	*276*	*443*	*358*	*1077*

* Includes a few smokers who did not say how many cigarettes a day they smoked.

Table 2.14 Length of time ex-smokers have stopped smoking by age and sex
Ex-smokers aged 16-74

Age	16-34	35-44	45-54	55-64	65-74	Total	HEMS 1995 Total
Length of time ex-smokers have stopped	%	%	%	%	%	%	%
Men							
Less than 6 months	25	4	2	3	1	5	3
Six months, less than 1 year	11	5	1	1	1	3	2
One year, less than 2 years	11	5	3	5	1	4	3
Two years, less than 5 years	14	16	12	6	9	11	13
Five years or more	39	70	81	85	89	76	79
Base = 100%	*68*	*93*	*130*	*138*	*171*	*600*	*635*
Women							
Less than 6 months	16	5	3	2	1	6	6
Six months, less than 1 year	10	1	3	1	2	4	4
One year, less than 2 years	10	4	3	3	1	4	5
Two years, less than 5 years	26	15	9	13	5	14	18
Five years or more	38	75	82	81	92	72	67
Base = 100%	*112*	*99*	*90*	*95*	*141*	*537*	*520*
All							
Less than 6 months	20	5	3	3	1	6	4
Six months, less than 1 year	10	4	2	1	1	3	3
One year, less than 2 years	11	4	3	4	1	4	4
Two years, less than 5 years	21	16	11	8	7	12	15
Five years or more	38	72	82	83	90	74	74
Base = 100%	*180*	*192*	*220*	*233*	*312*	*1137*	*1155*

Table 2.15 Main reason why ex-smokers stopped smoking by age and sex
Ex–smokers aged 16–74

Age Main reason for stopping smoking	16–34 %	35–44 %	45–54 %	55–64 %	65–74 %	Total %
Men						
Health reasons	59	53	70	60	56	60
Cost	13	14	15	21	23	18
Family reasons	13	21	4	8	7	10
Advised to by health professional	2	-	0	2	1	1
Did not like it/enjoy it	8	9	9	8	11	9
Other/None of these	5	3	0	2	2	2
Base = 100%	*64*	*93*	*120*	*128*	*171*	*576*
Women						
Health reasons	41	43	51	59	52	49
Cost	8	14	14	15	22	15
Family reasons	11	19	9	6	10	11
Pregnant	20	18	11	7	5	13
Advised to by health professional	-	2	2	4	1	2
Did not like it/enjoy it	17	5	10	7	6	9
Other/None of these	2	-	3	1	4	2
Base = 100%	*109*	*98*	*86*	*88*	*136*	*517*
All						
Health reasons	49	49	63	60	54	55
Cost	10	14	15	19	23	16
Family reasons	12	20	6	7	8	11
Pregnant	11	8	4	3	2	5
Advised to by health professional	1	1	1	3	1	1
Did not like it/enjoy it	13	7	9	8	9	9
Other/None of these	3	2	1	2	3	2
Base = 100%	*173*	*191*	*206*	*216*	*307*	*1093*

Table 2.16 Main reason why ex-smokers stopped smoking by number of cigarettes they used to smoke per day
Ex-smokers aged 16–74

Number of cigarettes per day Main reason for stopping smoking	0–9 %	10–19 %	20 or more %	All* %
Health reasons	43	54	60	55
Cost	11	18	17	16
Family reasons	11	8	12	11
Pregnant	11	8	2	5
Advised to by health professional	1	1	2	1
Did not like it/enjoy it	22	9	6	9
Other/None of these	1	4	2	2
Base = 100%	*185*	*362*	*543*	*1090*

* Includes a few smokers who did not say how many cigarettes a day they smoked.

Table 2.17 Methods smokers used to stop smoking by whether successful or not and number of cigarettes they (used to) smoke per day
Current smokers who have tried stopping and ex-smokers aged 16–74

Number of cigarettes per day	0–9	10–19	20 or more	All*	HEMS 1995 Total
Methods used to stop smoking	%	%	%	%	%
Ex-smokers					
Will power	94	90	90	91	90
Support from family	11	16	16	15	12
Nicotine chewing gum	0	4	7	5	4
Nicotine patch	1	4	6	5	3
Advice from doctor	4	6	7	6	7
Special clinic or stop smoking group	1	1	2	2	1
Quitline	-	1	0	0	0
Other	2	7	8	7	8
Base †	*149*	*326*	*510*	*985*	*1014*
Current smokers					
Will power	92	83	71	81	80
Support from family	22	19	15	18	19
Nicotine chewing gum	11	17	25	18	19
Nicotine patch	10	18	27	19	18
Advice from doctor	8	8	8	8	8
Special clinic or stop smoking group	2	2	3	2	2
Quitline	0	1	1	1	1
Other	4	5	7	5	8
Base †	*238*	*390*	*315*	*943*	*952*

* Includes a few smokers who did not say how many cigarettes a day they smoked.
† Percentages total more than 100% as some respondents used more than one method.

Table 2.18 When smokers intend to give up smoking by age
Current cigarette smokers aged 16–74

Age	16–24	25–34	35–44	45–54	55–64	65–74	Total
When smokers intend to give up smoking	%	%	%	%	%	%	%
Within the next month	10	9	6	3	2	4	6
Within the next six months	18	12	9	10	8	2	11
Within the next year	21	22	14	9	7	6	15
Intends to give up but not in the next year	27	24	28	20	15	11	23
Unlikely to give up smoking	24	33	43	59	68	77	45
Base = 100%	*201*	*345*	*284*	*209*	*189*	*151*	*1379*

Table 2.19 When smokers intend to give up smoking by number of cigarettes smoked per day
Current cigarette smokers aged 16–74

Number of cigarettes per day	0–9	10–19	20 or more	All*
When smokers intend to give up smoking	%	%	%	%
Within the next month	10	7	2	6
Within the next six months	14	12	7	11
Within the next year	16	17	11	15
Intends to give up but not in the next year	22	22	24	22
Unlikely to give up smoking	37	42	55	45
Base = 100%	387	544	441	1372

* Includes a few smokers who did not say how many cigarettes a day they smoked.

Table 2.20 When smokers intend to give up smoking by whether they want to give up smoking
Current cigarette smokers aged 16–74

Whether want to give up smoking	Want to give up smoking	Do not want to give up smoking	Total
When smokers intend to give up smoking	%	%	%
Within the next month	9	-	6
Within the next six months	16	2	11
Within the next year	20	4	15
Intends to give up but not in the next year	23	22	23
Unlikely to give up smoking	32	72	45
Base = 100%	895	427	1379

Table 2.21 Extent to which informant thinks the health of his/her children is affected by smoking in the home by age and sex
Parents of children aged under 16 where smoking is allowed in the home

Age	16–24	25–34	35–44	45–74	Total
How much health of children is affected by smoking	%	%	%	%	%
A great deal	28	15	14	10	15
Quite a lot	34	31	26	25	28
A little	25	36	35	38	35
Not at all	13	16	22	24	20
Don't smoke at home	-	2	3	4	3
Base = 100%	58	325	382	101	866

Table 2.22 Extent to which informant thinks the health of his/her children is affected by smoking in the home by social class
Parents of children aged under 16 where smoking is allowed in the home

Social class	I & II	III(NM)	III(M)	IV & V	Total*
How much health of children is affected by smoking	%	%	%	%	%
A great deal	9	18	19	16	15
Quite a lot	28	22	23	31	28
A little	39	34	35	35	35
Not at all	19	23	23	16	20
Don't smoke at home	4	3	-	2	3
Base = 100%	220	214	135	232	866

* Members of the Armed Forces, persons in inadequately described occupations and persons who have never worked are not shown as separate categories but are included in the figures for all persons.

Table 2.23 Extent to which informant thinks the health of his/her children is affected by smoking in the home by cigarette smoking status and sex
Parents of children aged under 16 where smoking is allowed in the home

Smoking status	Current smoker	Ex-smoker	Never smoked	Total
How much health of children is affected by smoking	%	%	%	%
A great deal	14	15	15	15
Quite a lot	32	23	26	28
A little	41	36	27	35
Not at all	13	21	26	20
Don't smoke at home	-	5	5	3
Base = 100%	408	155	303	866

Table 2.24 Informant's attitude to his/her children smoking by age and sex
Parents of children aged 9–15

Age	16–34	35–44	45–74	Total
Attitude to children smoking	%	%	%	%
Men				
Does not want them to smoke	87	95	95	93
It is up to them whether they smoke	13	5	6	7
Base = 100%	38	144	85	267
Women				
Does not want them to smoke	89	92	85	91
It is up to them whether they smoke	10	8	15	9
Base = 100%	100	271	53	424
All				
Does not want them to smoke	89	93	92	92
It is up to them whether they smoke	11	7	9	8
Base = 100%	138	415	138	691

Table 2.25 Informant's attitude to his/her children smoking by social class based on own current or last job and sex
Parents of children aged 9–15

Social class	I & II	III(NM)	III(M)	IV & V	Total*
Attitude to children smoking	%	%	%	%	%
Men					
Does not want them to smoke	98	[22]	91	88	93
It is up to them whether they smoke	2	[3]	9	12	7
Base = 100%	107	25	73	48	267
Women					
Does not want them to smoke	93	90	95	88	91
It is up to them whether they smoke	7	10	5	12	9
Base = 100%	107	134	39	120	424
All					
Does not want them to smoke	96	90	92	88	92
It is up to them whether they smoke	4	10	8	12	8
Base = 100%	214	159	112	168	691

* Members of the Armed Forces, persons in inadequately described occupations and persons who have never worked are not shown as separate categories but are included in the figures for all persons.

Table 2.26 Informant's attitude to his/her children smoking by cigarette smoking status and sex
Parents of children aged under 9–16

Smoking status	Current smoker	Ex-smoker	Never smoked	Total
Attitude to children smoking	%	%	%	%
Men				
Does not want them to smoke	91	94	95	93
It is up to them whether they smoke	9	6	5	7
Base = 100%	87	63	117	267
Women				
Does not want them to smoke	85	92	93	91
It is up to them whether they smoke	15	8	7	9
Base = 100%	143	85	196	424
All				
Does not want them to smoke	88	93	94	92
It is up to them whether they smoke	12	7	6	8
Base = 100%	230	148	313	691

Health in England 1996 : What people know, what people think, what people do

Table 2.27 Workplace smoking policy of respondents who had a job in the week before interview by age and sex
Adults aged 16–74 who had a job last week

Age	16–34	35–44	45–54	55–64	65–74	Total	HEMS 1995 Total
Workplace smoking policy	%	%	%	%	%	%	%
Men							
Smoking is banned	23	26	28	28	20	26	24
Smoking is allowed in special areas only	58	44	47	40	45	46	46
Smoking is allowed anywhere	17	27	19	23	26	22	24
Work at home	-	1	5	4	6	3	3
Don't know	3	2	1	5	4	3	2
Base = 100%	148	362	335	293	159	1320	1398
Women							
Smoking is banned	32	43	44	39	45	41	39
Smoking is allowed in special areas only	51	43	42	46	40	44	47
Smoking is allowed anywhere	15	9	9	10	11	10	9
Work at home	1	3	4	3	3	3	4
Don't know	0	2	2	2	1	2	1
Base = 100%	146	361	372	258	133	1294	1343
All							
Smoking is banned	27	33	35	33	30	32	31
Smoking is allowed in special areas only	55	44	44	43	43	45	47
Smoking is allowed anywhere	16	19	14	17	20	17	17
Work at home	0	2	5	4	5	3	4
Don't know	2	2	2	4	3	2	2
Base = 100%	294	723	707	551	292	2614	2741

* The total includes a small number of respondents aged 65–74 who were working last week.

Table 2.28 Workplace smoking policy of respondents who had a job in the week before interview by social class of job and sex
Adults aged 16–74 who had a job last week

Social class	I & II	III(NM)	III(M)	IV & V	Total*
Workplace smoking policy	%	%	%	%	%
Men					
Smoking is banned	35	32	15	18	26
Smoking is allowed in special areas only	45	53	38	50	46
Smoking is allowed anywhere	14	9	40	25	22
Work at home	4	4	3	2	3
Don't know	2	1	4	5	3
Base = 100%	*582*	*138*	*357*	*222*	*1319*
Women					
Smoking is banned	47	43	31	33	41
Smoking is allowed in special areas only	41	45	53	45	44
Smoking is allowed anywhere	5	10	15	16	10
Work at home	4	2	1	3	3
Don't know	3	1	-	3	2
Base = 100%	*441*	*439*	*106*	*306*	*1294*
All					
Smoking is banned	40	40	18	26	32
Smoking is allowed in special areas only	43	47	41	48	45
Smoking is allowed anywhere	10	10	35	20	17
Work at home	4	3	3	3	3
Don't know	2	1	4	4	2
Base = 100%	*1023*	*577*	*463*	*528*	*2613*

* Members of the Armed Forces and persons in inadequately described occupation are not shown as separate categories but are included in the figures for all persons.

Table 2.29 Workplace smoking policy of respondents who had a job in the week before interview by employment status and size of the establishment and sex
Adults aged 16-74 who had a job last week

Employment status and size of establishment	Employee 1-24 employees	Employee 25+ employees	Self-employed No employees	Self-employed With employees	Total
Workplace smoking policy	%	%	%	%	%
Men					
Smoking is banned	28	27	14	27	26
Smoking is allowed in special areas only	37	58	15	11	46
Smoking is allowed anywhere	30	13	42	52	22
Work at home	1	1	18	8	3
Don't know	3	1	12	1	3
Base = 100%	*294*	*782*	*177*	*66*	*1319*
Women					
Smoking is banned	46	39	29	[9]	41
Smoking is allowed in special areas only	31	54	18	[7]	44
Smoking is allowed anywhere	17	6	17	[3]	10
Work at home	3	0	32	[2]	3
Don't know	3	1	5	[0]	2
Base = 100%	*419*	*776*	*77*	*21*	*1294*
All					
Smoking is banned	38	32	17	31	32
Smoking is allowed in special areas only	34	57	16	15	45
Smoking is allowed anywhere	23	10	36	45	17
Work at home	2	1	21	8	3
Don't know	3	1	10	1	2
Base = 100%	*713*	*1558*	*254*	*87*	*2613*

Table 2.30 Whether visitors are allowed to smoke cigarettes in respondent's home by age and sex
Adults aged 16–74

Age	16–24	25–34	35–44	45–54	55–64	65–74	Total	Total HEMS 1995
Whether visitors are allowed to smoke in respondent's home	%	%	%	%	%	%	%	%
Men								
Yes, can smoke anywhere	38	35	39	47	52	47	42	46
Not when children are around	4	7	5	3	4	1	4	5
Yes, in some places only	30	21	22	23	24	22	23	24
No, smoking not allowed in the house	26	35	33	27	20	27	29	25
Don't know	3	1	1	1	1	3	1	1
Base = 100%	224	436	396	368	308	310	2042	2119
Women								
Yes, can smoke anywhere	40	28	36	39	42	45	37	38
Not when children are around	5	6	6	3	7	2	5	5
Yes, in some places only	29	29	26	26	22	23	26	27
No, smoking not allowed in the house	26	36	31	30	27	29	30	28
Don't know	-	1	1	2	2	1	1	1
Base = 100%	266	586	533	392	362	461	2600	2548
All								
Yes, can smoke anywhere	39	32	38	43	47	46	40	42
Not when children are around	4	7	5	3	6	1	5	5
Yes, in some places only	29	25	24	24	23	22	25	25
No, smoking not allowed in the house	26	36	32	28	23	28	30	27
Don't know	1	1	1	1	1	2	1	1
Base = 100%	490	1022	929	760	670	771	4642	4667

Health in England 1996 : What people know, what people think, what people do

Table 2.31 Whether visitors are allowed to smoke cigarettes in respondent's home by social class based on own current or last job and sex
Adults aged 16–74

Social class Whether visitors are allowed to smoke in respondent's home	I & II %	III(NM) %	III(M) %	IV & V %	Total* %
Men					
Yes, can smoke anywhere	38	34	48	48	42
Not when children are around	4	4	6	3	4
Yes, in some places only	21	31	22	23	23
No, smoking not allowed in the house	35	32	24	24	29
Don't know	1	–	1	2	1
Base = 100%	782	195	561	367	2041
Women					
Yes, can smoke anywhere	26	40	40	42	37
Not when children are around	6	4	5	6	5
Yes, in some places only	25	26	29	27	26
No, smoking not allowed in the house	41	30	25	24	30
Don't know	2	1	0	1	1
Base = 100%	677	862	224	680	2598
All					
Yes, can smoke anywhere	33	38	46	45	40
Not when children are around	5	4	6	5	5
Yes, in some places only	23	27	23	25	25
No, smoking not allowed in the house	37	30	24	24	30
Don't know	1	1	1	2	1
Base = 100%	1459	1057	785	1047	4639

* Members of the Armed Forces, persons in inadequately described occupations and persons who have never worked are not shown as separate categories but are included in the figures for all persons.

Table 2.32 Whether visitors are allowed to smoke cigarettes in respondent's home by whether respondent has any children under 16 in the household and sex
Adults aged 16–74

Whether visitors are allowed to smoke in respondent's home	Children under 16 in household %	No children under 16 in household %	Total %
Men			
Yes, can smoke anywhere	34	45	42
Not when children are around	8	3	4
Yes, in some places only	24	23	23
No, smoking not allowed in the house	34	27	29
Don't know	1	2	1
Base = 100%	513	1529	2042
Women			
Yes, can smoke anywhere	31	40	37
Not when children are around	8	4	5
Yes, in some places only	25	27	26
No, smoking not allowed in the house	35	28	30
Don't know	1	1	1
Base = 100%	859	1741	2600
All			
Yes, can smoke anywhere	32	43	40
Not when children are around	8	3	5
Yes, in some places only	25	25	25
No, smoking not allowed in the house	35	28	30
Don't know	1	1	1
Base = 100%	1372	3270	4642

Table 2.33 Whether visitors are allowed to smoke cigarettes in respondent's home by cigarette smoking status and sex
Adults aged 16–74

Whether visitors are allowed to smoke in respondent's home	Current smoker %	Ex-smoker %	Never smoked %	Total %
Men				
Yes, can smoke anywhere	59	44	29	42
Not when children are around	6	2	4	4
Yes, in some places only	24	24	23	23
No, smoking not allowed in the house	10	29	43	29
Don't know	1	1	2	1
Base = 100%	*642*	*600*	*799*	*2041*
Women				
Yes, can smoke anywhere	54	37	28	37
Not when children are around	8	4	4	5
Yes, in some places only	28	25	25	26
No, smoking not allowed in the house	9	33	41	30
Don't know	0	2	1	1
Base = 100%	*763*	*537*	*1300*	*2600*
All				
Yes, can smoke anywhere	57	41	28	40
Not when children are around	7	3	4	5
Yes, in some places only	26	24	24	25
No, smoking not allowed in the house	10	31	42	30
Don't know	0	1	2	1
Base = 100%	*1405*	*1137*	*2099*	*4641*

Table 2.34 Alcohol consumption level (AC rating) and mean weekly number of units by age and sex
Adults aged 16–74

Age	16–24	25–34	35–44	45–54	55–64	65–74	Total	Total HEMS 1995
Alcohol consumption in units per week	%	%	%	%	%	%	%	%
Men								
Non-drinker	9	7	6	5	10	3	7	6
Under one	6	5	6	8	8	11	7	6
1–10	23	35	34	28	32	36	31	34
11–21	20	25	25	26	28	21	24	23
22–35	20	16	17	19	13	15	17	16
36–50	11	7	7	8	4	7	7	8
51 and over	11	6	5	6	5	7	7	6
Mean weekly units	22.4	16.8	17.4	18.4	14.8	18	18	18.2
Standard error of the mean	0.9	0.6	0.7	0.7	0.8	1.3	0.3	0.4
Median	15.5	11.5	12	13.5	10	9.2	12.2	11.5
Base = 100%	221	430	389	365	302	300	2007	2119
Women								
Non-drinker	5	8	5	12	15	17	10	9
Under one	7	13	16	18	23	31	17	17
1–7	35	39	44	40	40	33	39	42
8–14	20	21	20	14	12	10	17	17
15–25	18	11	9	11	8	5	11	10
26–35	7	4	3	3	1	2	3	3
36 and over	8	3	3	2	1	2	3	2
Mean weekly units	14.4	8.1	7.9	6.4	4.6	4.3	7.7	7.0
Standard error of the mean	0.9	0.4	0.5	0.4	0.3	0.4	0.2	0.2
Median	7.6	4.5	3.8	2.7	1.5	0.7	3.1	3.1
Base = 100%	258	577	524	386	361	454	2560	2548

Table 2.35 Alcohol consumption level (AC rating) and mean weekly number of units by social class based on own current or last job and sex
Adults aged 16–74

Social class	I & II	III(NM)	III(M)	IV & V	Total*
Alcohol consumption in units per week	%	%	%	%	%
Men					
Non-drinker	5	8	6	7	7
Under one	6	8	6	11	7
1–10	31	32	35	26	31
11–21	28	25	23	21	24
22–35	19	15	16	14	17
36–50	7	8	7	9	7
51 and over	4	3	8	11	7
Mean weekly units	*16.8*	*15.1*	*18.9*	*20.9*	*18*
Standard error of the mean	*0.5*	*0.9*	*0.7*	*1*	*0.3*
Base = 100%	*769*	*193*	*549*	*361*	*2006*
Women					
Non-drinker	8	8	11	12	10
Under one	13	16	24	21	17
1–7	43	41	32	37	39
8–14	20	18	16	15	17
15–25	10	10	12	10	11
26–35	4	4	4	2	3
36 and over	3	3	2	3	3
Mean weekly units	*7.5*	*8*	*6.7*	*6.8*	*7.7*
Standard error of the mean	*0.3*	*0.4*	*0.5*	*0.4*	*0.2*
Base = 100%	*671*	*847*	*219*	*672*	*2558*

* Members of the Armed Forces, persons in inadequately described occupations and persons who have never worked are not shown as separate categories but are included in the figures for all persons.

Table 2.36 Frequency and mean weekly consumption of alcoholic soft drinks in the last 12 months by age and sex
Adults aged 16–74 who drank alcoholic soft drinks

Age	16–24	25–34	35–44	45–74	Total
Frequency of consuming alcoholic soft drinks	%	%	%	%	%
Men					
At least once a week	15	3	1	1	2
Once or twice a month	15	6	2	–	4
Once every couple of months	9	4	1	0	3
Once or twice a year	16	19	12	5	11
Not at all in the last 12 months	45	68	85	94	79
Mean consumption (weekly units)	*2.6*	*0.4*	*0.1*	*0.1*	*0.5*
Standard error of the mean	*0.3*	*0.1*	*0*	*0.1*	*0.1*
Base = 100%	*208*	*413*	*376*	*927*	*1924*
Women					
At least once a week	21	5	1	1	5
Once or twice a month	16	8	3	0	5
Once every couple of months	13	7	2	1	4
Once or twice a year	23	18	19	5	14
Not at all in the last 12 months	28	62	74	93	72
Mean consumption (weekly units)	*3*	*0.5*	*0.2*	*0.1*	*0.7*
Standard error of the mean	*0.3*	*0.1*	*0*	*0.1*	*0.1*
Base = 100%	*251*	*542*	*506*	*1035*	*2334*
All					
At least once a week	17	4	1	1	4
Once or twice a month	15	7	2	0	4
Once every couple of months	11	5	2	1	4
Once or twice a year	19	18	16	5	12
Not at all in the last 12 months	36	65	79	94	76
Mean consumption (weekly units)	*2.8*	*0.4*	*0.1*	*0.1*	*0.6*
Standard error of the mean	*0.2*	*0*	*0*	*0.1*	*0.04*
Base = 100%	*459*	*955*	*882*	*1962*	*4258*

Table 2.37 Frequency of consuming different types of alcoholic drinks by sex
Adults aged 16–24

Type of drink	'Alcopops'	Shandy	Beer	Spirits	Sherry	Wine
Frequency of consuming alcoholic drinks	%	%	%	%	%	%
Men						
At least once a week	15	11	73	22	2	17
Once or twice a month	15	12	13	22	4	21
Once every couple of months	9	10	5	14	3	23
Once or twice a year	16	14	5	17	14	12
Not at all in the last 12 months	45	50	4	25	77	27
Base = 100%	*208*	*208*	*208*	*208*	*208*	*208*
Women						
At least once a week	21	8	49	30	4	31
Once or twice a month	16	6	17	25	5	21
Once every couple of months	13	6	10	11	8	10
Once or twice a year	23	23	11	14	13	18
Not at all in the last 12 months	28	57	13	18	70	20
Base = 100%	*251*	*251*	*251*	*251*	*251*	*250*

Table 2.38 Mean weekly consumption of 'alcopops' as a proportion of total mean weekly alcohol consumption by age and sex
Adults aged 16–74 who drank alcoholic soft drinks

Age	16–24	25–34	35–44	45–74	Total
Men					
At least once a week	15	3	1	1	2
Mean consumption (weekly units) of 'alcopops'	2.6	0.4	0.1	0.1	0.5
Total mean consumption (weekly units) of all alcoholic drinks	22.4	16.8	17.4	17.2	18
Consumption of 'alcopops' as a proportion of total consumption	12%	2%	1%	1%	3%
Women					
Mean consumption (weekly units) of 'alcopops'	3	0.5	0.2	0.1	0.7
Total mean consumption (weekly units) of all alcoholic drinks	14.4	8.1	7.9	5.2	7.7
Consumption of 'alcopops' as a proportion of total consumption	21%	6%	3%	2%	9%

Table 2.39 Percentage who would like to drink less by age and social class based on own current or last job and sex
Current drinkers aged 16–74 who drank at least once or twice a week

Characteristic	Men	Women	All	Men (Base=100%)	Women (Base=100%)	All (Base=100%)
Age						
16–24	28	24	26	163	157	320
25–34	17	19	18	315	322	637
35–44	21	18	19	303	314	617
45–54	17	13	16	280	204	484
55–64	13	8	11	210	156	366
65–74	5	4	4	234	178	412
Total	17	16	17	1505	1331	2836
Social class						
I and II	19	18	19	610	410	1020
III (NM)	19	15	16	130	453	583
III (M)	15	12	14	418	94	512
IV and V	19	14	17	250	298	548
Total*	17	16	17	1504	1330	2834

* Members of the Armed Forces, persons in inadequately described occupations and persons who have never worked are not shown as separate categories but are included in the figures for all persons.

Table 2.40 Percentage who would like to drink less by the amount of alcohol consumed per week and sex
Current drinkers aged 16–74 who drank at least once or twice a week

Alcohol consumed (units per week)	1–10 (men)/ 1–7 (women)	11–21 (men)/ 8–14 (women)	22–35 (men)/ 15–25 (women)	36–50 (men)/ 26–35 (women)	51+ (men)/ 36+ (women)	Total*
Respondent's attitude to his/her drinking	%	%	%	%	%	%
Men						
Drinks about the right amount	95	87	80	61	56	83
Would like to drink less	5	13	20	39	45	17
Base = 100%	407	471	327	142	130	1479
Women						
Drinks about the right amount	96	87	75	61	46	84
Would like to drink less	4	13	25	39	54	16
Base = 100%	519	400	241	71	72	1305

* Total includes a small number of respondents who drank less than one unit per week.

Table 2.41 When respondents intend to cut down on drinking by age and sex
Current drinkers aged 16–74 who drank at least once or twice a week and would like to cut down on their drinking

Age When respondent intends to cut down on drinking	16–24 %	25–34 %	35–44 %	45–74 %	Total %
Men					
Within the next month	32	18	22	19	23
Within the next six months	4	15	19	7	11
Within the next year	15	19	8	6	12
Intends to cut down, but not in the next year	23	9	2	13	12
Unlikely to cut down	26	38	48	55	43
Base = 100%	46	62	68	90	266
Women					
Within the next month	16	13	21	17	16
Within the next six months	9	9	26	14	14
Within the next year	18	11	5	12	11
Intends to cut down, but not in the next year	18	6	8	2	9
Unlikely to cut down	40	62	41	55	49
Base = 100%	41	65	57	46	209
All					
Within the next month	25	16	22	19	20
Within the next six months	6	12	22	9	12
Within the next year	16	15	7	8	12
Intends to cut down, but not in the next year	21	8	5	9	11
Unlikely to cut down	32	49	45	55	45
Base = 100%	87	127	125	136	475

Table 2.42 When respondents intend to cut down on drinking by social class based on current or last job and sex
Current drinkers aged 16–74 who drank at least once or twice a week and would like to cut down on their drinking

Social class When respondent intends to cut down on drinking	I & II %	III(NM) %	III(M) %	IV & V %	Total* %
Men					
Within the next month	20	[6]	15	40	23
Within the next six months	15	[2]	6	7	11
Within the next year	8	[4]	17	14	12
Intends to cut down, but not in the next year	11	[6]	16	2	12
Unlikely to cut down	47	[7]	46	37	43
Base = 100%	120	25	62	45	266
Women					
Within the next month	17	13	[1]	21	16
Within the next six months	11	19	[1]	13	14
Within the next year	15	12	[1]	6	11
Intends to cut down, but not in the next year	14	6	[0]	4	9
Unlikely to cut down	43	50	[8]	57	49
Base = 100%	72	70	11	39	209
All					
Within the next month	19	14	14	33	20
Within the next six months	13	16	6	9	12
Within the next year	10	13	17	10	12
Intends to cut down, but not in the next year	12	11	14	3	11
Unlikely to cut down	46	44	49	45	45
Base = 100%	192	95	73	84	475

* Members of the Armed Forces, persons in inadequately described occupations and persons who have never worked are not shown as separate categories but are included in the figures for all persons.

Table 2.43 When respondents intend to cut down on drinking by the amount of alcohol consumed per week and sex
Current drinkers aged 16–74 who drank at least once or twice a week and would like to cut down on their drinking

Alcohol consumed (units per week)	1–21 (men)/ 1–14 (women)	22–35 (men)/ 15–25 (women)	36+ (men)/ 26+ (women)	Total*
When respondent intends to cut down on drinking	%	%	%	%
Men				
Within the next month	13	21	30	23
Within the next six months	16	8	9	11
Within the next year	12	9	13	12
Intends to cut down, but not in the next year	6	21	11	12
Unlikely to cut down	53	41	36	42
Base = 100%	80	67	115	262
Women				
Within the next month	14	20	16	17
Within the next six months	17	15	10	14
Within the next year	13	4	17	12
Intends to cut down, but not in the next year	5	13	10	9
Unlikely to cut down	51	49	46	49
Base = 100%	77	62	66	206

* Total includes a small number of respondents who drank less than one unit a week.

Table 2.45 Percentage who had heard of alcohol units and correctly identified the number in specified drinks by each type of drink
Adults aged 16–74 who had heard of alcohol units

Type of drink	Glass of wine	Pint of beer	Single pub measure of spirits
Estimated number	%	%	%
Less than one	0	0	0
One	43	9	34
Two	13	43	15
Three-five	6	10	9
More than five	2	3	4
Don't know	35	35	38
Haven't heard of units	-	-	-
Base = 100%	3777	3777	3777

Table 2.44 Percentage who have heard about measuring alcohol in units by age and sex
Adults aged 16–74

Age	16–24	25–34	35–44	45–54	55–64	65–74	Total	Total HEMS 1995
Whether heard of units	%	%	%	%	%	%	%	%
Men	87	89	87	86	75	75	84	83
Base = 100%	224	436	396	367	309	310	2042	2120
Women	89	87	88	85	72	58	81	77
Base = 100%	266	586	533	392	362	461	2600	2545
All 88	88	87	85	73	66	83	80	
Base = 100%	490	1022	929	759	671	771	4642	4665

Table 2.46 Percentage who had heard of alcohol units and correctly identified the number in specified drinks by age and sex
Adults aged 16–74 who had heard of alcohol units

Age	16–24	25–34	35–44	45–54	55–64	65–74	Total	Total HEMS 1995
Type of drink	\multicolumn{7}{c}{Percentage correctly identifying the number of units}	
Men								
Glass of wine	46	49	51	45	39	32	45	44
Pint of beer	47	54	62	53	43	36	51	50
Single pub measure of spirits	39	42	38	38	31	29	37	35
Base = 100%	*198*	*391*	*344*	*314*	*232*	*226*	*1705*	*1742*
Women								
Glass of wine	45	50	42	39	31	23	41	38
Pint of beer	45	44	35	31	19	12	34	30
Single pub measure of spirits	33	38	32	26	23	18	30	27
Base = 100%	*236*	*506*	*473*	*333*	*256*	*268*	*2072*	*1925*
All								
Glass of wine	45	50	46	42	35	27	43	41
Pint of beer	46	49	48	43	31	24	43	40
Single pub measure of spirits	36	40	35	32	27	24	34	31
Base = 100%	*434*	*897*	*817*	*647*	*488*	*494*	*3777*	*3667*

Table 2.47 Percentage who had heard of alcohol units and correctly identified the number in specified drinks by age and social class based on own current or last job and sex
Adults aged 16–74 who had heard of alcohol units

Social class	I & II	III(NM)	III(M)	IV & V	Total*
Type of drink	\multicolumn{5}{c}{Percentage correctly identifying the number of units}
Men					
Glass of wine	58	40	38	30	45
Pint of beer	63	49	42	34	51
Single pub measure of spirits	49	30	28	24	37
Base = 100%	*713*	*165*	*444*	*269*	*1704*
Women					
Glass of wine	55	37	31	29	41
Pint of beer	44	31	26	27	34
Single pub measure of spirits	39	27	25	25	30
Base = 100%	*617*	*720*	*163*	*457*	*2072*
All					
Glass of wine	57	38	36	29	43
Pint of beer	55	35	38	30	43
Single pub measure of spirits	45	28	27	25	34
Base = 100%	*1330*	*885*	*607*	*726*	*3777*

* Members of the Armed Forces, persons in inadequately described occupations and persons who have never worked are not shown as separate categories but are included in the figures for all persons.

Table 2.48 Percentage who had heard of alcohol units and correctly identified the number in specified drinks by alcohol consumption and sex
Adults aged 16–74 who had heard of alcohol units

Alcohol consumed	Abstainer/ non in last year	Under one	1–10 (men)/ 1–7 (women)	11–21 (men)/ 8–14 (women)	22–35 (men)/ 15–25 (women)	36–50 (men)/ 26–35 (women)	51+ (men)/ 36+ (women)	Total
Type of drink	%	%	%	%	%	%	%	%
Men								
Glass of wine	34	21	44	53	50	48	36	45
Pint of beer	34	22	48	58	61	50	53	51
Single pub measure of spirits	21	17	34	44	46	38	38	38
Base = 100%	84	105	507	429	297	129	121	1672
Women								
Glass of wine	24	20	40	50	57	48	49	41
Pint of beer	14	16	34	46	44	38	38	34
Single pub measure of spirits	15	15	28	35	48	47	35	30
Base = 100%	155	325	830	367	224	72	67	2040

Table 2.49 Attitude to changes in sensible drinking levels by age and sex
Adults aged 16–74

Age	16–24	25–34	35–44	45–54	55–64	65–74	Total
Attitudes to changes in sensible drinking levels	%	%	%	%	%	%	%
Men							
I haven't heard anything about the changes	33	27	23	18	24	24	24
I feel confused about the changes	13	12	16	17	12	13	14
I don't feel confused about the changes	24	26	30	26	22	21	25
It is of no interest to me	30	35	32	38	42	42	37
Base = 100%	224	434	396	367	307	307	2035
Women							
I haven't heard anything about the changes	42	34	25	19	25	24	28
I feel confused about the changes	14	17	19	14	11	10	14
I don't feel confused about the changes	17	22	24	24	14	10	19
It is of no interest to me	27	27	33	43	51	57	39
Base = 100%	266	585	530	391	361	457	2590
All							
I haven't heard anything about the changes	38	31	24	18	24	24	26
I feel confused about the changes	13	15	17	16	11	11	14
I don't feel confused about the changes	20	24	26	25	18	14	22
It is of no interest to me	28	31	32	41	47	51	38
Base = 100%	490	1019	926	758	668	764	4625

Table 2.50 Attitude to changes in sensible drinking levels by social class based on own current or last job and sex
Adults aged 16–74

Social class Attitude to changes in sensible drinking levels	I & II %	III(NM) %	III(M) %	IV & V %	Total* %
Men					
I haven't heard anything about the changes	17	24	29	34	24
I feel confused about the changes	14	17	13	13	14
I don't feel confused about the changes	35	21	18	15	25
It is of no interest to me	34	38	39	38	37
Base = 100%	*782*	*195*	*558*	*364*	*2034*
Women					
I haven't heard anything about the changes	20	27	29	36	28
I feel confused about the changes	17	15	10	13	14
I don't feel confused about the changes	29	19	16	11	19
It is of no interest to me	35	39	45	41	39
Base = 100%	*675*	*860*	*223*	*676*	*2588*
All					
I haven't heard anything about the changes	18	26	29	35	26
I feel confused about the changes	15	15	12	13	14
I don't feel confused about the changes	32	20	18	12	22
It is of no interest to me	34	39	41	40	38
Base = 100%	*1457*	*1055*	*781*	*1040*	*4622*

* Members of the Armed Forces, persons in inadequately described occupations and persons who have never worked are not shown as separate categories but are included in the figures for all persons.

Table 2.51 Attitudes to changes in sensible drinking levels by alcohol consumption level
Adults aged 16–74

Alcohol consumed	Abstainer/ non in last year	Under one	1–10 (men)/ 1–7 (women)	11–21 (men)/ 8–14 (women)	22–35 (men)/ 15–25 (women)	36–50 (men)/ 26–35 (women)	51+ (men)/ 36+ (women)	Total
Attitude to changes in sensible drinking levels	%	%	%	%	%	%	%	%
Men								
I haven't heard anything about the changes	23	23	25	23	25	22	29	24
I feel confused about the changes	6	11	15	15	15	16	9	14
I don't feel confused about the changes	7	10	21	31	33	36	23	25
It is of no interest to me	64	56	39	32	27	25	39	37
Base = 100%	*122*	*145*	*628*	*488*	*336*	*148*	*132*	*1999*
Women								
I haven't heard anything about the changes	22	27	27	28	30	38	27	27
I feel confused about the changes	5	13	16	17	19	9	14	14
I don't feel confused about the changes	6	8	20	28	26	36	35	19
It is of no interest to me	67	53	37	26	25	16	24	39
Base = 100%	*273*	*470*	*992*	*421*	*245*	*74*	*74*	*2549*

Health in England 1996 : What people know, what people think, what people do

Table 2.52 Attitude to changes in sensible drinking levels by whether heard of units of alcohol and sex
Adults aged 16–74

Whether heard of units of alcohol / Attitude to changes in sensible drinking levels	Yes %	No %	Don't know %	Total %
Men				
I haven't heard anything about the changes	20	47	34	24
I feel confused about the changes	15	9	12	14
I don't feel confused about the changes	29	6	6	25
It is of no interest to me	36	38	47	37
Base = 100%	1701	302	32	2035
Women				
I haven't heard anything about the changes	24	40	44	28
I feel confused about the changes	16	7	9	14
I don't feel confused about the changes	22	5	3	19
It is of no interest to me	37	49	44	39
Base = 100%	2066	492	32	2590
All				
I haven't heard anything about the changes	23	42	39	26
I feel confused about the changes	16	8	11	14
I don't feel confused about the changes	25	5	5	22
It is of no interest to me	37	45	45	38
Base = 100%	3767	794	64	4625

Table 2.53 Alcohol consumption by smoking status (HEMS 95 and HEMS 96 combined)
Adults aged 16–74

Smoking status / Alcohol consumption	Smoker %	Non-smoker %	Total %
None/less than 1 unit	19	21	20
1–21 units (men)/ 1–14 units (women)	48	59	56
22–50 units (men)/ 15–35 units (women)	24	17	19
51+ units (men)/ 36+ units (women)	9	3	5
Base = 100%	2777	6443	9220

Table 3.1 Frequency of at least moderate-intensity activity for 30 minutes or more by age and sex
Adults aged 16–74

Age	16–24	25–34	35–44	45–54	55–64	65–74	Total	Total HEMS 1995
Frequency of activity	%	%	%	%	%	%	%	%
Men								
Less than one day a week (sedentary)	9	19	20	26	38	42	24	25
1–2 days a week	21	20	25	25	23	29	23	25
3–4 days a week	14	12	12	11	7	14	12	13
5 or more days a week	56	48	43	39	32	14	41	38
Base = 100%	224	436	396	368	309	310	2043	2119
Women								
Less than one day a week (sedentary)	20	18	19	22	37	46	26	29
1–2 days a week	29	27	33	28	33	28	30	31
3–4 days a week	18	15	14	14	9	11	14	13
5 or more days a week	32	39	34	35	21	14	31	27
Base = 100%	265	586	533	392	362	461	2599	2547
All								
Less than one day a week (sedentary)	15	19	19	24	37	44	25	27
1–2 days a week	25	23	29	26	28	29	27	28
3–4 days a week	16	14	13	12	8	13	13	13
5 or more days a week	44	44	38	37	27	14	36	32
Base = 100%	489	1022	929	760	671	771	4642	4666

Table 3.2 Frequency of moderate-intensity activity for 30 minutes or more by social class based on last or current job and sex
Adults aged 16–74

Social class	I & II	III(NM)	III(M)	IV & V	Total*
Frequency of activity	%	%	%	%	%
Men					
Less than one day a week (sedentary)	26	28	23	22	24
1–2 days a week	28	23	21	18	23
3–4 days a week	14	14	10	5	12
5 or more days a week	32	35	47	55	41
Base = 100%	783	195	561	367	2042
Women					
Less than one day a week (sedentary)	23	26	21	28	26
1–2 days a week	30	33	28	25	30
3–4 days a week	16	16	12	10	14
5 or more days a week	31	25	39	37	31
Base = 100%	677	862	224	680	2597

* Members of the Armed Forces, persons in inadequately described occupations and persons who have never worked are not shown as separate categories but are included in the figures for all persons.

Table 3.3 Age-standardised ratios for at least moderate activity on five or more days a week by social class based on own current or last job and sex
Adults aged 16–74

Social class*	I & II	III(NM)	III(M)	IV & V
At least moderate activity on five or more days a week				
Men				
Observed %	32	35	47	54
Expected %[†]	40	45	40	42
Standardised ratio**	80[††]	79[††]	115[††]	128[††]
Standard error of the ratio	2.2	4.6	2.8	3.5
Base = 100%	783	195	561	367
Women				
Observed %	31	25	39	37
Expected % [†]	32	32	30	30
Standardised ratio**	96[††]	80[††]	128[††]	123[††]
Standard error of the ratio	3.6	2.8	7.5	3.9
Base = 100%	677	862	224	680

* Excludes members of the Armed Forces, persons in inadequately described occupations and persons who have never worked.
† Calculations of the expected numbers used age-specific rates for having self-reported good general health for all men and all women. The age-groups used were 16–24, 25–34, 35–44, 45–54, 55–64, and 65–74.
**The standardised ratio is given as the observed rate divided by the expected rate and the ratio multiplied by 100. A 2-tailed test was used to show whether the ratio was significantly different from 100. The resulting figure was multiplied by the square root of the mean of the weight to allow for weighting.
†† Significant at the 95% level.

Table 3.4 Percentage participating in vigorous activity for 20 minutes or more at least three times a week by age, social class based on own current or last job and sex
Adults aged 16–74

	Men	Women	All	Men	Women	All
	Percentage participating in vigorous activity for 20 minutes or more, at least three times a week			Base = 100%		
Characteristic						
Age						
16–24	36	13	25	224	265	489
25–34	23	13	18	436	586	1022
35–44	18	9	13	396	533	929
45–54	11	8	10	368	392	760
55–64	7	2	5	309	362	671
65–74	2	1	1	310	461	771
All	18	8	13	2043	2599	4642
All – HEMS 1995	18	7	12	2119	2547	4666
Social Class*						
I & II	14	11	13	783	677	1460
III (NM)	24	8	11	195	862	1057
III (M)	16	5	13	561	224	785
IV & V	22	7	13	367	680	1047
All	18	8	13	2042	2597	4639
All – HEMS 1995	17	7	11	2071	2474	4545

* Members of the Armed Forces, persons in inadequately described occupations and persons who have never worked are not shown as separate categories but are included in the figures for all persons.

Table 3.5 'How long people should be physically active' by age and sex
Adults aged 16–74

Age	16–24	25–34	35–44	45–54	55–64	65–74	Total
How long people should be physically active	%	%	%	%	%	%	%
Men							
Less than 20 minutes	8	7	10	10	13	11	9
20–30 minutes	12	16	15	12	10	9	13
30 minutes	32	36	36	37	34	33	35
More than 30 minutes	47	38	37	35	36	34	38
30 minutes or more	78	74	72	72	70	67	73
Don't know	1	3	2	6	7	13	5
Base = 100%	*220*	*430*	*389*	*364*	*296*	*295*	*1994*
Women							
Less than 20 minutes	10	8	13	9	12	11	10
20–30 minutes	15	16	19	18	15	12	16
30 minutes	34	35	39	41	33	37	37
More than 30 minutes	41	38	27	25	33	29	32
30 minutes or more	75	74	67	67	66	67	69
Don't know	1	2	2	6	6	11	4
Base = 100%	*262*	*579*	*522*	*385*	*345*	*436*	*2529*
All							
Less than 20 minutes	9	7	11	9	12	11	10
20–30 minutes	14	16	17	15	13	11	15
30 minutes	33	36	38	39	33	35	36
More than 30 minutes	44	38	32	31	35	32	35
30 minutes or more	77	74	70	70	68	67	71
Don't know	1	3	2	6	7	12	5
Base = 100%	*482*	*1009*	*911*	*749*	*641*	*731*	*4523*

Table 3.6 'How long people should be physically active' by social class based on own current or last job, and sex
Adults aged 16–74

Social class	I & II	III(NM)	III(M)	IV & V	Total*
How long people should be physically active	%	%	%	%	%
Men					
Less than 20 minutes	10	10	10	10	9
20–30 minutes	18	15	8	7	13
30 minutes	35	35	32	38	35
More than 30 minutes	33	36	44	40	38
30 minutes or more	68	71	76	78	73
Don't know	4	4	7	5	5
Base = 100%	*768*	*191*	*547*	*353*	*1993*
Women					
Less than 20 minutes	9	10	11	10	10
20–30 minutes	22	16	11	12	16
30 minutes	36	38	34	39	37
More than 30 minutes	30	33	37	32	33
30 minutes or more	66	70	71	71	69
Don't know	3	3	7	6	4
Base = 100%	*667*	*847*	*220*	*647*	*2528*

* Members of the Armed Forces, persons in inadequately described occupations and persons who have never worked are not shown as separate categories but are included in the figures for all persons.

Table 3.7 Number of days by 'how long people should be physically active', age and sex
Adults aged 16–74

Number of days	Fewer than 3	3–4	5–7	Depends on the person	Total*
How long people should be physically active	%	%	%	%	%
Men					
Less than 20 minutes	5	6	15	12	9
20–30 minutes	5	15	16	7	13
30 minutes	29	35	40	21	35
More than 30 minutes	58	42	25	24	38
Don't know	4	1	4	37	5
Base = 100%	*424*	*637*	*822*	*100*	*1994*
Women					
Less than 20 minutes	4	6	17	5	10
20–30 minutes	7	19	19	13	16
30 minutes	35	38	39	20	37
More than 30 minutes	52	35	21	19	4
Don't know	2	1	4	42	4
Base = 100%	*487*	*852*	*1070*	*109*	*2529*
All					
Less than 20 minutes	4	6	16	9	10
20–30 minutes	6	17	17	9	15
30 minutes	32	37	39	20	36
More than 30 minutes	55	39	23	22	35
Don't know	3	1	4	39	5
Base = 100%	*911*	*1489*	*1892*	*209*	*4523*

* Respondents who said 'it does not matter' or 'don't know' are not shown as separate categories but are included in the figures for all persons.

Health in England 1996 : What people know, what people think, what people do

Table 3.8 Number of days and length of time people should be physically active by age and sex
Adults aged 16-74

Age	16-24	25-34	35-44	45-54	55-64	65-74	Total
Number of days and length of time				Percentage giving this answer			
Men							
30 minutes or more on at least five days a week	16	21	25	28	31	37	25
20 minutes or more on at least three days a week	68	65	64	60	59	61	63
Fewer than three occasions or less than 20 minutes	31	31	34	33	33	26	32
Don't know	1	3	2	6	7	13	5
*Base = 100%**	*220*	*430*	*389*	*364*	*296*	*295*	*1994*
Women							
30 minutes or more on at least five days a week	14	19	23	28	32	36	25
20 minutes or more on at least three days a week	58	67	66	64	61	63	64
Fewer than three occasions or less than 20 minutes	41	31	32	30	33	27	32
Don't know	1	2	2	6	6	11	4
*Base = 100%**	*262*	*579*	*522*	*385*	*345*	*436*	*2529*
All							
30 minutes or more on at least five days a week	15	20	24	28	32	37	25
20 minutes or more on at least three days a week	63	66	65	62	60	62	63
Fewer than three occasions or less than 20 minutes	36	31	33	32	33	26	32
Don't know	1	3	2	6	7	12	5
*Base = 100%**	*482*	*1009*	*911*	*749*	*641*	*731*	*4523*

* Percentages add to more than 100% because respondents who said '30 minutes on five days a week' are also included in the category '20 minutes on three days a week'.

Table 3.9 Number of days and length of time people should be physically active by social class based on own current or last job, and sex
Adults aged 16–74

Social class	I & II	III(NM)	III(M)	IV & V	Total*
Number of days and length of time	\multicolumn{5}{l}{Percentage giving this answer}				

Men

	I & II	III(NM)	III(M)	IV & V	Total*
30 minutes or more on at least five days a week	26	23	26	27	25
20 minutes or more on at least three days a week	66	65	59	60	63
Fewer than three occasions or less than 20 minutes	30	31	34	34	32
Don't know	4	4	7	5	5
Base = 100%†	*768*	*191*	*547*	*353*	*1993*

Women

	I & II	III(NM)	III(M)	IV & V	Total*
30 minutes or more on at least five days a week	22	26	23	26	25
20 minutes or more on at least three days a week	69	64	53	61	64
Fewer than three occasions or less than 20 minutes	28	33	41	32	32
Don't know	3	3	7	6	4
Base = 100%†	*667*	*847*	*220*	*647*	*2528*

* Members of the Armed Forces, persons in inadequately described occupations and persons who have never worked are not shown as separate categories but are included in the figures for all persons.
† Percentages add to more than 100% because respondents who said '30 minutes on five days a week' are also included in the category '20 minutes on three days a week'.

Health in England 1996 : What people know, what people think, what people do

Table 3.10 Level of activity 'compared with others of the same age' by age and sex
Adults aged 16–74

Age Level of activity 'compared with others of the same age'	16–24 %	25–34 %	35–44 %	45–54 %	55–64 %	65–74 %	Total %	Total HEMS 1995 %
Men								
Very or fairly physically active	78	74	75	72	75	84	76	74
Not very physically active	20	21	20	23	19	12	20	21
Not at all physically active	1	5	6	5	6	5	5	5
Base = 100%	*224*	*436*	*395*	*364*	*305*	*308*	*2032*	*2116*
Women								
Very or fairly physically active	65	68	70	74	69	80	71	70
Not very physically active	27	27	25	21	24	14	23	23
Not at all physically active	8	5	5	6	7	6	6	6
Base = 100%	*264*	*585*	*531*	*385*	*362*	*460*	*2587*	*2541*
All								
Very or fairly physically active	72	71	72	73	72	81	73	72
Not very physically active	24	24	22	22	22	13	22	22
Not at all physically active	5	5	5	5	6	5	5	6
Base – 100%	*488*	*1021*	*926*	*749*	*667*	*768*	*4619*	*4657*

Table 3.11 Level of activity 'compared with others of the same age' by social class based on own current or last job, and sex
Adults aged 16–74

Social class	I & II	III(NM)	III(M)	IV & V	Total*
Level of activity 'compared with others of the same age'	%	%	%	%	%
Men					
Very or fairly physically active	71	71	81	80	76
Not very physically active	25	22	15	15	20
Not at all physically active	4	8	4	6	5
Base = 100%	777	195	560	363	2031
Women					
Very or fairly physically active	70	70	71	74	71
Not very physically active	24	25	23	21	23
Not at all physically active	6	5	7	5	6
Base = 100%	676	858	224	676	2585

* Members of the Armed Forces, persons in inadequately described occupations and persons who have never worked are not shown as separate categories but are included in the figures for all persons.

Table 3.13 Whether getting enough exercise to keep fit by social class based on own current or last job, and sex
Adults aged 16–74

Social class	I & II	III(NM)	III(M)	IV & V	Total*
Whether getting enough exercise to keep fit	%	%	%	%	%
Men					
Yes	44	53	59	65	54
No	54	46	38	33	44
Can't take exercise	2	1	3	2	2
Base = 100%	782	195	560	367	2038
Women					
Yes	45	45	55	59	49
No	54	53	41	39	48
Can't take exercise	1	2	4	3	2
Base = 100%	676	859	224	678	2590

* Members of the Armed Forces, persons in inadequately described occupations and persons who have never worked are not shown as separate categories but are included in the figures for all persons.

Table 3.12 Whether getting enough exercise to keep fit by age and sex
Adults aged 16–74

Age	16–24	25–34	35–44	45–54	55–64	65–74	Total	Total HEMS 1995
Whether getting enough exercise to keep fit	%	%	%	%	%	%	%	%
Men								
Yes	61	47	46	45	63	74	54	52
No	39	52	52	54	32	22	44	46
Can't take exercise	1	1	2	1	5	4	2	2
Base = 100%	223	436	396	368	307	309	2039	2113
Women								
Yes	40	47	43	50	57	65	49	48
No	59	52	56	48	39	27	48	49
Can't take exercise	1	1	1	1	5	8	2	2
Base = 100%	264	584	532	390	361	461	2529	2542
All								
Yes	51	47	45	48	60	69	52	50
No	49	52	54	51	35	25	46	47
Can't take exercise	1	1	1	1	5	6	2	2
Base = 100%	487	1020	928	758	668	770	4631	4655

Health in England 1996 : What people know, what people think, what people do

Table 3.14 Percentage who would like to take more exercise by age, social class based on own current or last job and sex
Adults aged 16–74*

	Men	Women	All	Men	Women	All
	\multicolumn{3}{c}{Percentage who would like to take more exercise}	\multicolumn{3}{c}{Base = 100%}
Characteristic						
Age						
16–24	69	83	76	219	261	480
25–34	77	76	76	432	580	1012
35–44	71	76	73	386	524	910
45–54	69	69	69	359	375	734
55–64	55	58	57	289	344	633
65–74	39	40	40	291	424	715
All	66	69	68	1976	2508	4484
Social Class†						
I & II	73	76	74	767	660	1427
III (NM)	69	71	70	191	832	1023
III (M)	63	65	64	537	214	751
IV & V	54	62	59	349	653	1002
All	66	69	68	1975	2506	4481

* Excludes respondents who can't take exercise.
† Members of the Armed Forces, persons in inadequately described occupations and persons who have never worked are not shown as separate categories but are included in the figures for all persons.

Table 3.15 When intends to take more exercise by age and sex
Adults aged 16–74*

Age	16–24	25–34	35–44	45–54	55–64	65–74	Total
When intends to take more exercise	%	%	%	%	%	%	%
Men							
Within the next month	34	34	24	24	12	14	25
Within the next six months	26	22	22	18	13	8	19
Within the next year	14	10	13	8	8	3	10
Intends to take more exercise but not in the next year	2	4	3	2	5	1	3
Unlikely to take more exercise	25	29	39	48	62	74	43
Base = 100%	221	434	388	360	288	293	1984
Women							
Within the next month	42	29	28	26	12	9	25
Within the next six months	32	27	23	17	16	8	22
Within the next year	8	13	9	7	8	9	9
Intends to take more exercise but not in the next year	2	5	6	4	4	2	4
Unlikely to take more exercise	17	25	34	46	60	71	39
Base = 100%	262	579	526	379	344	425	2515
All							
Within the next month	38	31	26	25	12	11	25
Within the next six months	29	25	23	18	15	8	20
Within the next year	11	12	11	8	8	6	10
Intends to take more exercise but not in the next year	2	5	4	3	4	2	4
Unlikely to take more exercise	21	27	36	47	61	73	41
Base = 100%	483	1013	914	739	632	718	4499

* Excludes respondents who did not know whether they wanted to take more exercise.

Table 3.16 When intends to take more exercise by social class based on own current or last job and sex
Adults aged 16–74*

Social class	I & II	III(NM)	III(M)	IV & V	Total†
When intends to take more exercise	%	%	%	%	%
Men					
Within the next month	25	29	22	20	25
Within the next six months	21	22	17	17	19
Within the next year	10	11	9	10	10
Intends to take more exercise but not in the next year	2	2	4	4	3
Unlikely to take more exercise	40	36	48	49	43
Base = 100%	*763*	*193*	*541*	*355*	*1983*
Women					
Within the next month	30	25	21	20	25
Within the next six months	24	22	18	19	22
Within the next year	9	11	10	9	9
Intends to take more exercise but not in the next year	4	4	6	4	4
Unlikely to take more exercise	32	38	45	47	39
Base = 100%	*662*	*834*	*213*	*656*	*2513*

* Excludes respondents who did not know whether they wanted to take more exercise.
† Members of the Armed Forces, persons in inadequately described occupations and persons who have never worked are not shown as separate categories but are included in the figures for all persons.

Table 3.17 When intends to take more exercise by whether would like to take more exercise and sex
Adults aged 16–74*

Whether would like to take more exercise	Yes	No	Total
When intends to take more exercise	%	%	%
Men			
Within the next month	34	7	25
Within the next six months	27	4	19
Within the next year	13	4	10
Intends to take more exercise but not in the next year	3	3	3
Unlikely to take more exercise	23	83	43
Base = 100%	*1266*	*704*	*1970*
Women			
Within the next month	34	6	25
Within the next six months	29	6	22
Within the next year	12	4	9
Intends to take more exercise but not in the next year	5	3	4
Unlikely to take more exercise	21	81	39
Base = 100%	*1686*	*812*	*2498*

* Excludes respondents who did not know whether they wanted to take more exercise.

Table 3.18 When intends to take more exercise by frequency of participation in at least moderate-intensity activity for 30 minutes or more by age and sex
Adults aged 16–74*

Frequency of activity	Less than one day a week (sedentary)	1–2 days a week	3–4 days a week	5 or more days a week	Total
When intends to take more exercise	%	%	%	%	%
Men					
Within the next month	18	29	36	24	25
Within the next six months	19	20	23	17	19
Within the next year	11	11	7	10	10
Intends to take more exercise but not in the next year	4	3	-	3	3
Unlikely to take more exercise	48	38	33	45	43
Base = 100%	476	481	233	794	1984
Women					
Within the next month	22	26	23	29	25
Within the next six months	19	23	27	19	22
Within the next year	10	11	9	8	9
Intends to take more exercise but not in the next year	5	4	6	3	4
Unlikely to take more exercise	45	35	34	41	39
Base = 100%	633	751	361	770	2515

* Excludes respondents who did not know whether they wanted to take more exercise.

Table 3.19 Barriers to exercise by age and sex
Adults aged 16–74

Age	16-24	25-34	35-44	45-54	55-64	65-74	Total
Barriers to exercise				Percentage mentioning each barrier			
Men							
I don't have the time	52	67	61	55	33	19	51
I'm not the sporty type	7	13	12	12	16	12	12
I have an injury or disability	14	9	10	18	16	23	14
My health is not good	5	3	5	8	12	19	8
I don't enjoy physical activity	4	6	8	6	6	4	6
Other	9	8	8	5	4	5	7
None of these	24	15	18	17	27	28	20
*Base = 100%**	*224*	*436*	*396*	*368*	*309*	*310*	*2043*
Women							
I don't have the time	67	63	64	56	36	20	53
I'm not the sporty type	16	13	18	26	22	18	18
I have an injury or disability	5	8	12	15	25	22	14
My health is not good	7	6	8	7	18	23	11
I don't enjoy physical activity	9	7	11	6	6	5	7
Other	11	11	8	6	5	8	8
None of these	10	15	12	14	13	23	14
*Base = 100%**	*265*	*586*	*532*	*392*	*362*	*459*	*2596*
All							
I don't have the time	60	65	63	55	34	19	52
I'm not the sporty type	11	13	15	18	19	15	15
I have an injury or disability	10	9	11	17	20	23	14
My health is not good	6	5	6	8	15	21	9
I don't enjoy physical activity	6	6	9	6	6	5	7
Other	10	9	8	5	5	6	7
None of these	17	15	15	16	20	25	17
*Base = 100%**	*489*	*1022*	*928*	*760*	*671*	*769*	*4639*

* Percentages add to more than 100% because respondents may have given more than one answer.

Table 3.20 Barriers to exercise by social class based on own current or last job and sex
Adults aged 16–74

Social class	I & II	III(NM)	III(M)	IV & V	Total*
Barriers to exercise	%	%	%	%	%
Men					
Within the next month	25	29	22	20	25
I don't have the time	57	50	54	44	51
I'm not the sporty type	11	14	13	10	12
I have an injury or disability	14	18	14	14	14
My health is not good	6	11	8	10	8
I don't enjoy physical activity	6	6	6	5	6
Other	7	7	6	6	7
None of these	18	22	17	25	20
Base = 100%†	*783*	*195*	*561*	*367*	*2042*
Women					
I don't have the time	63	53	54	46	53
I'm not the sporty type	15	19	23	20	18
I have an injury or disability	12	14	13	17	14
My health is not good	7	10	11	14	11
I don't enjoy physical activity	9	8	10	4	7
Other	9	7	8	8	8
None of these	15	14	13	13	14
Base = 100%†	*677*	*862*	*223*	*678*	*2594*

* Excludes respondents who did not know whether they wanted to take more exercise.
† Members of the Armed Forces, persons in inadequately described occupations and persons who have never worked are not shown as separate categories but are included in the figures for all persons.

Health in England 1996 : What people know, what people think, what people do

Table 4.1 Knowledge of what constitutes a healthy diet by age and sex
Adults aged 16–74

Age	16–24	25–34	35–44	45–54	55–64	65–74	Total
Knowledge of what constitutes a healthy diet			Percentage giving each answer				
Men							
Eat lots of fruit, vegetables or salad	59	61	61	60	61	58	60
Cut down on fatty or fried foods, eat grilled food	43	49	42	49	41	35	44
Eat lots of fibre, cereals, wholemeal food	24	27	28	33	25	26	27
Eat a balanced diet	35	30	35	26	21	22	29
Eat lots of starch, carbohydrates, potatoes, pasta or rice	27	23	22	14	14	9	19
Eat everything in moderation	18	15	19	19	22	24	19
Avoid red meat, eat white meat, fish	10	15	15	14	11	16	14
Cut down on sugar, cakes and confectionery	9	7	8	11	10	10	9
Eat lots of meat, eggs, cheese, drink lots of milk	9	8	8	3	9	7	7
Drink lots of water, fruit juice, liquid	7	4	2	3	2	3	4
Cut down on salt	3	3	3	3	2	3	3
Other*	14	11	9	10	8	12	11
Don't know	0	1	1	1	5	2	1
Identified at least three of 'eat less fat', 'eat more fruit','eat more starch', 'eat more fibre'	15	17	14	15	11	12	14
Base = 100%	*222*	*426*	*390*	*365*	*305*	*305*	*2013*
Women							
Eat lots of fruit, vegetables or salad	68	70	68	83	78	74	73
Cut down on fatty or fried foods, eat grilled food	48	53	46	46	41	40	46
Eat lots of fibre, cereals, wholemeal food	22	29	29	28	27	22	27
Eat a balanced diet	26	27	24	21	20	16	23
Eat lots of starch, carbohydrates, potatoes, pasta or rice	22	24	24	19	16	12	20
Eat everything in moderation	17	13	18	16	18	18	16
Avoid red meat, eat white meat, fish	17	16	15	21	22	19	18
Cut down on sugar, cakes and confectionery	17	17	12	14	11	13	14
Eat lots of meat, eggs, cheese, drink lots of milk	7	7	6	8	4	8	7
Drink lots of water, fruit juice, liquid	7	7	5	5	6	5	6
Cut down on salt	6	4	4	3	2	3	4
Other*	14	8	12	12	10	11	11
Don't know	0	1	1	0	1	1	1
Identified at least three of 'eat less fat', 'eat more fruit','eat more starch', 'eat more fibre'	14	20	19	18	17	12	17
Base = 100%	*262*	*581*	*526*	*387*	*356*	*457*	*2569*

* The answers given as 'other' were coded but the proportions in each category were too small to show separately.

Table 4.1 – continued
Adults aged 16–74

Age Knowledge of what constitutes a healthy diet	16–24	25–34	35–44	45–54	55–64	65–74	Total
	\multicolumn{7}{c}{Percentage giving each answer}						
All							
Eat lots of fruit, vegetables or salad	63	66	64	71	70	66	67
Cut down on fatty or fried foods, eat grilled food	45	51	44	48	41	38	45
Eat lots of fibre, cereals, wholemeal food	23	28	28	31	26	24	27
Eat a balanced diet	30	29	30	23	21	18	26
Eat lots of starch, carbohydrates, potatoes, pasta or rice	25	24	23	16	15	11	20
Eat everything in moderation	18	14	18	17	20	21	18
Avoid red meat, eat white meat, fish	13	15	15	18	17	17	16
Cut down on sugar, cakes and confectionery	13	12	10	12	11	12	12
Eat lots of meat, eggs, cheese, drink lots of milk	8	7	7	6	7	7	7
Drink lots of water, fruit juice, liquid	7	5	4	4	4	4	5
Cut down on salt	5	3	4	3	2	3	3
Other*	14	10	11	11	9	11	11
Don't know	0	1	1	1	3	1	1
Identified at least three of 'eat less fat', 'eat more fruit','eat more starch', 'eat more fibre'	15	18	17	17	14	12	16
Base = 100%	484	1007	916	752	661	762	4582

* The answers given as 'other' were coded but the proportions in each category were too small to show separately.

Table 4.2 Knowledge of what constitutes a healthy diet by social class based on own current or last job and sex
Adults aged 16–74

Social class	I & II	III (NM)	III (M)	IV & V	Total†
Knowledge of what constitutes a healthy diet			Percentage giving each answer		
Men					
Eat lots of fruit, vegetables or salad	59	58	61	63	60
Cut down on fatty or fried foods, eat grilled food	49	45	42	38	44
Eat lots of fibre, cereals, wholemeal food	32	29	25	20	27
Eat a balanced diet	36	32	20	21	29
Eat lots of starch, carbohydrates, potatoes, pasta or rice	18	22	16	24	19
Eat everything in moderation	21	23	16	17	19
Avoid red meat, eat white meat, fish	13	13	15	15	14
Cut down on sugar, cakes and confectionery	11	9	9	8	9
Eat lots of meat, eggs, cheese, drink lots of milk	8	8	7	8	7
Drink lots of water, fruit juice, liquid	3	9	3	4	4
Cut down on salt	3	4	2	2	3
Other*	11	9	11	10	11
Don't know	1	1	2	2	1
Identified at least three of 'eat less fat', 'eat more fruit','eat more starch', 'eat more fibre'	18	19	11	11	14
Base = 100%	778	193	548	360	2012
Women					
Eat lots of fruit, vegetables or salad	71	75	72	73	73
Cut down on fatty or fried foods, eat grilled food	48	46	43	45	46
Eat lots of fibre, cereals, wholemeal food	36	25	20	23	27
Eat a balanced diet	32	22	19	15	23
Eat lots of starch, carbohydrates, potatoes, pasta or rice	26	17	21	18	20
Eat everything in moderation	18	19	15	14	16
Avoid red meat, eat white meat, fish	16	18	19	20	18
Cut down on sugar, cakes and confectionery	15	14	13	15	14
Eat lots of meat, eggs, cheese, drink lots of milk	7	6	8	6	7
Drink lots of water, fruit juice, liquid	6	5	4	7	6
Cut down on salt	4	4	1	4	4
Other*	13	10	12	10	11
Don't know	0	0	1	1	1
Identified at least three of 'eat less fat', 'eat more fruit','eat more starch', 'eat more fibre'	23	15	13	15	17
Base = 100%	673	858	223	662	2568

* The answers given as 'other' were coded but the proportions in each category were too small to show separately.
† Members of the Armed Forces, persons in inadequately described occupations and persons who have never worked are not shown as separate categories but are included in the figures for all persons.

Table 4.3 Whether looks at ingredients when shopping and what looks for, by age and sex
Adults aged 16–74

Age Whether looks at ingredients when shopping, and what looks for	16–24 %	25–34 %	35–44 %	45–54 %	55–64 %	65–74 %	Total %	Total HEMS 1995 %
Men								
Total fat content	14	25	24	22	19	17	21	21
E-numbers, additives	8	15	19	14	10	9	13	14
Calories, energy	10	12	12	9	5	4	9	12
Sugar	5	7	10	10	8	7	8	7
Salt	1	3	4	5	5	6	4	5
Cholesterol	1	0	2	1	1	2	1	3
Suitable for vegetarians	1	4	3	0	1	1	2	-
Fibre content	2	5	4	4	3	2	3	-
Something else	10	11	9	12	6	6	9	10
Does not shop/never looks	73	60	57	62	72	71	65	63
Base = 100%*	*223*	*436*	*394*	*368*	*308*	*306*	*2035*	*2117*
Women								
Total fat content	31	41	44	43	39	29	39	37
E-numbers, additives	11	30	36	24	22	19	25	25
Calories, energy	33	29	28	25	16	10	25	27
Sugar	8	15	19	19	13	15	15	17
Salt	4	6	7	5	6	9	6	8
Cholesterol	0	1	2	2	3	4	2	3
Suitable for vegetarians	4	5	5	4	2	1	4	-
Fibre content	4	5	6	5	4	2	4	-
Something else	8	12	14	12	13	10	12	14
Does not shop/never looks	48	33	24	31	39	48	36	37
Base = 100%*	*265*	*586*	*531*	*389*	*360*	*451*	*2582*	*2537*
All								
Total fat content	23	33	34	32	29	23	30	29
E-numbers, additives	10	22	27	19	16	14	19	20
Calories, energy	21	20	21	16	11	7	17	19
Sugar	6	11	14	14	10	11	11	13
Salt	2	4	5	5	5	8	5	7
Cholesterol	1	1	2	2	2	3	2	3
Suitable for vegetarians	3	4	4	2	1	1	3	-
Fibre content	3	5	5	5	3	2	4	-
Something else	9	12	11	12	9	8	11	12
Does not shop/never looks	61	46	40	47	55	58	50	50
Base = 100%*	*488*	*1022*	*925*	*757*	*668*	*757*	*4617*	*4654*

* Percentages total more than 100% because respondents may look for more than one ingredient.

Health in England 1996 : What people know, what people think, what people do

Table 4.4 Whether looks at ingredients when shopping and what looks for, by social class based on own current or last job, and sex
Adults aged 16–74

Social class	I & II	III(NM)	III(M)	IV & V	Total*
Whether looks at ingredients when shopping, and what looks for	%	%	%	%	%
Men					
Total fat content	28	20	14	17	21
E-numbers, additives	18	15	9	6	13
Calories, energy	12	14	6	5	9
Sugar	11	5	6	6	8
Salt	5	2	3	4	4
Cholesterol	1	2	1	1	1
Suitable for vegetarians	2	2	1	2	2
Fibre content	4	5	1	2	3
Something else	11	9	7	9	9
Does not shop/ never looks	54	63	75	71	65
Base = 100%†	781	195	559	363	2034
Women					
Total fat content	49	37	35	32	39
E-numbers, additives	35	23	20	18	25
Calories, energy	30	25	20	21	25
Sugar	20	16	11	11	15
Salt	8	5	5	7	6
Cholesterol	2	2	1	2	2
Suitable for vegetarians	5	3	3	3	4
Fibre content	7	3	2	4	4
Something else	13	11	10	11	12
Does not shop/ never looks	23	37	41	45	36
Base = 100%†	676	858	220	674	2580

* Members of the Armed Forces, persons in inadequately described occupations and persons who have never worked are not shown as separate categories but are included in the figures for all persons.

† Totals add to more than 100% because respondents may look for more than one ingredient.

Table 4.5 Whether looks at ingredients when shopping and what looks for, by highest qualification level and sex
Adults aged 16–74

Highest qualification level	'A' level or above	Other qualifications	No qualifications	Total*
Whether looks at ingredients when shopping, and what looks for	%	%	%	%
Men				
Total fat content	30	17	12	21
E-numbers, additives	20	10	7	13
Calories, energy	15	7	5	9
Sugar	12	5	5	8
Salt	5	3	3	4
Cholesterol	1	1	2	1
Suitable for vegetarians	4	1	1	2
Fibre content	4	3	1	3
Something else	13	8	6	9
Does not shop/ never looks	49	72	78	65
Base = 100%*	773	734	522	2029
Women				
Total fat content	49	39	29	39
E-numbers, additives	33	26	15	25
Calories, energy	36	25	14	25
Sugar	20	15	10	15
Salt	8	7	4	6
Cholesterol	2	2	2	2
Suitable for vegetarians	7	3	1	4
Fibre content	7	4	2	4
Something else	16	10	9	12
Does not shop/ never looks	21	35	50	36
Base = 100%*	707	1023	850	2580

* Totals add to more than 100% because respondents may look for more than one ingredient.

Table 4.6 What looks for when shopping by sex
Adults aged 16–74 who bought food

Sex	Men		Women		All	
	1996	1995*	1996	1995*	1996	1995*
What looks for when shopping	%	%	%	%	%	%
Total fat content	24	21	40	37	33	29
E-numbers, additives	15	14	25	25	21	20
Calories, energy	11	12	25	27	19	19
Sugar	9	7	16	17	13	13
Salt	4	5	6	8	5	7
Cholesterol	1	3	2	3	2	3
Suitable for vegetarians	2	-	4	-	3	-
Fibre content	4	-	5	-	4	-
Something else	11	10	12	14	12	12
Does not look	59	63	34	37	45	50
Base = 100%	1794	2117	2514	2537	4308	4654

† Totals add to more than 100% because respondents may look for more than one ingredient.

* The proportions presented in the 1995 report were not based on respondents who bought food so these proportions were re-calculated. They therefore differ from the proportions presented in the 1995 report.

Table 4.7 Whether looks at ingredients when shopping and what looks for, by number correctly stated of 'eat less fat', 'eat more fruit', 'eat more starch' and 'eat more fibre', age and sex
Adults aged 16–74

	Number correctly stated of 'eat less fat', 'eat more fruit', 'eat more starch' and 'eat more fibre'			
Whether looks at ingredients when shopping, and what looks for	None to two	Three	Four	Total*
	%	%	%	%
Men				
Total fat content	19	34	[13]	21
E-numbers, additives	12	19	[4]	13
Calories, energy	8	14	[7]	9
Sugar	7	12	[3]	8
Salt	4	5	[2]	4
Cholesterol	1	1	[1]	1
Suitable for vegetarians	2	4	[0]	2
Fibre content	3	7	[3]	3
Something else	8	15	[5]	9
Does not shop/ never looks	67	48	[12]	64
Base = 100%*	1726	252	29	2007
Women				
Total fat content	36	51	55	39
E-numbers, additives	24	26	41	25
Calories, energy	24	30	27	25
Sugar	14	17	35	15
Salt	6	8	13	6
Cholesterol	2	3	4	2
Suitable for vegetarians	3	5	6	4
Fibre content	4	9	8	4
Something else	11	12	19	12
Does not shop/ never looks	37	30	22	35
Base = 100%*	2119	378	58	2555

* Totals add to more than 100% because respondents may look for more than one ingredient.

Table 4.8 Consumption of foods containing fibre and starchy carbohydrates by age and sex
Adults aged 16–74

Age	16–24	25–34	35–44	45–54	55–64	65–74	Total
Food			Percentage consuming each food				
Men							
Eats wholemeal bread	7	14	16	21	23	22	17
Eats bread daily	83	77	87	84	89	92	84
Eats fruit, vegetables and salad daily	43	51	56	69	72	73	59
Eats potatoes, pasta or rice daily	35	51	55	56	63	66	53
Eats bread; fruit, vegetables and salad; and potatoes, pasta or rice daily	19	31	34	41	45	51	36
Base = 100%	*222*	*435*	*395*	*364*	*306*	*308*	*2030*
Women							
Eats wholemeal bread	16	23	24	30	29	34	25
Eats bread daily	76	75	79	83	83	93	81
Eats fruit, vegetables and salad daily	57	60	74	81	86	83	72
Eats potatoes, pasta or rice daily	44	51	55	62	67	64	56
Eats bread; fruit, vegetables and salad; and potatoes, pasta or rice daily	24	32	38	45	53	53	40
Base = 100%	*263*	*582*	*532*	*389*	*355*	*456*	*2577*
All							
Eats wholemeal bread	12	19	20	25	26	29	21
Eats bread daily	79	76	83	83	86	93	83
Eats fruit, vegetables and salad daily	50	56	65	75	79	78	66
Eats potatoes, pasta or rice daily	39	51	55	59	65	65	55
Eats bread; fruit, vegetables and salad; and potatoes, pasta or rice daily	22	31	36	43	49	52	38
Base = 100%	*485*	*1017*	*927*	*753*	*661*	*764*	*4607*

Table 4.9 Consumption of foods containing fibre and starchy carbohydrates by social class based on own current or last job, and sex
Adults aged 16–74

Social class	I & II	III(NM)	III(M)	IV & V	Total*
Food	\multicolumn{5}{c}{Percentage consuming each food}				
Men					
Eats wholemeal bread	21	15	15	14	17
Eats bread daily	84	84	86	83	84
Eats fruit, vegetables and salad daily	66	51	59	52	59
Eats potatoes, pasta or rice daily	56	46	58	47	53
Eats bread; fruit, vegetables and salad; and potatoes, pasta or rice daily	41	28	37	29	36
Base = 100%	778	191	560	364	2029
Women					
Eats wholemeal bread	30	25	29	23	25
Eats bread daily	78	80	81	84	81
Eats fruit, vegetables and salad daily	81	71	66	68	72
Eats potatoes, pasta or rice daily	60	54	52	59	56
Eats bread; fruit, vegetables and salad; and potatoes, pasta or rice daily	45	38	33	42	40
Base = 100%	666	859	222	676	2575

* Members of the Armed Forces, persons in inadequately described occupations and persons who have never worked are not shown as separate categories but are included in the figures for all persons.

Table 4.10 Consumption of foods containing fibre and starchy carbohydrates by highest qualification level and sex
Adults aged 16–74

Highest qualification level	'A' level or above	Other qualifications	No qualifications	Total*
Food	%	%	%	%
Men				
Eats wholemeal bread	20	14	16	17
Eats bread daily	83	86	86	84
Eats fruit, vegetables and salad daily	65	55	57	59
Eats potatoes, pasta or rice daily	56	51	54	54
Eats bread; fruit, vegetables and salad; and potatoes, pasta or rice daily	39	32	36	36
Base = 100%	772	731	521	2024
Women				
Eats wholemeal bread	30	24	23	25
Eats bread daily	78	79	86	81
Eats fruit, vegetables and salad daily	81	67	71	72
Eats potatoes, pasta or rice daily	57	55	59	56
Eats bread; fruit, vegetables and salad; and potatoes, pasta or rice daily	43	36	42	40
Base = 100%	698	1022	854	2574

Table 4.11 Consumption of foods containing fibre and starchy carbohydrates by standard region and sex
Adults aged 16–74

Region	North	Yorkshire & Humberside	North West	East Midlands	West Midlands
Food		Percentage consuming each food			
Men					
Eats wholemeal bread	16	14	17	17	14
Eats bread daily	87	87	85	91	84
Eats fruit, vegetables and salad daily	50	60	51	63	66
Eats potatoes, pasta or rice daily	39	56	50	53	55
Eats bread; fruit, vegetables and salad; and potatoes, pasta or rice daily	21	36	31	39	40
Base = 100%	*123*	*219*	*271*	*187*	*215*
Women					
Eats wholemeal bread	21	25	24	25	29
Eats bread daily	82	84	84	85	84
Eats fruit, vegetables and salad daily	72	67	71	69	70
Eats potatoes, pasta or rice daily	49	60	50	56	48
Eats bread; fruit, vegetables and salad; and potatoes, pasta or rice daily	36	41	35	35	36
Base = 100%	*178*	*306*	*361*	*235*	*283*

Region	East Anglia	Greater London	Outer Metropolitan & SE	South West	Total
Food		Percentage consuming each food			
Men					
Eats wholemeal bread	12	19	18	21	17
Eats bread daily	83	78	83	86	84
Eats fruit, vegetables and salad daily	68	53	61	63	59
Eats potatoes, pasta or rice daily	67	48	55	60	53
Eats bread; fruit, vegetables and salad; and potatoes, pasta or rice daily	45	26	40	43	36
Base = 100%	*84*	*266*	*452*	*213*	*2030*
Women					
Eats wholemeal bread	25	21	27	30	25
Eats bread daily	77	74	80	77	81
Eats fruit, vegetables and salad daily	83	71	75	75	72
Eats potatoes, pasta or rice daily	71	50	64	59	56
Eats bread; fruit, vegetables and salad; and potatoes, pasta or rice daily	52	35	45	44	40
Base = 100%	*116*	*310*	*540*	*248*	*2577*

Table 4.12 Consumption of foods containing fibre and starchy carbohydrates by number correctly stated of 'eat less fat', 'eat more fruit', 'eat more starch' and 'eat more fibre' and sex
Adults aged 16–74

	Number correctly stated of 'eat less fat', 'eat more fruit', 'eat more starch' and 'eat more fibre'			
Food	None to two	Three	Four	Total
	Percentage consuming each food			
Men				
Eats wholemeal bread	16	24	[8]	17
Eats bread daily	84	87	[25]	85
Eats fruit, vegetables and salad daily	58	69	[21]	60
Eats potatoes, pasta or rice daily	53	53	[21]	54
Eats bread; fruit, vegetables and salad; and potatoes, pasta or rice daily	35	43	[15]	36
Base = 100%	*1721*	*250*	*29*	*2000*
Women				
Eats wholemeal bread	24	31	44	26
Eats bread daily	80	81	85	81
Eats fruit, vegetables and salad daily	71	80	80	72
Eats potatoes, pasta or rice daily	55	61	73	56
Eats bread; fruit, vegetables and salad; and potatoes, pasta or rice daily	38	46	64	40
Base = 100%	*2113*	*377*	*58*	*2548*

Table 4.13 Consumption of fats by age and sex
Adults aged 16–74

Age	16-24	25-34	35-44	45-54	55-64	65-74	Total	Total HEMS 1995
Food			Percentage consuming each food					
Men								
Drinks skimmed, semi-skimmed milk	69	71	60	72	64	67	67	67
Eats chips less than once a week	20	33	37	36	49	41	35	31
Uses oil for cooking	92	92	90	93	86	79	90	88
Uses no fat, low- or reduced fat spread	48	56	54	53	52	44	52	49
Uses low-fat varieties of milk, cooking fat and spread, and eats chips less than once a week*	9	16	16	18	24	18	17	14
Base = 100%	208	417	374	343	293	299	1934	2118
Women								
Drinks skimmed, semi-skimmed milk	77	73	76	77	78	64	74	73
Eats chips less than once a week	41	52	52	59	57	58	53	48
Uses oil for cooking	89	93	93	89	89	84	90	89
Uses no fat, low- or reduced fat spread	50	59	58	57	55	50	56	59
Uses low-fat varieties of milk, cooking fat and spread, and eats chips less than once a week*	20	29	29	30	30	23	27	25
Base = 100%	251	556	509	370	338	450	2474	2545
All								
Drinks skimmed, semi-skimmed milk	73	72	68	75	71	65	71	71
Eats chips less than once a week	30	42	45	47	53	50	44	40
Uses oil for cooking	90	93	92	91	87	81	90	89
Uses no fat, low- or reduced fat spread	49	58	56	55	53	47	54	54
Uses low-fat varieties of milk, cooking fat and spread, and eats chips less than once a week*	14	23	23	24	27	21	22	20
Base = 100%	459	973	883	713	631	749	4408	4663

* Skimmed or semi-skimmed milk, low- or reduced-fat spread and cooking oil.

Table 4.14 Consumption of fats by social class based on own current or last job, and sex
Adults aged 16–74

Social class	I & II	III(NM)	III(M)	IV & V	Total*
Food	\multicolumn{5}{l}{Percentage consuming each food}				
Men					
Drinks skimmed, semi-skimmed milk	74	75	65	58	67
Eats chips less than once a week	43	41	28	27	35
Uses oil for cooking	94	90	86	85	90
Uses no fat, low- or reduced fat spread	55	56	52	46	52
Uses low-fat varieties of milk, cooking fat and spread, and eats chips less than once a week	22	19	14	9	17
Base = 100%	741	183	539	340	1933
Women					
Drinks skimmed, semi-skimmed milk	84	76	74	64	74
Eats chips less than once a week	69	51	51	43	53
Uses oil for cooking	95	90	88	86	90
Uses no fat, low- or reduced fat spread	57	57	59	53	56
Uses low-fat varieties of milk, cooking fat and spread, and eats chips less than once a week	38	26	28	19	27
Base = 100%	636	826	213	652	2472

* Members of the Armed Forces, persons in inadequately described occupations and persons who have never worked are not shown as separate categories but are included in the figures for all persons.

Table 4.15 Consumption of fats by highest qualification level and sex
Adults aged 16–74

Highest qualification level	'A' level or above	Other qualifications	No qualifications	Total*
Food	\multicolumn{4}{l}{Percentage consuming each food}			
Men				
Drinks skimmed, semi-skimmed milk	73	66	62	67
Eats chips less than once a week	42	31	31	35
Uses oil for cooking	94	89	84	90
Uses no fat, low- or reduced fat spread	55	53	46	52
Uses low-fat varieties of milk, cooking fat and spread, and eats chips less than once a week	21	14	13	17
Base = 100%	738	693	497	1928
Women				
Drinks skimmed, semi-skimmed milk	84	75	65	74
Eats chips less than once a week	65	51	45	53
Uses oil for cooking	95	90	85	90
Uses no fat, low- or reduced fat spread	59	57	52	56
Uses low-fat varieties of milk, cooking fat and spread, and eats chips less than once a week	38	26	19	27
Base = 100%	663	987	823	2473

Table 4.16 Consumption of fats by standard region and sex
Adults aged 16–74

Region	North	Yorkshire & Humberside	North West	East Midlands	West Midlands
Food		Percentage consuming each food			
Men					
Drinks skimmed, semi-skimmed milk	68	64	69	66	58
Eats chips less than once a week	33	29	30	35	39
Uses oil for cooking	84	83	89	90	88
Uses no fat, low- or reduced fat spread	41	51	51	50	52
Uses low-fat varieties of milk, cooking fat and spread, and eats chips less than once a week	14	14	14	17	16
Base = 100%	*112*	*214*	*262*	*178*	*204*
Women					
Drinks skimmed, semi-skimmed milk	76	70	73	73	70
Eats chips less than once a week	53	44	49	55	48
Uses oil for cooking	90	88	88	86	91
Uses no fat, low- or reduced fat spread	59	56	48	50	58
Uses low-fat varieties of milk, cooking fat and spread, and eats chips less than once a week	30	22	21	28	28
Base = 100%	*171*	*296*	*348*	*227*	*271*

Region	East Anglia	Greater London	Outer Metropolitan & SE	South West	Total
Food		Percentage consuming each food			
Men					
Drinks skimmed, semi-skimmed milk	68	64	75	67	67
Eats chips less than once a week	35	39	38	35	35
Uses oil for cooking	91	92	93	90	90
Uses no fat, low- or reduced fat spread	62	51	58	48	52
Uses low-fat varieties of milk, cooking fat and spread, and eats chips less than once a week	18	21	18	14	17
Base = 100%	*82*	*249*	*430*	*203*	*1934*
Women					
Drinks skimmed, semi-skimmed milk	82	77	76	77	74
Eats chips less than once a week	45	60	59	55	53
Uses oil for cooking	96	93	89	93	90
Uses no fat, low- or reduced fat spread	72	53	58	57	56
Uses low-fat varieties of milk, cooking fat and spread, and eats chips less than once a week	29	26	31	29	27
Base = 100%	*10*	*292*	*516*	*243*	*2474*

Table 4.17 Consumption of confectionery and biscuits or cakes by age and sex
Adults aged 16–74

Age	16–24	25–34	35–44	45–54	55–64	65–74	Total
Food			Percentage consuming each food				
Men							
Eats confectionery less than once a week	13	26	32	44	51	43	34
Eats biscuits or cakes less than once a week	22	28	25	28	22	14	24
Base = 100%	224	436	396	368	309	308	2041
Women							
Eats confectionery less than once a week	20	25	29	39	45	45	33
Eats biscuits or cakes less than once a week	30	32	29	30	23	24	28
Base = 100%	265	586	533	392	361	460	2597
All							
Eats confectionery less than once a week	16	26	31	42	48	44	33
Eats biscuits or cakes less than once a week	26	30	27	29	22	20	26
Base = 100%	489	1022	929	760	670	768	4638

Table 4.18 Consumption of confectionery and biscuits or cakes by social class based on own current or last job, and sex
Adults aged 16–74

Social class	I & II	III(NM)	III(M)	IV & V	Total*
Food		Percentage consuming each food			
Men					
Eats confectionery less than once a week	34	29	38	31	34
Eats biscuits or cakes less than once a week	25	19	23	26	24
Base = 100%	783	195	561	365	2040
Women					
Eats confectionery less than once a week	32	29	38	37	33
Eats biscuits or cakes less than once a week	31	26	35	26	28
Base = 100%	677	862	224	680	2595

* Members of the Armed Forces, persons in inadequately described occupations and persons who have never worked are not shown as separate categories but are included in the figures for all persons.

Table 4.19 Consumption of confectionery and biscuits or cakes by highest qualification level and sex
Adults aged 16–74

Highest qualification level	'A' level or above	Other qualifications	No qualifications	Total*
Food		Percentage consuming each food		
Men				
Eats confectionery less than once a week	31	30	46	34
Eats biscuits or cakes less than once a week	27	20	26	24
Base = 100%	776	735	524	2035
Women				
Eats confectionery less than once a week	29	30	40	33
Eats biscuits or cakes less than once a week	30	29	26	28
Base = 100%	707	1028	860	2595

* Totals add to more than 100% because respondents may look for more than one ingredient.

Health in England 1996 : What people know, what people think, what people do

Table 4.20 Consumption of confectionery and biscuits or cakes by standard region and sex
Adults aged 16–74

Region	North	Yorkshire & Humberside	North West	East Midlands	West Midlands
Food			Percentage consuming each food		
Men					
Eats confectionary less than once a week	29	34	43	39	34
Eats biscuits or cakes less than once a week	20	25	27	24	30
Base = 100%	*124*	*220*	*272*	*187*	*218*
Women					
Eats confectionary less than once a week	32	28	33	33	31
Eats biscuits or cakes less than once a week	29	19	30	29	24
Base = 100%	*179*	*308*	*361*	*235*	*285*

Region	East Anglia	Greater London	Outer Metropolitan & SE	South West	Total
Food			Percentage consuming each food		
Men					
Eats confectionary less than once a week	33	35	30	27	34
Eats biscuits or cakes less than once a week	19	25	25	15	24
Base = 100%	*84*	*269*	*455*	*212*	*2041*
Women					
Eats confectionary less thanonce a week	35	34	33	37	33
Eats biscuits or cakes less than once a week	25	36	29	32	28
Base = 100%	*118*	*317*	*544*	*250*	*2597*

Table 4.21 Attitudes to diet by age and sex
Adults aged 16–74

Age	16–24	25–34	35–44	45–54	55–64	65–74	Total
Attitudes to diet	%	%	%	%	%	%	%
Men							
As healthy as it could be	4	11	10	21	35	44	18
Quite good but could improve	81	82	81	72	60	53	74
Not very healthy	15	7	8	6	4	3	7
Don't know	-	1	1	1	1	-	1
Base = 100%	*224*	*436*	*396*	*368*	*309*	*308*	*2041*
Women							
As healthy as it could be	6	15	12	19	34	44	20
Quite good but could improve	81	76	83	76	60	54	73
Not very healthy	12	9	5	4	6	2	6
Don't know	-	-	-	1	1	1	0
Base = 100%	*265*	*586*	*532*	*392*	*360*	*460*	*2595*
All							
As healthy as it could be	5	13	11	20	34	44	19
Quite good but could improve	81	79	82	74	60	54	73
Not very healthy	14	8	6	5	5	2	7
Don't know	-	0	0	1	1	0	0
Base = 100%	*489*	*1022*	*928*	*760*	*669*	*768*	*4636*

Table 4.22 Attitudes to diet by frequency of consumption of bread; fruit, vegetables or salad; and potatoes, pasta or rice, and sex
Adults aged 16–74

Frequency of consumption Attitudes to diet	Eats foods from all three groups every day %	Frequency of eating foods from all three groups varies %	Total* %
Men			
As healthy as it could be	26	14	18
Quite good but could improve	72	75	74
Not very healthy	2	10	7
Don't know	0	1	1
Base = 100%	726	1304	2041
Women			
As healthy as it could be	26	16	20
Quite good but could improve	71	75	73
Not very healthy	2	9	6
Don't know	0	0	0
Base = 100%	1033	1548	2595
All			
As healthy as it could be	26	15	19
Quite good but could improve	71	75	73
Not very healthy	2	10	7
Don't know	0	1	0
Base = 100%	1759	2852	4636

* Includes a small number of respondents who ate food from all three groups 1-2 days a week.

Table 4.23 Attitudes to diet by type of fats consumed and sex
Adults aged 16–74

Type of fat Attitudes to diet	Saturated fat content varied %	Low in saturated fats %	Total* %
Men			
As healthy as it could be	17	24	18
Quite good but could improve	75	72	74
Not very healthy	8	3	7
Don't know	1	-	1
Base = 100%	1588	326	1933
Women			
As healthy as it could be	18	26	20
Quite good but could improve	74	72	74
Not very healthy	7	2	6
Don't know	0	0	0
Base = 100%	1780	684	2471
All			
As healthy as it could be	17	25	19
Quite good but could improve	75	72	74
Not very healthy	8	3	7
Don't know	1	0	0
Base = 100%	3368	1010	4404

* Includes a small number of respondents who ate all foods high in saturated fats.

Table 4.24 Intentions to change diet by age and sex
Adults aged 16–74 who say their diet is not as healthy as it could be

Age	16–24	25–34	35–44	45–54	55–64	65–74	Total
Intentions to change diet	%	%	%	%	%	%	%
Men							
Intends to change in next month	12	9	8	6	4	5	8
Intends to change in next 6 months	21	18	16	11	8	2	15
Intends to change in next year	10	11	7	5	4	0	7
Want to change but thinks it unlikely	18	28	31	40	30	38	30
Does not want to change	39	35	38	38	55	54	40
Base = 100%	*212*	*377*	*341*	*280*	*194*	*159*	*1563*
Women							
Intends to change in next month	20	18	18	9	11	5	15
Intends to change in next 6 months	27	20	18	11	6	4	16
Intends to change in next year	8	9	9	6	6	2	7
Want to change but thinks it unlikely	23	26	30	36	37	36	30
Does not want to change	22	26	25	40	40	52	31
Base = 100%	*242*	*491*	*457*	*307*	*238*	*246*	*1981*
All							
Intends to change in next month	16	13	13	8	8	5	11
Intends to change In next 6 months	24	19	17	11	7	3	15
Intends to change in next year	9	10	8	6	5	2	7
Want to change but thinks it unlikely	20	27	30	38	34	37	30
Does not want to change	31	31	31	38	47	53	36
Base = 100%	*454*	*868*	*798*	*587*	*432*	*405*	*3544*

Table 4.25 Intentions to change diet by social class based on own current or last job, and sex
Adults aged 16–74 who say their diet is not as healthy as it could be

Social class	I & II	III (NM)	III (M)	IV & V	Total*
Intentions to change diet	%	%	%	%	%
Men					
Intends to change in next month	6	11	9	6	8
Intends to change in next 6 months	16	20	13	14	15
Intends to change in next year	7	7	6	9	7
Want to change but thinks it unlikely	28	27	33	30	30
Does not want to change	43	35	38	40	40
Base = 100%	*613*	*158*	*410*	*268*	*1562*
Women					
Intends to change in next month	16	15	19	11	15
Intends to change in next 6 months	16	16	17	14	16
Intends to change in next year	6	8	6	8	7
Want to change but thinks it unlikely	34	28	31	32	30
Does not want to change	28	32	27	35	31
Base = 100%	*524*	*671*	*155*	*513*	*1981*
All					
Intends to change in next month	10	14	12	9	11
Intends to change in next 6 months	16	17	14	14	15
Intends to change in next year	7	8	6	8	7
Want to change but thinks it unlikely	31	28	33	32	30
Does not want to change	37	33	36	37	36
Base = 100%	*1137*	*829*	*565*	*781*	*3543*

* Members of the Armed Forces, persons in inadequately described occupations and persons who have never worked are not shown as separate categories but are included in the figures for all persons.

Table 4.26 Whether agrees that 'I get confused over what's supposed to be healthy and what isn't' by age and sex
Adults aged 16–74

Age	16–24	25–34	35–44	45–54	55–64	65–74	Total	Total HEMS 1995
Whether agrees	%	%	%	%	%	%	%	%
Men								
Strongly agrees	1	2	3	3	5	3	3	5
Agrees	25	25	29	36	37	40	31	39
Neither agrees nor disagrees	19	20	13	11	12	12	15	9*
Disagrees	43	47	51	44	43	40	45	43
Strongly disagrees	13	6	5	5	3	4	6	4
Base = 100%	224	436	395	367	308	305	2035	2119
Women								
Strongly agrees	4	2	2	3	4	4	3	3
Agrees	24	25	25	27	28	33	27	33
Neither agrees nor disagrees	14	12	11	7	8	10	10	7*
Disagrees	54	51	54	55	56	49	53	50
Strongly disagrees	4	9	9	7	4	4	7	6
Base = 100%	265	586	532	392	360	460	2595	2544
All								
Strongly agrees	2	2	2	3	4	4	3	4
Agrees	24	25	27	32	32	36	29	36
Neither agrees nor disagrees	16	16	12	9	10	11	13	8*
Disagrees	48	49	53	50	50	45	49	47
Strongly disagrees	9	7	7	6	4	4	6	5
Base = 100%	489	1022	927	759	668	765	4630	4663

* 'Don't know' in 1995.

Table 4.27 Whether agrees that 'I get confused over what's supposed to be healthy and what isn't' by social class based on own current or last job, and sex
Adults aged 16–74

Social class	I & II	III(NM)	III(M)	IV & V	Total*
Whether agrees	%	%	%	%	%
Men					
Strongly agrees	2	2	4	2	3
Agrees	26	28	35	41	31
Neither agrees nor disagrees	13	16	16	15	15[†]
Disagrees	51	48	41	39	45
Strongly disagrees	7	6	4	4	6
Base = 100%	783	195	560	360	2034
Women					
Strongly agrees	1	3	4	4	3
Agrees	18	25	28	37	27
Neither agrees nor disagrees	7	11	11	12	10[†]
Disagrees	60	56	52	44	53
Strongly disagrees	14	5	5	3	7
Base = 100%	677	862	224	678	2594
All					
Strongly agrees	2	3	4	3	3
Agrees	23	26	33	39	29
Neither agrees nor disagrees	11	12	14	13	13[†]
Disagrees	55	54	44	42	49
Strongly disagrees	10	5	5	3	6
Base = 100%	1460	1057	784	1038	4628

* Members of the Armed Forces, persons in inadequately described occupations and persons who have never worked are not shown as separate categories but are included in the figures for all persons.
† 'Don't know' in 1995.

Table 4.28 Percentage agreeing that 'I get confused over what's supposed to be healthy and what isn't' by number of ways of achieving a healthier diet correctly identified
Adults aged 16–74

				Base = 100%		
	Men	Women	All	Men	Women	All
Number correctly stated of 'eat less fat', 'eat more fruit', 'eat more starch' and 'eat more fibre'	%	%	%			
None to two	35	32	33	1726	2129	3855
Three	27	17	22	252	380	632
Four	[6]	26	23	29	58	87
Total	34	29	31	2007	2567	4574

Table 4.29 Percentage agreeing that 'experts never agree what foods are good for you' by age
Adults aged 16–74

Age	16–24	25–34	35–44	45–54	55–64	65–74	Total	Total HEMS 1995
Whether agrees	%	%	%	%	%	%	%	%
Strongly agrees	6	12	15	14	16	17	13	11
Agrees	49	49	54	59	61	64	55	59
Neither agrees nor disagrees	27	21	14	12	11	10	16	12*
Disagrees	16	16	15	14	11	8	14	16
Strongly disagrees	2	2	1	2	1	1	1	1
Base = 100%	486	1021	922	757	662	763	4611	4658

Table 4.30 Percentage 'strongly agreeing' or 'agreeing' that 'eating healthy food is expensive' by selected characteristics
Adults aged 16–74

Characteristic	HEMS 1996 %	HEMS 1995 %	Base = 100% HEMS 1996	Base = 100% HEMS 1995
Age				
16–24	30	32	485	515
25–34	39	41	1020	1039
35–44	37	37	925	900
45–54	36	38	758	789
55–64	41	41	667	716
65–74	42	49	766	704
Social class				
I & II	29	31	1458	1519
III (NM)	33	36	1052	1072
III (M)	41	46	776	907
IV & V	49	48	1043	1046
Income				
Under £5,000	51	57	619	607
£5,000–£9,999	48	51	914	887
£10,000–£19,999	38	43	1342	1392
£20,000 or more	29	28	1550	1547
Number correctly stated of 'eat less fat', 'eat more fruit', 'eat more starch' and 'eat more fibre'				
None to two	38	54	3849	220
Three	29	45	628	1735
Four	30	35	87	2708
All	37	39	4564	4663

Health in England 1996 : What people know, what people think, what people do

Table 4.31 Percentage agreeing that 'healthy foods are enjoyable' by age and sex
Adults aged 16–74

Age	16–24	25–34	35–44	45–54	55–64	65–74	Total	Total HEMS 1995
Whether agrees	%	%	%	%	%	%	%	%
Men								
Strongly agrees	6	9	8	10	10	8	9	9
Agrees	62	60	63	61	54	70	61	66
Neither agrees nor disagrees	24	26	24	22	27	17	24	14
Disagrees	8	5	5	7	8	5	6	10
Strongly disagrees	-	0	-	0	1	-	0	1
Base = 100%	224	436	396	367	307	306	2036	2119
Women								
Strongly agrees	8	11	12	8	8	10	10	11
Agrees	64	66	70	70	75	74	69	75
Neither agrees nor disagrees	20	17	15	15	12	13	15	8
Disagrees	8	6	4	6	5	3	5	7
Strongly disagrees	0	0	-	0	0	-	0	0
Base = 100%	265	586	532	391	360	461	2595	2543
All								
Strongly agrees	7	10	10	9	9	9	9	10
Agrees	63	63	67	65	65	72	65	71
Neither agrees nor disagrees	22	21	19	18	19	15	19	11
Disagrees	8	5	4	7	7	4	6	8
Strongly disagrees	0	0	-	0	1	-	0	0
Base = 100%	489	1022	928	758	667	767	4631	4662

Table 4.32 Percentage 'strongly agreeing' or 'agreeing' that 'healthy foods are enjoyable' by selected characteristics
Adults aged 16–74

	Men	Women	All	Men	Women	All
					Base = 100%	
Characteristic	%	%	%			
Social class						
I & II	71	84	77	782	676	1458
III (NM)	73	79	78	195	862	1057
III (M)	68	78	70	560	223	783
IV & V	70	77	74	363	679	1042
Number correctly stated of 'eat less fat', 'eat more fruit', 'eat more starch' and 'eat more fibre'						
None to two	70	79	74	1727	2128	3855
Three	72	83	78	252	380	632
Four	[23]	86	82	29	58	87
All	70	79	75	2008	2566	4574

* Members of the Armed Forces, persons in inadequately described occupations and persons who have never worked are not shown as separate categories but are included in the figures for all persons.

Table 4.33 Percentage 'strongly agreeing' or 'agreeing' that 'the tastiest foods are the ones that are bad for you' by selected characteristics
Adults aged 16–74

	HEMS 1996	HEMS 1995	Base = 100% HEMS 1996	HEMS 1995
Characteristic	%	%		
Age				
16–24	44	46	489	516
25–34	34	48	1021	1038
35–44	36	38	926	900
45–54	38	39	758	788
55–64	41	44	668	716
65–74	40	49	760	704
Social class				
I & II	29	35	1457	1519
III (NM)	40	42	1055	1073
III (M)	44	49	778	907
IV & V	44	51	1041	1044
Number correctly stated of 'eat less fat', 'eat more fruit', 'eat more starch' and 'eat more fibre'				
None to two	39	50	3850	220
Three	33	49	629	1734
Four	39	40	87	2708
All	38	44	4566	4662

* Members of the Armed Forces, persons in inadequately described occupations and persons who have never worked are not shown as separate categories but are included in the figures for all persons.

Table 5.1 Percentage who had ever used drugs, had used drugs in the past year or had used drugs in the past month by sex
Adults aged 16–54

Drug use	Ever	Past year	Past month
Drugs		Percentage using each drug	
Men			
Any drug	38	17	12
Cannabis	34	16	11
Amphetamines	16	6	3
Amyl nitrate	12	4	2
LSD	10	2	1
Magic mushrooms	10	2	0
Ecstasy	6	3	2
Cocaine	6	2	1
Solvents or glue	3	0	-
Tranquilisers	4	1	0
Heroin	2	0	0
Anabolic steroids	1	1	0
Crack	1	0	0
Methadone	1	0	0
Other	2	1	0
*Base = 100%**	1398	1398	1398
Women			
Any drug	26	11	6
Cannabis	22	10	6
Amphetamines	9	3	1
Amyl nitrate	5	1	0
LSD	5	0	0
Magic mushrooms	4	0	0
Ecstasy	3	2	1
Cocaine	3	2	1
Solvents or glue	2	0	0
Tranquilisers	3	0	0
Heroin	0	-	-
Anabolic steroids	-	-	-
Crack	0	0	0
Methadone	0	0	0
Other	1	0	0
*Base = 100%**	1745	1745	1745
All			
Any drug	32	14	9
Cannabis	28	13	8
Amphetamines	13	4	2
Amyl nitrate	9	2	1
LSD	7	1	0
Magic mushrooms	7	1	0
Ecstasy	5	2	1
Cocaine	4	2	1
Solvents or glue	2	0	0
Tranquilisers	3	1	0
Heroin	1	0	0
Anabolic steroids	1	0	0
Crack	1	0	0
Methadone	0	0	0
Other	1	0	0
*Base = 100%**	3143	3143	3143

* Percentages add to more than 100% because respondents may have taken more than one drug.

Table 5.2 Percentage who had ever used drugs by age and sex
Adults aged 16–54

Age	16–29	30–54	Total
Drugs		Percentage using each drug	
Men			
Any drug	54	29	38
Cannabis	49	26	34
Amphetamines	26	10	16
Amyl nitrate	23	6	12
LSD	16	7	10
Magic mushrooms	14	8	10
Ecstasy	13	2	6
Cocaine	9	4	6
Solvents or glue	7	1	3
Tranquilisers	6	2	4
Heroin	2	1	2
Anabolic steroids	3	1	1
Crack	1	1	1
Methadone	1	0	1
Other	3	1	2
*Base = 100%**	417	981	1398
Women			
Any drug	41	19	26
Cannabis	36	15	22
Amphetamines	15	6	9
Amyl nitrate	11	2	5
LSD	9	2	5
Magic mushrooms	7	3	4
Ecstasy	8	1	3
Cocaine	6	1	3
Solvents or glue	4	0	2
Tranquilisers	2	3	3
Heroin	1	0	0
Anabolic steroids	-	-	-
Crack	1	0	0
Methadone	0	0	0
Other	1	0	1
*Base = 100%**	540	1205	1745
All			
Any drug	48	24	32
Cannabis	42	21	28
Amphetamines	21	8	13
Amyl nitrate	17	4	9
LSD	13	4	7
Magic mushrooms	11	6	7
Ecstasy	11	1	5
Cocaine	7	3	4
Solvents or glue	6	1	2
Tranquilisers	4	2	3
Heroin	2	1	1
Anabolic steroids	1	0	1
Crack	1	0	1
Methadone	1	0	0
Other	2	1	1
*Base = 100%**	957	2186	3143

* Percentages add to more than 100% because respondents may have taken more than one drug.

Table 5.3 Percentage who had ever used drugs, had used drugs in the past year or in the past month by drug category, age and sex
Adults aged 16–54

Age	16–29			30–54			All		
Drug use	Ever	Past year	Past month	Ever	Past year	Past month	Ever	Past year	Past month
Drug category			Percentage using each category of drug						
Men									
Any drug	54	34	24	29	8	6	38	17	12
Cannabis	49	32	21	26	8	5	34	16	11
Hallucinants	36	18	9	15	3	1	23	8	4
Opiates	9	5	2	5	1	0	7	3	1
Other	15	4	2	4	1	0	8	2	1
*Base = 100%**	*417*	*417*	*417*	*981*	*981*	*981*	*1398*	*1398*	*1398*
Women									
Any drug	41	23	14	19	4	2	26	11	6
Cannabis	36	20	12	15	4	2	22	10	6
Hallucinants	23	9	5	9	1	0	14	4	2
Opiates	6	4	2	2	0	0	3	2	1
Other	6	1	0	3	1	0	4	1	0
*Base = 100%**	*540*	*540*	*540*	*1205*	*1205*	*1205*	*1745*	*1745*	*1745*
All									
Any drug	48	29	19	24	6	4	32	14	9
Cannabis	42	26	17	21	6	4	28	13	8
Hallucinants	29	14	7	12	2	1	18	6	3
Opiates	8	5	2	3	1	0	5	2	1
Other	11	2	1	4	1	0	6	1	0
*Base = 100%**	*957*	*957*	*957*	*2186*	*2186*	*2186*	*3143*	*3143*	*3143*

* Percentages add to more than 100% because respondents may have taken drugs from more than one category.

Health in England 1996 : What people know, what people think, what people do

Table 5.4 Whether had ever used drugs by drug category, age and sex
Adults aged 16–54

Age	16–19	20–24	25–29	30–34	35–39	40–44	45–54	Total
Drug category			Percentage using each category of drug					
Men								
Any drug	42	70	50	39	34	36	18	38
Cannabis	38	64	44	36	30	32	14	34
Hallucinants	28	46	33	19	17	20	10	23
Opiates	4	14	9	8	5	7	2	7
Other	6	20	17	4	5	6	2	8
Base = 100%*	86	134	197	229	217	176	359	1398
Women								
Any drug	47	46	32	26	26	16	11	26
Cannabis	42	41	28	23	21	13	7	22
Hallucinants	33	24	16	13	13	8	4	14
Opiates	6	9	4	2	3	1	0	3
Other	10	3	7	4	5	2	3	4
Base = 100%*	76	185	279	300	277	251	377	1745
All								
Any drug	44	57	41	33	30	25	14	32
Cannabis	39	52	36	30	25	22	11	28
Hallucinants	31	34	25	16	15	13	7	18
Opiates	5	11	6	5	4	4	1	5
Other	8	11	12	4	5	3	2	6
Base = 100%*	162	319	476	529	494	427	736	3143

* Percentages add to more than 100% because respondents may have taken drugs from more than one category.

Table 5.5 Whether had used drugs in the past year by drug category, age and sex
Adults aged 16–54

Age	16–19	20–24	25–29	30–34	35–39	40–44	45–54	Total
Drug category			Percentage using each category of drug					
Men								
Any drug	36	46	23	13	10	8	5	17
Cannabis	33	43	22	12	10	8	4	16
Hallucinants	17	28	10	4	3	3	2	8
Opiates	3	8	4	2	1	2	1	3
Other	1	7	4	1	0	1	0	2
Base = 100%*	86	134	197	229	217	176	359	1398
Women								
Any drug	41	26	11	8	6	2	1	11
Cannabis	40	23	8	7	6	2	1	10
Hallucinants	21	8	5	1	2	0	0	4
Opiates	6	5	2	1	0	0	0	2
Other	0	1	1	1	0	1	0	1
Base = 100%*	76	185	279	300	277	251	377	1745
All								
Any drug	38	35	17	11	8	5	3	14
Cannabis	36	32	15	10	8	5	3	13
Hallucinants	19	17	7	3	2	1	1	6
Opiates	4	7	3	1	0	1	0	2
Other	1	4	2	1	0	1	0	1
Base = 100%*	162	319	476	529	494	427	736	3143

* Percentages add to more than 100% because respondents may have taken drugs from more than one category.

Table 5.6 Whether had used drugs in the past month by drug category, age and sex
Adults aged 16–54

Age	16–19	20–24	25–29	30–34	35–39	40–44	45–54	Total
Drug category			Percentage using each category of drug					
Men								
Any drug	27	35	12	9	6	6	3	12
Cannabis	24	32	10	8	6	6	3	11
Hallucinants	8	16	5	2	0	3	1	4
Opiates	1	2	2	1	-	1	0	1
Other	-	3	2	0	0	1	-	1
*Base = 100%**	*86*	*134*	*197*	*229*	*217*	*176*	*359*	*1398*
Women								
Any drug	24	17	7	4	3	2	1	6
Cannabis	23	14	5	4	3	1	1	6
Hallucinants	11	5	3	0	-	0	-	2
Opiates	3	2	1	0	-	-	-	1
Other	-	0	0	-	-	-	-	-
*Base = 100%**	*76*	*185*	*279*	*300*	*277*	*251*	*377*	*1745*
All								
Any drug	26	25	10	7	5	4	2	9
Cannabis	24	23	7	6	4	3	2	8
Hallucinants	9	10	4	1	0	1	0	3
Opiates	2	2	1	1	-	1	0	1
Other	-	2	1	0	0	0	-	0
*Base = 100%**	*162*	*319*	*476*	*529*	*494*	*427*	*736*	*3143*

* Percentages add to more than 100% because respondents may have taken drugs from more than one category.

Table 5.7 Whether had ever used drugs by drug category, age and sex
Adults aged 16–54

Age	16–18	19–21	22–24	25–29	30–54	Total
Drug category		Percentage using each category of drug				
Men						
Any drug	39	74	64	50	29	38
Cannabis	37	69	55	44	26	34
Hallucinants	25	55	38	33	15	23
Opiates	3	15	13	9	5	7
Other	6	26	12	17	4	8
*Base = 100%**	*73*	*57*	*90*	*197*	*981*	*1398*
Women						
Any drug	47	50	42	32	19	26
Cannabis	42	47	36	28	15	22
Hallucinants	35	22	25	16	9	14
Opiates	8	9	6	4	2	3
Other	13	3	2	7	3	4
*Base = 100%**	*57*	*80*	*124*	*279*	*1205*	*1745*
All						
Any drug	42	61	53	41	24	32
Cannabis	39	57	45	36	21	28
Hallucinants	29	37	31	25	12	18
Opiates	5	12	9	6	3	5
Other	9	14	7	12	4	6
*Base = 100%**	*130*	*137*	*214*	*476*	*2186*	*3143*

* Percentages add to more than 100% because respondents may have taken drugs from more than one category.

Health in England 1996 : What people know, what people think, what people do

Table 5.8 Whether had used drugs in the last year by drug category, age and sex
Adults aged 16–54

Age	16–18	19–21	22–24	25–29	30–54	Total
Drug category			Percentage using each category of drug			
Men						
Any drug	35	57	36	23	8	17
Cannabis	31	53	34	22	8	16
Hallucinants	17	36	19	10	3	8
Opiates	2	11	5	4	1	3
Other	1	9	4	4	1	2
*Base = 100%**	73	57	90	197	981	1398
Women						
Any drug	41	31	25	11	4	11
Cannabis	41	27	23	8	4	10
Hallucinants	22	12	7	5	1	4
Opiates	8	3	6	2	0	2
Other	0	0	1	1	1	1
*Base = 100%**	57	80	124	279	1205	1745
All						
Any drug	37	43	30	17	6	14
Cannabis	35	39	28	15	6	13
Hallucinants	19	23	13	7	2	6
Opiates	4	7	6	3	1	2
Other	1	4	2	2	1	1
*Base = 100%**	130	137	214	476	2186	3143

* Percentages add to more than 100% because respondents may have taken drugs from more than one category.

Table 5.9 Whether had used drugs in the last month by drug category, age and sex
Adults aged 16–54

Age	16–18	19–21	22–24	25–29	30–54	Total
Drug category			Percentage using each category of drug			
Men						
Any drug	24	50	25	12	6	12
Cannabis	21	46	24	10	5	11
Hallucinants	7	27	6	5	1	4
Opiates	1	4	0	2	0	1
Other	-	5	1	2	0	1
*Base = 100%**	73	57	90	197	981	1398
Women						
Any drug	24	20	15	7	2	6
Cannabis	22	20	12	5	2	6
Hallucinants	10	7	4	3	0	2
Opiates	5	2	1	1	0	1
Other	-	0	-	0	-	0
*Base = 100%**	57	80	124	279	1205	1745
All						
Any drug	24	34	20	10	4	9
Cannabis	21	32	18	7	4	8
Hallucinants	9	16	5	4	1	3
Opiates	2	3	1	1	0	1
Other	-	3	0	1	0	0
*Base = 100%**	130	137	214	476	2186	3143

* Percentages add to more than 100% because respondents may have taken drugs from more than one category.

Table 5.10 Respondents who had used any drug in the past year or in the past month as a proportion of those who had ever used any drug, by age and sex
Adults aged 16–54

Age	16–18	19–21	22–24	25–29	30–54	Total
Ever use, use in the past year and use in the past month, as a proportion of those who had ever used any drug			*Percentage using any drug*			
Men						
Ever used any drug	39	74	64	50	29	38
Used last year (of ever used any drug)	88	78	56	47	29	46
Used last month (of ever used any drug)	61	68	38	24	19	31
Base = 100%* (All respondents)	73	57	90	197	981	1398
Base = 100%* (Respondents who had ever used a drug)	33	43	58	99	312	545
Women						
Ever used any drug	47	50	42	32	19	26
Used last year (of ever used)	[22]	61	59	34	23	41
Used last month (of ever used)	[13]	40	36	23	12	24
Base = 100%* (All respondents)	57	80	124	279	1205	1745
Base = 100%* (Respondents who had ever used a drug)	26	43	52	102	251	474
All						
Ever used any drug	42	61	53	41	24	32
Used last year (of ever used)	88	70	57	42	27	44
Used last month (of ever used)	56	56	38	24	16	28
Base = 100%* (All respondents)	130	137	214	476	2186	3143
Base = 100%* (Respondents who had ever used a drug)	59	86	110	201	563	1019

* Percentages add to more than 100% because respondents may have taken drugs from more than one category.

Health in England 1996 : What people know, what people think, what people do

Table 5.11 Respondents who had used cannabis in the past year or in the past month as a proportion of those who had ever used any drug, by age and sex
Adults aged 16–54

Age	16–18	19–21	22–24	25–29	30–54	Total
Ever use of cannabis, use in the past year and use in the past month, as a proportion of those who had ever used cannabis			Percentage using any drug			
Men						
Ever used cannabis	37	69	55	44	26	34
Used last year (of ever used cannabis)	84	78	62	50	30	47
Used last month (of ever used cannabis)	57	67	42	22	20	32
Base = 100%* (All respondents)	73	57	90	197	981	1398
Base = 100%* (Respondents who had ever used cannabis)	31	40	50	86	275	482
Women						
Ever used cannabis	42	47	36	28	15	22
Used last year (of ever used cannabis)	[22]	57	62	30	25	43
Used last month (of ever used cannabis)	[12]	42	33	19	14	25
Base = 100%* (All respondents)	57	80	124	279	1205	1745
Base = 100%* (Respondents who had ever used cannabis)	23	40	45	88	206	402
All						
Ever used cannabis	39	57	45	36	21	28
Used last year (of ever used cannabis)	90	69	62	42	28	45
Used last month (of ever used cannabis)	55	56	39	21	18	29
Base = 100%* (All respondents)	130	137	214	476	2186	3143
Base = 100%* (Respondents who had ever used cannabis)	54	80	95	174	481	884

* Percentages add to more than 100% because respondents may have taken drugs from more than one category.

Table 5.12 Number of different drugs used, by whether used any drugs ever, in the past year or in the past month, and sex

Adults aged 16–54 who had ever used drugs

Sex	Men			Women			All		
Use of any drug	Ever used any drug	Used a drug in the past year	Used a drug in the past month	Ever used any drug	Used a drug in the past year	Used a drug in the past month	Ever used any drug	Used a drug in the past year	Used a drug in the past month
Number of different drugs used	%	%	%	%	%	%	%	%	%
1	43	55	69	51	66	77	46	59	72
2	20	15	11	20	20	12	20	17	12
3	10	12	11	10	5	4	10	9	8
4	7	6	6	8	5	5	8	5	6
5	7	7	2	5	2	-	6	5	1
6 or more	14	6	1	6	2	2	11	5	1
Base = 100%*	534	235	155	469	177	109	1003	412	264

* Excludes those who responded 'Don't want to answer' about any drug.

Table 5.13 Respondents who had used cannabis and/or other drugs, by recency of use and sex

Adults aged 16–54 who had ever used drugs

Sex	Men			Women			All		
Use of any drug	Ever used any drug	Used a drug in the past year	Used a drug in the past month	Ever used any drug	Used a drug in the past year	Used a drug in the past month	Ever used any drug	Used a drug in the past year	Used a drug in the past month
Number of drugs used and use of cannabis	%	%	%	%	%	%	%	%	%
Cannabis only	35	51	62	38	57	69	36	53	64
Cannabis and one other drug	18	14	10	19	18	8	18	15	9
Cannabis and two or more other drugs	37	28	18	28	14	11	33	23	16
One drug only, not cannabis	7	4	7	13	9	7	10	6	7
Two drugs, neither cannabis	2	1	1	1	2	4	2	1	2
Three or more drugs, none cannabis	1	2	1	1	1	-	1	2	1
Base = 100%*	534	235	155	469	177	109	1003	412	264

* Excludes those who responded 'Don't want to answer' about any drug.

Table 5.14 Whether knows people who use drugs, by age and sex
Adults aged 16–54

Age	16–19	20–24	25–29	30–34	35–39	40–44	45–54	Total
Whether knows people who use drugs	%	%	%	%	%	%	%	%
Men								
Yes	84	82	68	62	49	40	29	55
No	13	12	27	33	44	52	64	39
Don't know	1	3	3	5	6	6	5	5
Don't want to answer	2	2	3	-	1	1	1	1
Base = 100%	86	134	197	229	217	176	359	1398
Women								
Yes	86	79	52	43	41	32	21	45
No	12	16	43	53	55	61	70	49
Don't know	0	5	4	2	4	7	8	5
Don't want to answer	1	0	1	1	0	0	1	1
Base = 100%	76	185	279	300	277	251	377	1745
All								
Yes	85	80	60	52	45	35	26	50
No	13	14	35	43	49	57	67	44
Don't know	1	4	3	4	5	7	7	5
Don't want to answer	2	1	2	1	1	1	1	1
Base = 100%	162	319	476	529	494	427	736	3143

* Percentages add to more than 100% because respondents may have taken drugs from more than one category.

Table 5.15 Whether respondents know people who use drugs by whether had used a drug in the past month, year, more than a year or never, age and sex
Adults aged 16–54

				Base = 100%		
Age	15–29	30–54	Total	15–29	30–54	All
Whether knows people who use drugs	Percentage knowing people who use drugs					
Men						
Used a drug in the past month	97	96	97	90	65	155
Used a drug in the past year, but not in the past month	97	93	95	46	32	78
Used a drug more than 12 months ago	81	69	73	88	212	300
Never used a drug/Never heard of it	60	29	37	180	667	847
Women						
Last used in the past month	98	95	97	74	35	109
Last used in the past year, but not in the past month	93	[28]	94	39	29	68
Last used more than 12 months ago	80	61	68	107	183	290
Never used a drug/Never heard of it	56	24	33	313	948	1261
All						
Last used in the past month	97	96	97	164	100	264
Last used in the past year, but not in the past month	95	95	95	85	61	146
Last used more than 12 months ago	80	66	71	195	395	590
Never used a drug/Never heard of it	58	27	35	493	1615	2108

* Percentages add to more than 100% because respondents may belong to more than one category.

Table 5.16 Whether would like to stop using drugs, by age and sex
Adults aged 16–54, who had used one or more drugs in the last month

Age	16–29	30–54	Total
Whether would like to stop using drugs	%	%	%
Men			
Would like to stop using drugs altogether	35	26	32
See no need to stop using drugs at the moment	57	57	57
Don't see the need to ever stop using drugs	8	17	11
Base = 100%	*89*	*63*	*152*
Women			
Would like to stop using drugs altogether	25	36	27
See no need to stop using drugs at the moment	69	45	64
Don't see the need to ever stop using drugs	6	19	9
Base = 100%	*73*	*34*	*107*
All			
Would like to stop using drugs altogether	31	29	31
See no need to stop using drugs at the moment	62	54	59
Don't see the need to ever stop using drugs	7	17	10
Base = 100%	*162*	*97*	*259*

Table 5.17 Intentions to stop using drugs by sex
Adults aged 16–54, who had used one or more drugs in the last month

Sex	Men	Women	Total
Intention to stop using drugs	%	%	%
Within the next month	19	17	18
Within 6 months	10	8	9
Within the next year	5	13	8
Not in the next year	36	39	37
Unlikely ever to stop	19	14	18
See no need ever to stop	11	9	10
Base = 100%	*151*	*106*	*257*

Table 5.18 Percentage who had used each method of taking drugs, by age and sex
Adults aged 16–54

Age	16-19	20-24	25-29	30-34	35-39	40-44	45-54	Total
Methods			Percentage using each method					
Men								
Smoked	90	87	87	93	85	86	80	87
Sniffed	21	33	26	18	21	16	9	22
Inhaled	10	20	14	10	10	12	8	13
Swallowed/eaten/drunk	23	45	39	31	41	36	23	36
Injected	-	2	1	4	-	3	1	2
Other	-	-	-	-	1	2	4	1
*Base = 100%**	*41*	*93*	*99*	*95*	*79*	*67*	*71*	*545*
Women								
Smoked	76	82	77	88	72	74	70	78
Sniffed	28	23	18	15	12	6	1	17
Inhaled	7	12	10	12	8	8	2	9
Swallowed/eaten/drunk	36	35	22	33	27	36	40	32
Injected	4	-	3	-	-	-	-	1
Other	-	-	2	2	5	4	7	2
*Base = 100%**	*35*	*86*	*102*	*84*	*74*	*47*	*45*	*473*
All								
Smoked	84	85	83	91	79	82	77	84
Sniffed	24	29	23	17	17	13	7	20
Inhaled	8	16	12	11	9	10	6	11
Swallowed/eaten/drunk	29	41	32	32	35	36	29	34
Injected	2	1	2	3	-	2	0	1
Other	-	-	1	1	2	3	5	1
*Base = 100%**	*76*	*179*	*201*	*179*	*153*	*114*	*116*	*1018*

* Percentages add to more than 100% because respondents may have taken drugs from more than one category.

Table 5.19 Percentage who had used drugs in combination by age and sex
Adults aged 16–54, who had used one or more drugs in the last month

Age	16-29	30-54	Total
	Percentage who had used two or more drugs in combination in one session in the past 12 months		
Men	55	[16]	55
Women	36	[7]	36
All	49	48	49
Base = 100%			
Men	68	29	97
Women	45	15	60
All	113	44	157

Table 5.20 Percentage who had used drugs in combination with alcohol by age and sex
Adults aged 16–54, who had used one or more drugs in the last 12 months

Age	16-29	30-54	Total
	Percentage who had used one or more drugs in combination with alcohol in one session in the past 12 months		
Men	71	52	65
Women	52	34	47
All	64	46	58
Base = 100%			
Men	138	97	235
Women	113	64	177
All	251	161	412

Table 5.21 Whether agrees that 'All use of drugs is wrong unless with a doctor's prescription or bought from a chemist' by age and sex
Adults aged 16–54

Age	16–19	20–24	25–29	30–34	35–39	40–44	45–54	Total
Whether agrees	%	%	%	%	%	%	%	%
Men								
Agrees	56	44	55	65	67	75	83	66
Disagrees	24	31	29	18	20	17	10	20
Neither agrees nor disagrees	20	25	16	17	12	8	7	14
Base = 100%	86	134	197	229	217	176	359	1398
Women								
Agrees	52	55	69	72	79	81	88	74
Disagrees	32	20	15	15	11	10	7	14
Neither agrees nor disagrees	17	25	16	14	10	9	5	13
Base = 100%	76	185	279	299	276	251	376	1742
All								
Agrees	54	50	62	68	73	79	85	70
Disagrees	27	25	22	16	16	13	9	17
Neither agrees nor disagrees	18	25	16	16	11	8	6	13
Base = 100%	162	319	476	528	493	427	735	3140

Table 5.22 Whether agrees that 'All use of drugs is wrong unless with a doctor's prescription or bought from a chemist' by whether had used any drug in the past month, year, longer than a year or never, and sex
Adults aged 16–54

Use of any drug	Used a drug in the past month	Used a drug in the past year, but not in past month	Used a drug, but not in past year	Never used any drug	Total
Whether agrees	%	%	%	%	%
Men					
Agrees	20	33	48	85	66
Disagrees	59	40	28	7	20
Neither agrees nor disagrees	21	27	23	8	14
Base = 100%	155	78	300	847	1398
Women					
Agrees	12	32	52	86	74
Disagrees	56	45	23	6	14
Neither agrees nor disagrees	32	23	25	7	13
Base = 100%	109	68	290	1258	1742
All					
Agrees	17	33	50	86	70
Disagrees	58	42	26	7	17
Neither agrees nor disagrees	25	25	24	8	13
Base = 100%	264	146	590	2105	3140

Health in England 1996 : What people know, what people think, what people do

Table 5.23 Whether agrees that 'I don't mind other people using drugs' by age and sex
Adults aged 16–54

Age	16–19	20–24	25–29	30–34	35–39	40–44	45–54	Total
Whether agrees	%	%	%	%	%	%	%	%
Men								
Agrees	40	45	33	20	15	11	12	23
Disagrees	33	30	43	49	58	66	70	53
Neither agrees nor disagrees	27	25	24	31	27	23	18	24
Base = 100%	86	134	197	229	217	176	357	1396
Women								
Agrees	34	32	23	18	12	11	11	18
Disagrees	31	33	49	60	65	69	72	57
Neither agrees nor disagrees	34	34	29	22	24	20	17	24
Base = 100%	76	185	279	300	276	251	374	1741
All								
Agrees	37	38	28	19	13	11	12	21
Disagrees	32	32	46	54	61	67	71	55
Neither agrees nor disagrees	30	30	26	26	25	21	18	24
Base = 100%	162	319	476	529	493	427	731	3137

Table 5.24 Whether agrees that 'I don't mind other people using drugs' by whether had used any drug in the past month, year, longer than a year or never, and sex
Adults aged 16–54

Use of any drug	Used a drug in the past month	Used a drug in the past year, but not in past month	Used a drug, but not in past year	Never used any drug	Total
Whether agrees	%	%	%	%	%
Men					
Agrees	52	37	30	13	23
Disagrees	9	23	38	69	53
Neither agrees nor disagrees	39	40	32	18	24
Base = 100%	155	78	299	846	1396
Women					
Agrees	52	43	22	13	18
Disagrees	13	18	42	67	57
Neither agrees nor disagrees	35	39	37	20	24
Base = 100%	109	68	289	1258	1741
All					
Agrees	52	40	26	13	21
Disagrees	10	21	40	68	55
Neither agrees nor disagrees	38	40	34	19	24
Base = 100%	264	146	588	2104	3137

Table 5.25 Whether agrees that drugs are safe to use by age and sex
Adults aged 16–54

Age	16-19	20-24	25-29	30-34	35-39	40-44	45-54	Total
Whether agrees	%	%	%	%	%	%	%	%
Men								
All drugs are safe to use (as long as you know what you're doing)	-	2	2	2	-	0	1	1
Some drugs are safe to use (as long as you know what you're doing)	49	47	37	34	29	27	20	32
No drugs are safe to use	46	38	52	52	61	60	66	56
I don't know whether drugs are safe to use or not	6	13	9	12	10	13	13	11
Base = 100%	86	134	196	229	216	176	358	1395
Women								
All drugs are safe to use (as long as you know what you're doing)	2	0	0	1	1	1	1	1
Some drugs are safe to use (as long as you know what you're doing)	38	27	27	27	20	16	12	22
No drugs are safe to use	54	63	62	61	70	73	77	67
I don't know whether drugs are safe to use or not	6	9	10	11	9	11	10	10
Base = 100%	76	185	279	300	275	251	377	1743
All								
All drugs are safe to use (as long as you know what you're doing)	1	1	1	1	1	1	1	1
Some drugs are safe to use (as long as you know what you're doing)	44	37	32	31	25	21	16	27
No drugs are safe to use	49	51	57	57	65	67	71	61
I don't know whether drugs are safe to use or not	6	11	10	11	9	12	11	10
Base = 100%	162	319	475	529	491	427	735	3138

Table 5.26 Whether agrees that drugs are safe to use by whether had used any drug in the past month, year, longer than a year or never, and sex
Adults aged 16–54

Use of any drug	Used a drug in the past month	Used a drug in the past year, but not in past month	Used a drug, but not in past year	Never used any drug	Total
Whether agrees	%	%	%	%	%
Men					
All drugs are safe to use (as long as you know what you're doing)	1	-	1	1	1
Some drugs are safe to use (as long as you know what you're doing)	74	65	48	16	32
No drugs are safe to use	20	28	39	71	56
I don't know whether drugs are safe to use or not	4	8	12	12	11
Base = 100%	*155*	*78*	*298*	*846*	*1395*
Women					
All drugs are safe to use (as long as you know what you're doing)	0	-	-	1	1
Some drugs are safe to use (as long as you know what you're doing)	70	57	34	13	22
No drugs are safe to use	23	36	60	75	67
I don't know whether drugs are safe to use or not	7	7	6	11	10
Base = 100%	*109*	*68*	*290*	*1259*	*1743*
All					
All drugs are safe to use (as long as you know what you're doing)	1	-	1	1	1
Some drugs are safe to use (as long as you know what you're doing)	73	61	42	14	27
No drugs are safe to use	21	31	48	73	61
I don't know whether drugs are safe to use or not	5	7	10	11	10
Base = 100%	*264*	*146*	*588*	*2105*	*3138*

Table 5.27 Percentage who had ever used any drug, by selected characteristics
Adults aged 16–54

	Men	Women	All	Men	Women	All
Characteristic	Percentage who had ever used any drug			Base = 100%*		
Age						
16–24	57	46	52	220	261	481
25–34	44	29	37	426	579	1005
35–44	35	21	28	393	528	921
45–54	18	11	14	359	377	736
Social class						
I & II	39	29	35	559	492	1051
III (NM)	45	24	29	135	585	720
III (M)	33	21	30	344	135	479
IV & V	41	25	32	245	411	656
Marital status						
Married	26	16	21	696	858	1554
Cohabiting	64	34	48	133	181	314
Single	51	45	48	442	429	871
Widowed, separated or divorced	34	30	31	127	277	404
Highest qualification level						
'A' level or above	42	36	40	640	580	1220
Other qualifications	39	25	31	516	784	1300
No qualifications	26	14	19	238	380	618
Economic activity status						
Working	36	26	32	1151	1188	2339
Unemployed	58	41	52	97	73	170
Economically inactive	37	24	28	150	484	634
Total household income						
Under £5,000	44	36	39	86	222	308
£5,000–£9,999	40	22	30	155	288	443
£10,000–£19,999	31	20	25	425	505	930
£20,000 or more	41	30	36	679	667	1346
Tenure						
Owner-occupied	35	23	30	980	1154	2134
Rented from local authority/ housing association	38	24	30	192	315	507
Privately rented	51	42	46	224	274	498
All	38	26	32	1398	1745	3143

* Members of the Armed Forces, persons in inadequately described occupations and persons who have never worked are not shown as separate categories, but are included in the figures for all persons.

Table 5.28 Percentage who had used any drug in the past year, by selected characteristics
Adults aged 16–54

	Men	Women	All	Men	Women	All
Characteristic	Percentage who used any drug in the past year			Base = 100%*		
Age						
16–24	41	31	36	220	261	481
25–34	18	10	14	426	579	1005
35–44	9	4	7	393	528	921
45–54	5	1	3	359	377	736
Social class						
I & II	13	9	11	559	492	1051
III (NM)	26	10	14	135	585	720
III (M)	14	8	12	344	135	479
IV & V	23	10	16	245	411	656
Marital status						
Married	6	2	4	696	858	1554
Cohabiting	29	14	21	133	181	314
Single	33	27	30	442	429	871
Widowed, separated or divorced	12	12	12	127	277	404
Highest qualification level						
'A' level or above	17	14	16	640	580	1220
Other qualifications	21	11	15	516	784	1300
No qualifications	11	5	8	238	380	618
Economic activity status						
Working	15	10	13	1151	1188	2339
Unemployed	31	25	29	97	73	170
Economically inactive	22	11	14	150	484	634
Total household income						
Under £5,000	23	18	20	86	222	308
£5,000–£9,999	21	8	14	155	288	443
£10,000–£19,999	14	8	11	425	505	930
£20,000 or more	18	11	15	679	667	1346
Housing tenure						
Owner-occupied	15	9	12	980	1154	2134
Rented from local authority/ housing association	17	9	13	192	315	507
Privately rented	30	21	26	224	274	498
All	17	11	14	1398	1745	3143

* Members of the Armed Forces, persons in inadequately described occupations and persons who have never worked are not shown as separate categories, but are included in the figures for all persons.

Table 5.29 Percentage who had used any drug in the past month, by selected characteristics
Adults aged 16-54

	Men	Women	All	Men	Women	All
Characteristic	Percentage who used any drug in the past month			Base = 100%*		
Age						
16–24	32	19	26	220	261	481
25–34	10	6	8	426	579	1005
35–44	6	2	4	393	528	921
45–54	3	1	2	359	377	736
Social class						
I & II	7	5	6	559	492	1051
III (NM)	15	5	7	135	585	720
III (M)	10	5	9	344	135	479
IV & V	19	8	13	245	411	656
Marital status						
Married	4	1	2	696	858	1554
Cohabiting	17	8	12	133	181	314
Single	24	17	21	442	429	871
Widowed, separated or divorced	7	7	7	127	277	404
Highest qualification level						
'A' level or above	11	9	10	640	580	1220
Other qualifications	16	6	10	516	784	1300
No qualifications	7	3	5	238	380	618
Economic activity status						
Working	10	6	8	1151	1188	2339
Unemployed	28	17	24	97	73	170
Economically inactive	15	7	9	150	484	634
Total household income						
Under £5,000	18	13	15	86	222	308
£5,000–£9,999	14	4	9	155	288	443
£10,000–£19,999	8	4	6	425	505	930
£20,000 or more	13	7	10	679	667	1346
Housing tenure						
Owner-occupied	9	5	7	980	1154	2134
Rented from local authority/ housing association	14	6	10	192	315	507
Privately rented	24	13	19	224	274	498
All	12	6	9	1398	1745	3143

* Members of the Armed Forces, persons in inadequately described occupations and persons who have never worked are not shown as separate categories, but are included in the figures for all persons.

Table 6.1 Number of sexual partners in the last 12 months by sex and age
Adults aged 16–54

Age	16–19	20–24	25–34	35–44	45–54	Total	Total HEMS 1995
Number of sexual partners in the last 12 months	%	%	%	%	%	%	%
Men							
None	47	10	11	10	14	14	16
One	22	48	73	81	81	69	67
Two	14	20	6	5	4	7	7
Three to four	12	13	6	3	1	5	6
Five to nine	3	7	3	1	0	2	2
Ten or more	2	3	2	1	0	1	2
Base = 100%	85	133	419	384	354	1375	1341
Median	2	1	1	1	1	1	1
95th percentile	5	7	5	3	2	4	5
Base = 100%[†]	48	120	372	340	293	1173	1114
Women							
None	27	8	10	9	17	12	14
One	39	68	82	87	80	78	77
Two	21	10	5	3	2	5	6
Three to four	10	9	2	1	1	3	2
Five to nine	1	4	1	-	-	1	0
Ten or more	2	1	0	-	-	0	0
Base = 100%	74	185	564	522	371	1716	1596
Median	1	1	1	1	1	1	1
95th percentile	4	4	2	1	1	2	2
Base = 100%[†]	54	171	512	459	288	1484	1353
All							
None	39	9	10	9	15	13	15
One	29	59	77	84	81	74	72
Two	17	14	6	4	3	6	7
Three to four	12	11	4	2	1	4	4
Five to nine	2	5	2	0	0	1	1
Ten or more	2	5	2	0	0	1	1
Base = 100%	159	318	983	906	725	3091	3078
Median	2	1	1	1	1	1	1
95th percentile	5	5	3	2	2	3	3
Base = 100%[†]	102	291	884	799	581	2657	2467

* Proportions differ from those shown in the 1995 report because they exclude married, cohabiting, widowed, divorced and separated respondents who said they had never had a sexual partner.
† Excludes respondents who did not report a sexual partner in the last year.

Table 6.2 Number of sexual partners in the last 12 months by social class based on own current or last job, age and sex

Adults aged 16–54

	Men					Women				
Social Class	I & II	III(NM)	III(M)	IV & V	Total*	I & II	III(NM)	III(M)	IV & V	Total*
Age and number of sexual partners in the last 12 months	%	%	%	%	%	%	%	%	%	%
16–34										
None	12	16	11	19	17	6	12	18	12	12
One	70	49	64	50	57	81	71	74	70	72
Two or more	18	35	25	31	25	13	17	9	17	16
35–54										
None	8	8	15	16	12	14	10	13	13	12
One	84	86	79	74	81	83	87	84	84	84
Two or more	8	6	6	10	8	3	3	3	4	3
All										
None	10	14	13	18	14	11	11	15	13	12
One	78	61	72	61	69	82	79	79	77	78
Two or more	12	25	15	21	16	7	10	6	10	10
Bases = 100%										
16–34	213	78	151	115	637	200	281	66	198	823
35–54	338	53	191	122	738	286	296	67	206	893
All	551	131	342	237	1375	486	577	133	404	1716
Median	1	1	1	1	1	1	1	1	1	1
95th percentile	3	5	4	10	4	2	2	2	3	2
Base = 100%†	485	114	295	195	1173	422	510	114	344	1484

* Members of the Armed Forces, persons in inadequately described occupations and persons who have never worked are not shown as separate categories but are included in the figures for all persons.

† Excludes respondents who did not report a sexual partner in the last year.

Table 6.3 Age-standardised ratios for reporting two or more sexual partners in the last year by social class based on own current or last job and sex
Adults aged 16–54

Social class*	I & II	III(NM)	III(M)	IV & V
Reported two or more sexual partners in the last year				
Men				
Observed %	12	25	15	21
Expected %†	13	21	15	18
Standardised ratio**	95	117	97	119
Standard error of the ratio	5.7	9.3	6.5	7.8
Base = 100%	*551*	*131*	*342*	*237*
Women				
Observed %	7	10	6	10
Expected %†	7	10	10	10
Standardised ratio**	99	103	59	106
Standard error of the ratio	10.0	6.5	14.0	9.3
Base = 100%	*486*	*577*	*133*	*404*

* Excludes members of the Armed Forces, persons in inadequately described occupations and persons who have never worked.

† Calculations of the expected numbers used age-specific rates for having self-reported good general health for all men and all women. The age-groups used were 16–24, 25–34, 35–44 and 45–54.

**The standardised ratio is given as the observed rate divided by the expected rate and the ratio multiplied by 100. A 2-tailed test was used to show whether the ratio was significantly different from 100. The resulting figure was multiplied by the square root of the mean of the weight to allow for weighting.

Table 6.4 Number of sexual partners in the last 12 months by marital status, age and sex
Adults aged 16–54

	Men					Women				
Marital status	Single	Married	Co-habiting	Widowed, divorced or separated	Total	Single	Married	Co-habiting	Widowed, divorced or separated	Total
Age and number of sexual partners in the last 12 months	%	%	%	%	%	%	%	%	%	%
16–34										
None	5	2	28	[2]	17	3	-	22	13	12
One	91	80	33	[6]	57	95	94	50	55	72
Two or more	4	17	39	[8]	25	2	6	28	32	16
35–54										
None	6	4	41	33	12	5	1	47	43	12
One	91	92	34	39	81	94	97	45	44	84
Two or more	3	4	25	27	8	1	2	8	14	3
All										
None	6	3	30	31	14	4	1	25	34	12
One	91	84	33	39	69	94	95	49	47	78
Two or more	3	13	37	30	16	2	4	26	19	10
Bases = 100%										
16–34	212	85	324	16	637	293	110	341	79	823
35–54	473	47	108	110	738	555	68	81	189	893
All	685	132	432	126	1375	848	178	422	268	1716
Median	1	1	2	1	1	1	1	1	1	1
95th percentile	1	3	7	5	4	1	1	4	3	2
Base = 100%[†]	650	128	306	89	1173	810	177	315	182	1484

[†] Excludes respondents who did not report a sexual partner in the last year.

Table 6.5 Age-standardised ratios for reporting two or more sexual partners in the last year by marital status and sex
Adults aged 16–54

Marital status	Married	Co-habiting	Single	Widowed, divorced or separated
Reported two or more sexual partners in the last year				
Men				
Observed %	3	13	37	31
Expected %*	10	17	27	8
Standardised ratio†	33**	73	135**	363**
Standard error of the ratio	3.7	10.1	3.5	36.9
Base = 100%	685	132	432	126
Women				
Observed %	2	4	26	19
Expected %*	6	11	20	5
Standardised ratio†	28**	37**	133**	363**
Standard error of the ratio	4.7	9.2	4.4	33.5
Base = 100%	040	178	422	268

* Calculations of the expected numbers used age-specific rates for having self-reported good general health for all men and all women. The age-groups used were 16–24, 25–34, 35–44 and 45–54.
† The standardised ratio is given as the observed rate divided by the expected rate and the ratio multiplied by 100. A 2-tailed test was used to show whether the ratio was significantly different from 100. The resulting figure was multiplied by the square root of the mean of the weight to allow for weighting.
**Significant at the 95% level.

Table 6.6 Respondents' assessment of the likelihood of 'someone like me getting HIV (the AIDS virus)' by age and sex
Adults aged 16–54

Age	16–24	25–34	35–44	45–54	Total	Total HEMS 1995
Likelihood of 'someone like me getting HIV (the AIDS virus)'	%	%	%	%	%	%
Men						
Very high	3	2	2	3	2	3
Quite high	21	6	3	3	8	8
Low	51	59	59	48	55	60
No risk	15	28	31	43	30	25
Don't know	11	5	5	3	6	5
Base = 100%	*222*	*426*	*393*	*358*	*1399*	*1429*
Women						
Very high	3	4	1	3	3	2
Quite high	11	4	2	2	5	7
Low	62	62	55	48	57	59
No risk	14	25	37	44	31	28
Don't know	10	5	5	3	5	4
Base = 100%	*262*	*577*	*524*	*375*	*1738*	*1721*
All						
Very high	3	3	2	3	3	3
Quite high	16	5	3	2	6	7
Low	56	61	57	48	56	59
No risk	14	27	34	44	30	26
Don't know	11	5	5	3	6	4
Base = 100%	*484*	*1003*	*917*	*733*	*3137*	*3150*

Health in England 1996 : What people know, what people think, what people do

Table 6.7 Respondents' assessment of the likelihood of 'someone like me getting another sexually transmitted disease' by age and sex
Adults aged 16–54

Age	16–24	25–34	35–44	45–54	Total	Total HEMS 1995
Likelihood of 'someone like me getting another sexually transmitted disease'	%	%	%	%	%	%
Men						
Very high	3	2	1	2	2	3
Quite high	21	6	2	2	7	7
Low	51	56	56	50	53	61
No risk	16	33	38	42	33	26
Don't know	9	3	3	4	5	3
Base = 100%	222	426	393	358	1399	1431
Women						
Very high	3	3	1	1	2	2
Quite high	13	3	2	2	5	6
Low	60	59	57	45	56	58
No risk	16	32	38	51	34	31
Don't know	7	3	3	2	4	4
Base = 100%	262	577	524	375	1738	1722
All						
Very high	3	2	1	1	2	2
Quite high	17	5	2	2	6	6
Low	55	57	56	48	54	60
No risk	16	32	38	46	34	28
Don't know	8	3	3	3	4	3
Base = 100%	484	1003	917	733	3137	3153

Table 6.8 Respondents' assessment of the likelihood of 'someone like me getting HIV (the AIDS virus)' by marital status and sex
Adults aged 16–54

Marital status	Single	Married	Cohabiting	Widowed, divorced or separated	Total
Likelihood of 'someone like me getting HIV (the AIDS virus)'	%	%	%	%	%
Men					
Very high	2	3	3	2	2
Quite high	2	5	17	9	8
Low	53	52	57	55	55
No risk	39	34	12	28	30
Don't know	3	6	10	6	6
Bases = 100%	*694*	*133*	*445*	*127*	*1399*
Women					
Very high	2	1	5	4	3
Quite high	2	5	9	7	5
Low	51	67	65	54	57
No risk	40	23	14	31	31
Don't know	5	4	8	5	5
Bases = 100%	*854*	*180*	*430*	*274*	*1738*

Table 6.9 Respondents' assessment of the likelihood of 'someone like me getting another sexually transmitted disease' by marital status and sex
Adults aged 16–54

Marital status	Single	Married	Cohabiting	Widowed, divorced or separated	Total
Likelihood of 'someone like me getting another sexually transmitted disease'	%	%	%	%	%
Men					
Very high	1	2	3	4	2
Quite high	2	6	17	7	7
Low	49	57	58	60	53
No risk	46	31	14	24	33
Don't know	3	4	8	5	5
Base = 100%	*694*	*133*	*445*	*127*	*1399*
Women					
Very high	1	1	4	3	2
Quite high	1	3	11	6	5
Low	51	64	62	56	56
No risk	44	30	17	31	34
Don't know	3	2	6	4	4
Base = 100%	*854*	*180*	*430*	*274*	*1738*

Table 6.10 Respondents' assessment of the likelihood of 'someone like me getting HIV (the AIDS virus)' by number of sexual partners in the last 12 months and sex
Adults aged 16–54

Number of sexual partners in the last 12 months	Never had a sexual partner	No sexual partner in the last 12 months	One	Two or more	Total
Likelihood of 'someone like me getting HIV (the AIDS virus)'	%	%	%	%	%
Men					
Very high	-	3	2	6	2
Quite high	15	6	4	20	8
Low	48	52	55	56	55
No risk	25	28	35	11	30
Don't know	13	11	4	8	6
Bases = 100%	*84*	*118*	*933*	*239*	*1374*
Women					
Very high	2	2	2	5	2
Quite high	5	1	4	15	5
Low	47	51	58	63	57
No risk	27	41	32	10	31
Don't know	19	5	4	7	5
Bases = 100%	*63*	*168*	*1311*	*172*	*1714*

Table 6.11 Respondents' assessment of the likelihood of 'someone like me getting another sexually transmitted disease' by number of sexual partners in the last 12 months and sex
Adults aged 16–54

Number of sexual partners in the last 12 months	Never had a sexual partner	No sexual partner in the last 12 months	One	Two or more	Total
Likelihood of 'someone like me getting another sexually transmitted disease'	%	%	%	%	%
Men					
Very high	3	1	1	4	2
Quite high	14	4	3	23	7
Low	43	53	53	58	53
No risk	30	28	39	10	33
Don't know	10	14	3	5	4
Bases = 100%	*84*	*118*	*933*	*239*	*1374*
Women					
Very high	1	2	1	6	2
Quite high	9	1	3	18	5
Low	41	47	56	66	56
No risk	32	48	36	10	34
Don't know	17	2	3	1	3
Bases = 100%	*63*	*168*	*1311*	*172*	*1714*

Table 6.12 Age-standardised ratios for likelihood of 'someone like me getting HIV (the AIDS virus)' by number of sexual partners in the last 12 months and sex
Adults aged 16–54

Number of sexual partners in the last 12 months	Never had a sexual partner	No partner in the last 12 months	One	Two or more
Likelihood of 'someone like me getting HIV (the AIDS virus)'*	%	%	%	%
Men				
Observed %	15	8	6	26
Expected %†	18	7	8	15
Standardised ratio**	83	114	72 ††	175 ††
Standard error of the ratio	11.3	24.1	4.3	10.8
Base = 100%	84	118	933	239
Women				
Observed %	7	3	6	20
Expected %†	10	6	7	10
Standardised ratio**	72	56	88	192 ††
Standard error of the ratio	21.6	18.9	4.1	19.6
Base = 100%	63	168	1311	172

* Respondents assessing themselves as 'very likely' or 'quite likely' to get HIV (the AIDS) virus.
† Calculations of the expected numbers used age-specific rates for having self-reported good general health for all men and all women. The age-groups used were 16–24, 25–34, 35–44 and 45–54.
**The standardised ratio is given as the observed rate divided by the expected rate and the ratio multiplied by 100. A 2-tailed test was used to show whether the ratio was significantly different from 100. The resulting figure was multiplied by the square root of the mean of the weight to allow for weighting.
†† Significant at the 95% level.

Table 6.13 Age-standardised ratios for likelihood of 'someone like me getting another sexually transmitted disease' by number of sexual partners in the last 12 months and sex
Adults aged 16–54

Number of sexual partners in the last 12 months	Never had a sexual partner	No partner in the last 12 months	One	Two or more
Likelihood of 'someone like me getting another sexually transmitted disease'*	%	%	%	%
Men				
Observed %	17	4	4	28
Expected %†	19	6	7	15
Standardised ratio**	90	72	62 ††	187 ††
Standard error of the ratio	11.2	21.6	4.8	11.6
Base = 100%	84	118	933	239
Women				
Observed %	11	3	5	23
Expected %†	11	5	6	11
Standardised ratio**	101	64	78 ††	205 ††
Standard error of the ratio	22.6	22.9	4.6	19.3
Base = 100%	63	168	1311	172

* Respondents assessing themselves as 'very likely' or 'quite likely' to get another sexually transmitted disease.
† Calculations of the expected numbers used age-specific rates for having self-reported good general health for all men and all women. The age-groups used were 16–24, 25–34, 35–44 and 45–54.
**The standardised ratio is given as the observed rate divided by the expected rate and the ratio multiplied by 100. A 2-tailed test was used to show whether the ratio was significantly different from 100. The resulting figure was multiplied by the square root of the mean of the weight to allow for weighting.
†† Significant at the 95% level.

Table 6.14 Whether would find it difficult to raise the subject of using a condom with a new partner by age and sex
Adults aged 16–54

Age	16–24	25–34	35–44	45–54	Total	Total HEMS 1995
Whether would find it difficult	%	%	%	%	%	%
Men						
Strongly agrees	4	5	7	9	6	5
Agrees	10	9	10	9	10	12
Neither agrees nor disagrees	16	20	17	23	19	22
Disagrees	47	46	49	46	47	53
Strongly disagrees	23	20	17	12	18	9
Base = 100%	222	425	388	353	1388	1428
Women						
Strongly agrees	3	7	8	11	7	6
Agrees	10	12	12	14	12	11
Neither agrees nor disagrees	6	14	12	17	13	21
Disagrees	50	42	46	41	45	50
Strongly disagrees	30	24	21	16	23	12
Base = 100%	261	574	520	365	1720	1718
All						
Strongly agrees	4	6	7	10	7	5
Agrees	10	10	11	12	11	12
Neither agrees nor disagrees	11	17	15	20	16	21
Disagrees	48	45	47	44	46	51
Strongly disagrees	26	22	19	14	20	10
Base = 100%	483	999	908	718	3108	3146

Table 6.15 Percentage 'strongly agreeing' or 'agreeing' that 'it would be difficult to raise the subject of using a condom with a new partner' by selected characteristics
Adults aged 16–54

	Men	Women	All	Men	Women	All
	\multicolumn{3}{c|}{Percentage agreeing}	\multicolumn{3}{c}{Base = 100%}
Characteristic						
Social class*						
I & II	11	13	12	554	487	1041
III (NM)	13	19	17	134	581	715
III (M)	20	16	19	343	133	476
IV & V	23	24	24	242	402	644
Marital status						
Married	16	21	18	684	837	1521
Cohabiting	19	17	18	133	180	313
Single	14	16	15	445	430	875
Widowed, divorced or separated	19	25	23	126	273	399
Highest qualification level						
'A' level or above	10	13	11	635	572	1207
Other qualifications	18	19	19	514	777	1291
No qualifications	26	31	29	235	370	605
Number of sexual partners						
Never had a sexual partner	21	29	24	84	63	147
None in the last year	32	24	28	117	165	282
One	14	19	17	925	1299	2224
Two or more	14	13	13	239	172	411
All	16	20	18	1388	1720	3108

* Members of the Armed Forces, persons in inadequately described occupations and persons who have never worked are not shown as separate categories but are included in the figures for all persons.

Table 6.16 Whether would use a condom if 'in the near future they did have sex with a new partner' by age and sex
Adults aged 16–54

Age	16–24	25–34	35–44	45–54	Total	Total HEMS 1995
Whether would use a condom	%	%	%	%	%	%
Men						
Would always use a condom	65	60	55	51	58	54
It would depend	32	30	33	30	31	34
Would never use a condom	1	1	1	3	1	2
Wouldn't contemplate having sex	3	10	10	17	10	11
Base = 100%	*222*	*426*	*390*	*354*	*1392*	*1421*
Women						
Would always use a condom	75	71	65	56	67	64
It would depend	20	16	18	13	17	18
Would never use a condom	-	1	1	2	1	1
Wouldn't contemplate having sex	6	11	16	28	15	18
Base = 100%	*261*	*574*	*522*	*372*	*1729*	*1716*
All						
Would always use a condom	70	65	60	53	62	59
It would depend	26	23	26	22	24	25
Would never use a condom	0	1	1	2	1	1
Wouldn't contemplate having sex	4	10	13	22	13	14
Base = 100%	*483*	*1000*	*912*	*726*	*3121*	*3137*

Table 6.17 Whether would use a condom with a new partner by number of sexual partners in the last 12 months and sex
Adults aged 16–54

Number of sexual partners in the last 12 months	Never had a sexual partner	No sexual partner in the last 12 months	One	Two or more	Total
Whether would use a condom	%	%	%	%	%
Men					
Would always use a condom	73	57	56	57	58
It would depend	17	37	30	41	31
Would never use a condom	-	2	1	2	1
Wouldn't contemplate having sex	10	4	13	1	10
Base = 100%	*83*	*116*	*930*	*239*	*1368*
Women					
Would always use a condom	58	71	67	66	67
It would depend	21	16	15	30	17
Would never use a condom	2	-	1	2	1
Wouldn't contemplate having sex	18	13	16	2	15
Base = 100%	*63*	*168*	*1305*	*172*	*1708*

Table 6.18 Whether would use a condom with a new partner by whether would find it difficult to raise the subject of using a condom with a new partner, and sex
Adults aged 16–54

Whether would find it difficult to raise the subject of using a condom	Agree	Disagree	Neither agree nor disagree	Total
Whether would use a condom with a new partner	%	%	%	%
Men				
Would always use a condom	58	64	38	58
It would depend	30	29	38	31
Would never use a condom	3	1	2	1
Wouldn't contemplate having sex	9	6	21	10
Base = 100%	*218*	*902*	*266*	*1386*
Women				
Would always use a condom	56	74	48	67
It would depend	22	15	20	17
Would never use a condom	2	0	4	1
Wouldn't contemplate having sex	20	11	28	15
Base = 100%	*333*	*1159*	*226*	*1718*

Table 6.19 Percentage using a condom with a new partner by selected characteristics
Adults aged 16–54, reporting a new partner in the last year

	Men	Women	All	Men	Women	All
Characteristic	Percentage using a condom with a new partner			Base = 100%		
Age						
16–24	66	75	70	109	94	203
25–34	58	59	59	109	102	211
35–44	58	48	53	56	63	119
45–54	44	[12]	41	41	28	69
Social class*						
I & II	63	60	62	105	75	180
III (NM)	70	71	71	34	98	132
III (M)	48	[12]	51	80	21	101
IV & V	59	56	58	66	62	128
Marital status						
Married	42	51	45	42	30	72
Cohabiting	[10]	[10]	43	25	22	47
Single	69	73	71	198	152	350
Widowed, divorced or separated	47	45	46	50	83	133
Highest qualification level						
'A' level or above	65	69	67	144	114	258
Other qualifications	58	60	59	132	131	263
No qualifications	52	56	54	39	42	81
Number of sexual partners in the last year						
One	58	58	58	117	140	257
Two or more	62	69	65	198	146	344
Whether would use a condom with a new partner						
Would always use a condom	79	80	79	175	176	351
It would depend	40	31	37	124	89	213
Never	–	–	–	6	5	11
Wouldn't contemplate having sex	–	[7]	[7]	9	17	26
Whether would find it difficult to raise the subject of using a condom with a new partner						
Agree	47	37	42	43	49	92
Disagree	68	73	70	231	212	443
Neither agree nor disagree	37	[6]	32	40	26	66
All	60	63	62	315	287	602
All : 1995	66	55	61	296	283	579

* Members of the Armed Forces, persons in inadequately described occupations and persons who have never worked are not shown as separate categories but are included in the figures for all persons.

Table 7.1 Number of occasions of sunburn in the 12 months prior to interview by age and sex
Adults aged 16–74

Age	16–24	25–34	35–44	45–54	55–64	65–74	Total	Total HEMS 1995
Number of occasions of sunburn in the last 12 months	%	%	%	%	%	%	%	%
Men								
Sunburnt in last 12 months:	40	37	30	27	19	12	29	26
Once	24	22	20	17	10	6	17	17
Twice	9	9	7	6	5	4	7	5
Three times	4	3	1	3	2	1	2	2
Four or more	2	3	2	2	2	1	2	2
Not sunburnt	60	63	70	73	81	88	71	73
Can't remember	-	-	-	0	0	0	0	0
Base = 100%	224	436	396	368	308	310	2042	2120
Women								
Sunburnt in last 12 months:	43	34	23	16	13	4	23	22
Once	22	20	16	12	9	4	15	17
Twice	13	8	5	3	3	0	5	4
Three times	4	2	0	1	1	0	1	1
Four or more	4	4	1	1	1	0	2	1
Not sunburnt	57	66	77	84	87	95	77	78
Can't remember	-	-	0	-	-	0	0	0
Base = 100%	266	585	533	392	362	461	2599	2548
All								
Sunburnt in last 12 months:	41	35	26	22	16	8	26	24
Once	23	21	18	14	9	5	16	17
Twice	11	8	6	4	4	2	6	4
Three times	4	2	1	2	1	1	2	2
Four or more	3	3	2	1	1	1	2	1
None	59	65	74	78	84	92	74	75
Can't remember	-	-	0	0	0	0	0	0
Base = 100%	490	1021	929	760	670	771	4641	4668

* HEMS 1995 data was presented differently in the 1995 report.

Table 7.2 Number of occasions of sunburn in the 12 months prior to interview by social class based on own current or last job and sex
Adults aged 16–74

Social class	I & II	III(NM)	III(M)	IV & V	Total[†]
Number of occasions of sunburn in the last 12 months	%	%	%	%	%
Men					
Sunburnt in last 12 months:	26	35	33	28	29
Once	16	23	19	16	17
Twice	6	10	9	6	7
Three times	2	1	1	4	2
Four or more	2	2	3	2	2
Not sunburnt	74	64	67	72	71
Can't remember	0	0	-	-	0
Base = 100%	782	195	561	367	2041
Women					
Sunburnt in last 12 months:	23	26	16	21	23
Once	15	15	11	14	15
Twice	5	7	0	5	5
Three times	1	1	4	1	1
Four or more	2	2	1	1	2
Not sunburnt	77	74	84	79	77
Can't remember	0	-	-	-	0
Base = 100%	677	862	224	680	2597
All					
Sunburnt in last 12 months:	25	28	29	24	26
Once	16	17	17	15	16
Twice	6	8	7	5	6
Three times	2	1	2	2	2
Four or more	2	2	3	1	2
Not sunburnt	75	72	71	76	74
Can't remember	0	0	-	-	0
Base = 100%	1459	1057	785	1047	4638

* Members of the Armed Forces, persons in inadequately described occupations and persons who have never worked are not shown as separate categories but are included in the figures for all persons.

Table 7.3 Skin type by sex
Adults aged 16–74

Sex	Men	Women	All
Skin type	%	%	%
Always burns and never tans	8	14	11
Burns at first and tans with difficulty	18	23	21
Burns at first then tans easily	31	28	29
Rarely burns and tans easily	29	23	26
Never burns and always tans	11	9	10
Other	3	4	3
Refused	0	0	0
Base = 100%	2032	2583	4615

Table 7.4 Number of occasions of sunburn in the 12 months prior to interview by skin type and sex
Adults aged 16–74

Skin type Number of occasions of sunburn in the last 12 months	Always burns and never tans %	Burns at first and tans with difficulty %	Burns at first then tans easily %	Rarely burns and tans easily %	Never burns and always tans %	Other %	Total %
Men							
Sunburnt in last 12 months:	48	40	37	21	3	3	29
Once	25	24	21	15	3	3	18
Twice	13	9	10	4	-	-	7
Three times	7	3	3	1	-	-	2
Four or more times	3	3	3	2	0	-	2
Not sunburnt	52	60	63	79	97	97	71
Can't remember	-	0	0	0	-	-	0
Base = 100%	*160*	*358*	*639*	*604*	*214*	*56*	*2032*
Women							
Sunburnt in last 12 months:	26	32	32	14	1	7	23
Once	14	18	22	11	1	6	15
Twice	9	9	6	2	-	1	5
Three times	2	2	1	0	-	-	1
Four or more times	2	3	3	0	-	-	2
Not sunburnt	74	68	68	86	99	93	77
Can't remember	-	0	0	-	-	-	0
Base = 100%	*354*	*572*	*716*	*599*	*240*	*100*	*2582*
All							
Sunburnt in last 12 months:	34	36	35	18	2	5	26
Once	18	21	21	13	2	4	16
Twice	10	9	8	3	-	1	6
Three times	4	3	2	1	-	-	2
Four or more times	2	3	3	1	0	-	2
Not sunburnt	66	64	65	82	98	95	74
Can't remember	-	0	0	0	-	-	0
Base = 100%	*514*	*930*	*1355*	*1203*	*454*	*156*	*4614*

Health in England 1996 : What people know, what people think, what people do

Table 7.5 Occasions on which respondents use suncream by age and sex
Adults aged 16-74

Age	16-24	25-34	35-44	45-54	55-64	65-74	Total	Total HEMS 1995
Occasions on which respondents use suncream				Percentage using a suncream				
Men								
Uses suncream:	61	68	70	65	53	39	61	61
Sunbathing abroad	44	50	46	44	32	17	41	39
Outdoors abroad, but not sunbathing	30	29	32	27	18	16	27	32
Sunbathing in this country	36	38	40	34	24	12	32	25
Outdoors in this country doing something else	27	29	30	23	23	21	26	26
Does not use suncream	39	31	30	34	46	59	38	38
Never goes out in the sun	0	1	0	1	1	3	1	1
Base = 100%	*224*	*435*	*396*	*368*	*308*	*310*	*2041*	*2115*
Women								
Uses suncream:	77	83	82	79	67	48	74	76
Sunbathing abroad	56	58	52	49	34	19	47	44
Outdoors abroad, but not sunbathing	42	40	38	36	26	21	35	41
Sunbathing in this country	52	59	60	53	35	19	49	43
Outdoors in this country doing something else	34	43	43	40	37	25	38	43
Does not use suncream	23	16	17	17	30	45	23	21
Never goes out in the sun	0	1	1	3	3	8	2	3
Base =100%	*266*	*586*	*533*	*392*	*362*	*461*	*2600*	*2547*
All								
Uses suncream:	69	75	76	72	60	44	68	69
Sunbathing abroad	50	54	49	46	33	18	44	41
Outdoors abroad, but not sunbathing	36	35	35	31	22	18	31	36
Sunbathing in this country	44	48	51	43	29	16	41	34
Outdoors in this country doing something else	30	36	37	31	30	23	32	34
Does not use suncream	31	24	23	26	38	51	30	29
Never goes out in the sun	0	1	1	2	2	5	2	2
Base = 100%	*490*	*1021*	*929*	*760*	*670*	*771*	*4641*	*4662*

Totals add to more than 100 because respondents could have given more than one answer.

* HEMS 1995 data was presented differently in the 1995 report.

Table 7.6 Occasions on which respondents use suncream by social class based on own current or last job, and sex
Adults aged 16–74

Social class	I & II	III(NM)	III(M)	IV & V	Total*
Occasion on which respondents use suncream			Percentage using a suncream		
Men					
Uses suncream:	72	65	55	51	61
Sunbathing abroad	49	46	36	29	41
Outdoors abroad, but not sunbathing	35	32	20	14	27
Sunbathing in this country	41	35	26	25	32
Outdoors in this country doing something else	31	27	22	20	26
Does not use suncream	27	34	45	48	38
Never goes out in the sun	1	0	0	1	1
Base = 100%	*782*	*195*	*561*	*366*	*2040*
Women					
Uses suncream:	84	79	66	64	74
Sunbathing abroad	58	51	40	33	47
Outdoors abroad, but not sunbathing	48	36	25	25	35
Sunbathing in this country	55	54	43	40	49
Outdoors in this country doing something else	44	39	33	32	38
Does not use suncream	14	18	31	34	23
Never goes out in the sun	2	3	3	3	2
Base = 100%	*677*	*862*	*224*	*680*	*2598*
All					
Uses suncream:	77	76	58	58	68
Sunbathing abroad	53	50	37	31	44
Outdoors abroad, but not sunbathing	40	35	21	20	31
Sunbathing in this country	47	50	30	34	41
Outdoors in this country doing something else	36	36	25	27	32
Does not use suncream	22	21	41	40	30
Never goes out in the sun	1	2	1	2	2
Base = 100%	*1459*	*1057*	*785*	*1046*	*4638*

Totals add to more than 100 because respondents could have given more than one answer.

* Members of the Armed Forces, persons in inadequately described occupations and persons who have never worked are not shown as separate categories but are included in the figures for all persons.

Table 7.7 Factor level of suncream used by age and sex
Adults aged 16–74

Age	16–24	25–34	35–44	45–54	55–64	65–74	Total	Total HEMS 1995
Factor levels of suncream used	%	%	%	%	%	%	%	%
Men								
2–5	7	12	9	9	8	4	9	11
6–10	25	24	27	21	18	11	22	22
11–16	16	16	19	14	9	7	14	13
17 or over	8	8	7	10	7	6	8	6
Don't know	5	8	8	11	11	9	9	10
Does not use suncream	39	32	30	35	46	60	38	38
Never goes out in the sun	0	1	0	1	1	3	1	1
Base = 100%	*223*	*432*	*395*	*361*	*308*	*307*	*2026*	*2107*
Women								
2–5	14	11	13	11	14	6	12	12
6–10	27	35	29	30	22	14	27	29
11–16	23	21	23	24	18	11	20	18
17 or over	10	13	14	10	8	5	10	10
Don't know	4	3	3	4	6	11	5	7
Does not use suncream	23	16	17	17	30	45	23	21
Never goes out in the sun	0	1	1	3	3	8	3	3
Base = 100%	*266*	*584*	*532*	*391*	*359*	*458*	*2590*	*2545*
All								
2–5	10	12	11	10	11	5	10	11
6–10	26	29	28	25	20	13	24	25
11–16	19	18	21	19	13	9	17	15
17 or over	9	10	10	10	7	6	9	8
Don't know	4	6	6	8	9	10	7	8
Does not use suncream	31	24	23	27	38	52	31	29
Never goes out in the sun	0	1	1	2	2	5	2	2
Base = 100%	*489*	*1016*	*927*	*752*	*667*	*765*	*4616*	*4652*

* HEMS 1995 data was presented differently in the 1995 report.

Table 7.8 Factor level of suncream used by sex
Adults aged 16–74 who used a suncream

Sex	Men	Women	All
Factor levels of suncream used	%	%	%
2–5	14	16	15
6–10	35	36	36
11–16	23	27	26
17 or over	13	14	13
Don't know	14	7	10
Base = 100%	*1193*	*1849*	*3042*

Table 7.9 Factor level of suncream used by skin type and sex
Adults aged 16–74

Skin type Factor level of suncream used	Always burns and never tans %	Burns at first and tans with difficulty %	Burns at first then tans easily %	Rarely burns and tans easily %	Never burns and always tans %	Other %	Total %
Men							
2–5	4	4	13	11	5	-	9
6–10	16	24	29	21	8	10	22
11–16	17	22	15	12	8	2	14
17 or over	18	11	9	4	4	2	8
Don't know	8	10	11	7	5	6	9
Does not use suncream	33	28	24	44	69	79	38
Never goes out in the sun	3	1	1	0	1	2	1
Base = 100%	*159*	*354*	*633*	*599*	*214*	*56*	*2016*
Women							
2–5	2	8	15	20	9	5	12
6–10	15	32	36	27	13	10	27
11–16	25	26	24	15	9	9	21
17 or over	19	15	10	4	5	10	10
Don't know	6	4	3	6	6	10	5
Does not use suncream	25	13	11	27	57	53	23
Never goes out in the sun	6	3	1	2	1	3	2
Base = 100%	*354*	*568*	*716*	*596*	*238*	*100*	*2573*
All							
2–5	3	6	14	15	7	3	10
6–10	16	28	32	23	10	10	24
11–16	22	24	19	13	8	6	17
17 or over	19	13	9	4	4	7	9
Don't know	7	7	7	7	5	8	7
Does not use suncream	28	20	18	37	64	65	30
Never goes out in the sun	5	2	1	1	1	2	2
Base = 100%	*513*	*922*	*1349*	*1195*	*452*	*156*	*4589*

Health in England 1996 : What people know, what people think, what people do

Table 7.10 Whether sunburnt in the last 12 months by whether uses a suncream or not and sex
Adults aged 16–74

Whether uses a suncream	Yes	No	Never go out in the sun	Total
Whether sunburnt in the last 12 months				
Men				
Yes	34	21	[3]	29
No	66	79	[20]	71
Can't remember	0	0	[1]	0
Base = 100%	1209	809	24	2042
Women				
Yes	27	12	3	23
No	73	88	97	77
Can't remember	0	0	0	0
Base = 100%	1859	665	76	2600
All				
Yes	30	17	5	26
No	69	82	94	74
Can't remember	0	0	1	0
Base = 100%	3068	1474	100	4642

Table 7.11 Whether having a suntan is important by age and sex
Adults aged 16–74

Age	16–24	25–34	35–44	45–54	55–64	65–74	Total	Total HEMS 1995
Respondents' attitudes towards the importance of having a suntan	%	%	%	%	%	%	%	%
Men								
Important	24	22	18	22	16	14	20	23
Not important	76	78	81	78	84	86	80	77
Don't know	-	0	0	-	0	0	0	0
Base = 100%	193	379	347	328	275	277	1799	1934
Women								
Important	44	38	32	29	23	12	31	32
Not important	56	62	67	71	76	88	69	67
Don't know	0	-	0	-	0	1	0	0
Base = 100%	232	525	478	358	328	426	2347	2363
All								
Important	34	30	26	26	20	13	25	28
Not important	66	70	74	74	80	87	74	72
Don't know	0	0	0	-	0	0	0	0
Base = 100%	425	904	825	686	603	703	4146	4297

Table 7.12 Whether agrees that 'having a suntan makes me feel healthier' by age and sex
Adults aged 16–74

Age	16–24	25–34	35–44	45–54	55–64	65–74	Total
Whether agrees that 'having a suntan makes me feel healthier'	%	%	%	%	%	%	%
Men							
Agrees	40	45	41	44	39	31	41
Disagrees	39	36	40	41	44	50	41
Neither agrees nor disagrees	21	20	19	16	16	19	18
Base = 100%	193	379	347	328	274	277	1798
Women							
Agrees	54	58	56	49	40	26	49
Disagrees	29	32	30	37	49	63	38
Neither agrees nor disagrees	17	11	14	14	11	11	13
Base = 100%	233	524	478	358	328	425	2346
All							
Agrees	47	51	49	46	40	28	45
Disagrees	34	34	35	39	47	57	40
Neither agrees nor disagrees	19	15	16	15	13	15	16
Base = 100%	426	903	825	686	602	702	4144

Table 7.13 Whether agrees that 'having a suntan makes me feel healthier' by social class based on own current or last job, and sex
Adults aged 16–74

Social class	I & II	III(NM)	III(M)	IV & V	Total[*]
Whether agrees that 'having a suntan makes me feel healthier'	%	%	%	%	%
Men					
Agrees	44	47	41	35	41
Disagrees	34	33	47	49	41
Neither agrees nor disagrees	22	21	12	15	18
Base = 100%	696	172	485	326	1797
Women					
Agrees	51	52	43	41	49
Disagrees	35	35	42	47	38
Neither agrees nor disagrees	14	13	15	11	13
Base = 100%	611	802	203	598	2344
All					
Agrees	47	51	41	39	45
Disagrees	34	34	46	48	40
Neither agrees nor disagrees	19	15	13	13	16
Base = 100%	1307	974	688	924	4141

* Members of the Armed Forces, persons in inadequately described occupations and persons who have never worked are not shown as separate categories but are included in the figures for all persons.

Table 7.14 Whether agrees that 'having a suntan makes me look more attractive' by age and sex
Adults aged 16–74

Age	16–24	25–34	35–44	45–54	55–64	65–74	Total
Whether agrees that 'having a suntan makes me look more attractive'	%	%	%	%	%	%	%
Men							
Agrees	47	46	43	36	37	27	40
Disagrees	24	28	32	36	37	50	34
Neither agrees nor disagrees	29	26	25	27	26	24	26
Base = 100%	*193*	*379*	*347*	*328*	*273*	*275*	*1795*
Women							
Agrees	51	54	54	55	45	30	49
Disagrees	32	29	28	26	39	53	33
Neither agrees nor disagrees	17	17	18	19	16	17	17
Base = 100%	*233*	*524*	*478*	*358*	*327*	*424*	*2344*
All							
Agrees	49	50	49	45	41	28	45
Disagrees	28	29	30	31	38	51	33
Neither agrees nor disagrees	23	21	21	23	21	20	22
Base = 100%	*426*	*903*	*825*	*686*	*600*	*699*	*4139*

Table 7.15 Whether agrees that 'having a suntan makes me look more attractive' by social class based on own current or last job, and sex
Adults aged 16–74

Social class	I & II	III(NM)	III(M)	IV & V	Total[*]
Whether agrees that 'having a suntan makes me look more attractive'	%	%	%	%	%
Men					
Agrees	43	42	39	35	40
Disagrees	28	33	39	40	34
Neither agrees nor disagrees	29	26	22	26	26
Base = 100%	*695*	*172*	*484*	*325*	*1794*
Women					
Agrees	55	51	44	41	49
Disagrees	26	32	41	42	33
Neither agrees nor disagrees	19	17	15	17	17
Base = 100%	*611*	*801*	*203*	*598*	*2342*
All					
Agrees	48	49	40	38	45
Disagrees	27	32	40	41	33
Neither agrees nor disagrees	25	19	20	21	22
Base = 100%	*1306*	*973*	*687*	*923*	*4136*

* Members of the Armed Forces, persons in inadequately described occupations and persons who have never worked are not shown as separate categories but are included in the figures for all persons.

Table 7.16 Whether agrees that 'having a suntan makes me look more attractive' by skin type and sex
Adults aged 16–74

Skin type	Always burns and never tans	Burns at first and tans with difficulty	Burns at first then tans easily	Rarely burns and tans easily	Never burns and always tans	Other	Total
Whether agrees that 'having a suntan makes me look more attractive'	%	%	%	%	%	%	%
Men							
Agrees	28	42	46	38	36	21	40
Disagrees	56	31	29	31	38	54	34
Neither agrees nor disagrees	16	27	25	31	26	25	26
Base = 100%	*158*	*348*	*584*	*514*	*149*	*33*	*1786*
Women							
Agrees	33	50	60	48	47	34	49
Disagrees	55	31	23	33	34	43	33
Neither agrees nor disagrees	13	19	17	19	20	23	17
Base = 100%	*350*	*561*	*674*	*504*	*155*	*88*	*2332*
All							
Agrees	31	47	53	43	41	29	45
Disagrees	55	31	26	32	36	47	33
Neither agrees nor disagrees	14	22	21	25	23	24	22
Base = 100%	*508*	*909*	*1258*	*1018*	*304*	*121*	*4118*

Table 8.1 Self-reported general health by sex and age
Adults aged 16–74

Age	16–24	25–34	35–44	45–54	55–64	65–74	Total	Total HEMS 1995
Self-reported general health	%	%	%	%	%	%	%	%
Men								
Very good	37	46	41	36	30	27	37	36
Good	48	41	45	44	40	38	43	42
Fair	14	12	12	12	21	28	15	17
Bad	1	1	2	5	7	6	3	3
Very bad	-	1	1	3	2	1	1	1
Base = 100%	224	436	394	367	308	309	2038	2121
Women								
Very good	34	43	41	35	29	26	36	35
Good	48	42	42	44	39	39	42	42
Fair	15	12	13	16	22	29	17	18
Bad	2	2	3	4	9	6	4	4
Very bad	1	0	0	1	2	1	1	1
Base = 100%	266	586	533	392	361	460	2598	2548
All								
Very good	35	45	41	36	29	27	37	36
Good	48	41	43	44	39	39	43	42
Fair	15	12	12	14	22	28	16	18
Bad	2	2	3	5	8	6	4	4
Very bad	0	0	1	2	2	1	1	1
Base = 100%	490	1022	927	759	669	769	4636	4669

Table 8.2 Self-reported general health by social class based on own current or last job, age and sex
Adults aged 16–74

Social class	I & II	III(NM)	III(M)	IV & V	Total†
Age	\multicolumn{5}{c}{Percentage reporting good* general health}
Men					
16–44	89	82	86	78	86
45–64	80	75	74	68	76
65–74	77	74	57	58	66
All	84	80	78	72	80
Bases= 100%					
16–44	393	116	257	186	1053
45–64	277	48	201	118	675
65–74	111	31	103	61	309
All	781	195	561	365	2037
Women					
16–44	90	83	78	80	84
45–64	80	79	72	64	74
65–74	73	69	59	56	64
All	85	80	73	71	78
Bases = 100%					
16–44	386	463	111	314	1385
45–64	195	240	63	226	752
65–74	95	159	50	140	459
All	676	862	224	680	2596

* Respondents were classified as having good health if they reported their general health as 'very good' or 'good'.
† Members of the Armed Forces, persons in inadequately described occupations and persons who have never worked are not shown as separate categories but are included in the figures for all persons.

Table 8.3 Age-standardised ratios for self-reported good* health by social class based on own current or last job and sex
Adults aged 16–74

Social class†	I & II	III(NM)	III(M)	IV & V
Self-reported good health	%	%	%	%
Men				
Observed %	84	80	78	72
Expected %**	80	80	79	80
Standardised ratio††	106***	99	98	91***
Standard error of the ratio	0.9	2.2	1.2	1.7
Base = 100%	781	195	561	365
Women				
Observed %	85	80	73	78
Expected %**	79	78	77	77
Standardised ratio††	107***	102	94	92***
Standard error of the ratio	1.2	1.0	2.7	1.4
Base = 100%	676	862	224	680

* Respondents were classified as having good health if they reported their general health as 'very good' or 'good'.
† Excludes members of the Armed Forces, persons in inadequately described occupations and persons who have never worked.
**Calculations of the expected numbers used age-specific rates for having self-reported good general health for all men and all women. The age-groups used were 16–24, 25–34, 35–44, 45–54, 55–64, and 65–74.
†† The standardised ratio is given as the observed rate divided by the expected rate and the ratio multiplied by 100. A 2-tailed test was used to show whether the ratio was significantly different from 100. The resulting figure was multiplied by the square root of the mean of the weight to allow for weighting.
*** Significant at the 95% level.

Table 8.4 Self-reported long-standing illness or disability by sex and age: HEMS, GHS 1995 and Health Survey 1994
Adults aged 16–74

Age	16–24	25–34	35–44	45–54	55–64	65–74	Total	Total* HEMS 1995
Self-reported general health								
	Percentage with self-reported long-standing illness or disability†							
Men								
HEMS	28	24	29	42	48	53	35	33
GHS 1995	21	21	28	37	51	55	34	34
Health Survey 1994	22	24	34	41	53	62	-	38
Women								
HEMS	24	23	32	40	56	57	37	37
GHS 1995	20	21	25	33	46	54	32	33
Health Survey 1994	25	24	29	40	52	59	-	38
All								
HEMS	26	23	31	41	52	55	36	3
GHS 1995	21	21	27	35	48	54	33	34
Health Survey 1994	24	24	32	41	52	60	-	38
	Percentage with self-reported limiting long-standing illness or disability							
Men								
HEMS	10	10	12	23	30	31	18	18
GHS 1995	8	11	15	22	34	38	20	20
Women								
HEMS	9	12	17	24	36	36	21	20
GHS 1995	11	11	15	21	31	37	20	20
All								
HEMS	10	11	14	23	33	34	19	19
GHS 1995	9	11	15	22	32	37	20	20
Bases = 100%								
Men								
HEMS	224	435	395	368	309	310	2041	2120
GHS	969	1366	1400	1290	1013	859	6897	6818
Health Survey	967	1434	1328	1125	1001	877	-	7209
Women								
HEMS	266	586	533	392	362	461	2600	2547
GHS	922	1636	1399	1384	1069	973	7383	7341
Health Survey	1080	1722	1518	1300	1059	1120	-	8044
All								
HEMS	490	1021	928	760	671	771	4641	4667
GHS	1891	3002	2799	2674	2082	1832	14280	14159
Health Survey	2047	3156	2846	2425	2060	1997	-	15253

* General Household Survey 1994; Health Survey for England 1993.
† Includes limiting and non-limiting illnesses.

Table 8.5 Self-reported long–standing illness by social class based on own current or last job, age and sex
Adults aged 16–74

Social class	I & II	III (NM)	III (M)	IV & V	Total*
Sex, age and self-reported long-standing illness			**Percentage reporting a long-standing illness**		
Men					
16–44					
Self-reported long-standing illness†	25	31	26	29	27
Self-reported limiting long-standing illness	10	10	11	13	11
45–64					
Self-reported long-standing illness†	44	46	46	42	44
Self-reported limiting long-standing illness	25	31	26	27	26
65–74					
Self-reported long-standing illness†	46	57	54	61	53
Self-reported limiting long-standing illness	19	39	37	38	31
All					
Self-reported long-standing illness†	34	37	37	37	35
Self-reported limiting long-standing illness	16	18	20	20	18
Bases = 100%					
16–44	392	116	257	187	1053
45–64	278	48	201	118	677
65–74	111	31	103	62	310
All	781	195	561	367	2040
Women					
16–44					
Self-reported long-standing illness†	27	28	27	25	27
Self-reported limiting long-standing illness	11	15	8	13	13
45–64					
Self-reported long-standing illness†	41	45	55	51	47
Self-reported limiting long-standing illness	21	27	35	36	29
65–74					
Self-reported long-standing illness†	48	60	51	62	57
Self-reported limiting long-standing illness	32	36	32	40	36
All					
Self-reported long-standing illness†	34	37	39	40	37
Self-reported limiting long-standing illness	17	21	20	25	21
Bases = 100%					
16–44	386	463	111	314	1385
45–64	195	240	63	226	753
65–74	96	159	50	140	460
All	677	862	224	680	2598

* Members of the Armed Forces, persons in inadequately described occupations and persons who have never worked are not shown as separate categories but are included in the figures for all persons.

† Includes limiting and non-limiting long-standing illnesses.

Table 8.6 Age-standardised ratios for self-reported long-standing illness by social class based on own current or last job and sex
Adults aged 16–74

Social class†	I & II	III(NM)	III(M)	IV & V
Self-reported long-standing illness				
Men				
Observed %	34	37	37	37
Expected %†	36	34	37	35
Standardised ratio**	95	111	100	105
Standard error of the ratio	2.5	6.3	3.0	4.1
Base = 100%	*781*	*195*	*561*	*367*
Women				
Observed %	34	37	39	40
Expected %†	36	36	38	38
Standardised ratio**	93	102	102	103
Standard error of the ratio	3.3	2.6	6.0	3.0
Base = 100%	*677*	*862*	*224*	*680*

* Excludes members of the Armed Forces, persons in inadequately described occupations and persons who have never worked.

† Calculations of the expected numbers used age-specific rates for having self-reported good general health for all men and all women. The age-groups used were 16–24, 25–34, 35–44, 45–54, 55–64, and 65–74.

**The standardised ratio is given as the observed rate divided by the expected rate and the ratio multiplied by 100. A 2-tailed test was used to show whether the ratio was significantly different from 100. The resulting figure was multiplied by the square root of the mean of the weight to allow for weighting.

Table 8.7 Self-reported general health by self-reported long-standing illness or disability age and sex
Adults aged 16–74

	Men				Women			
Age and self-reported general health	Has limiting long-standing illness or disability %	Has long-standing illness or disability* %	No long-standing illness or disability %	Total %	Has limiting long-standing illness or disability %	Has long-standing illness or disability* %	No long-standing illness or disability %	Total %
16–44								
Good	52	69	92	86	51	67	90	84
Not good	48	31	8	14	49	33	10	16
45–64								
Good	34	53	93	76	36	52	94	74
Not good	66	47	7	24	64	49	6	26
65–74								
Good	31	48	87	66	28	45	90	64
Not good	69	52	14	34	72	55	10	36
All								
Good	40	59	92	80	39	56	91	78
Not good	60	41	8	20	61	44	9	22
Bases = 100%								
16–44	111	279	773	1052	189	373	1012	1385
45–64	183	306	369	675	235	366	387	753
65–74	97	165	144	309	168	262	198	460
All	391	750	1286	2036	592	1001	1597	2598

* Includes limiting and non-limiting long-standing illnesses.

Health in England 1996 : What people know, what people think, what people do

Table 8.8 Self-reported stress in the last 12 months by age and sex
Adults aged 16–74

Age	16–24	25–34	35–44	45–54	55–64	65–74	Total	Total HEMS 1995
Self-reported stress	%	%	%	%	%	%	%	%
Men								
Completely free of stress	10	4	4	4	7	22	7	11
Small amount of stress	38	27	25	25	36	43	31	36
Moderate amount of stress	35	42	40	41	37	23	38	34
Large amount of stress	18	26	31	30	19	12	24	18
Don't know	-	0	-	-	0	0	0	0
Base = 100%	224	436	396	368	308	309	2041	2121
Women								
Completely free of stress	3	4	2	5	6	11	5	7
Small amount of stress	27	24	23	23	30	34	26	33
Moderate amount of stress	44	39	36	32	34	31	36	36
Large amount of stress	26	33	38	39	30	24	32	23
Don't know	-	1	-	0	-	0	0	0
Base = 100%	266	586	532	392	362	460	2598	2548
All								
Completely free of stress	6	4	3	4	7	16	6	9
Small amount of stress	32	26	24	24	33	38	29	35
Moderate amount of stress	39	41	38	37	36	27	37	35
Large amount of stress	22	29	35	35	24	18	28	21
Don't know	-	0	-	-	0	1	0	0
Base = 100%	490	1022	928	760	670	769	4639	4669

Table 8.9 Self-reported stress in the last 12 months by social class based on own current or last job, age and sex
Adults aged 16–74

Social class	I & II	III(NM)	III(M)	IV & V	Total*
Age	\multicolumn{5}{c}{Percentage reporting a large or moderate amount of stress}
Men					
16–44	76	62	60	55	65
45–64	74	55	62	50	65
65–74	31	21	36	48	35
All	71	56	57	52	62
Bases = 100%					
16–44	394	116	257	187	1055
45–64	277	48	201	118	676
65–74	111	31	102	62	309
All	782	195	560	367	2040
Women					
16–44	81	68	74	67	72
45–64	73	66	69	65	68
65–74	62	54	47	53	55
All	76	66	68	64	69
Bases = 100%					
16–44	386	463	111	313	1384
45–64	195	240	63	226	753
65–74	96	158	50	140	459
All	677	861	224	679	2596

* Members of the Armed Forces, persons in inadequately described occupations and persons who have never worked are not shown as separate categories but are included in the figures for all persons.

Table 8.10 Age-standardised ratios for self-reported stress* by social class based on own current or last job and sex
Adults aged 16–74

Social class[†]	I & II	III(NM)	III(M)	IV & V
Self-reported stress*				
Men				
Observed %	71	56	57	52
Expected %**	63	59	60	60
Standardised ratio[††]	112***	95	94	87
Standard error of the ratio	1.4	3.6	1.9	2.6
Base = 100%	782	195	560	367
Women				
Observed %	76	66	68	64
Expected %**	69	68	68	68
Standardised ratio[††]	110***	96	101	95
Standard error of the ratio	1.6	1.4	3.3	1.8
Base = 100%	677	861	224	679

* Respondents reporting a large or moderate amount of stress.
[†] Excludes members of the Armed Forces, persons in inadequately described occupations and persons who have never worked.
**Calculations of the expected numbers used age-specific rates for having self-reported good general health for all men and all women. The age-groups used were 16–24, 25–34, 35–44, 45–54, 55–64, and 65–74.
[††] The standardised ratio is given as the observed rate divided by the expected rate and the ratio multiplied by 100. A 2-tailed test was used to show whether the ratio was significantly different from 100. The resulting figure was multiplied by the square root of the mean of the weight to allow for weighting.
*** Significant at the 95% level.

Health in England 1996 : What people know, what people think, what people do

Table 8.11 Self-reported effect of stress on health by age and sex
Adults aged 16–74

Age	16–24	25–34	35–44	45–54	55–64	65–74	Total
Self-reported effect of stress on health	%	%	%	%	%	%	%
Men							
Very harmful	4	2	6	12	7	4	6
Quite harmful	32	37	39	39	32	24	35
Not harmful	54	55	50	44	52	49	51
Completely free of stress	10	4	4	4	7	22	7
Don't know	1	2	1	2	3	1	2
Base = 100%	*224*	*436*	*396*	*367*	*308*	*308*	*2039*
Women							
Very harmful	10	10	10	11	13	7	10
Quite harmful	40	43	50	45	40	37	43
Not harmful	45	42	37	38	40	44	41
Completely free of stress	3	4	2	5	6	11	5
Don't know	1	1	0	2	1	2	1
Base = 100%	*266*	*586*	*530*	*390*	*362*	*460*	*2594*
All							
Very harmful	7	6	8	12	10	5	8
Quite harmful	36	40	45	42	36	31	39
Not harmful	50	49	44	41	46	46	46
Completely free of stress	6	4	3	4	7	16	6
Don't know	1	1	1	2	2	2	1
Base = 100%	*490*	*1022*	*926*	*757*	*670*	*768*	*4633*

Table 8.12 Self-reported effect of stress on health by a) self-reported general health b) self-reported long-standing illness or disability and sex
Adults aged 16–74

	Self-reported general health		Self-reported long-standing illness		Total
	Good*	Not good	Long-standing illness†	No long-standing illness	
Self-reported effect of stress on health	%	%	%	%	%
Men					
Very harmful	4	16	11	3	6
Quite harmful	32	43	39	32	35
Not harmful	55	33	42	55	51
Completely free of stress	7	7	5	8	7
Don't know	2	2	2	1	2
Base = 100%	*1599*	*435*	*752*	*1285*	*2037*
Women					
Very harmful	6	26	18	6	10
Quite harmful	42	46	47	41	43
Not harmful	46	23	31	46	41
Completely free of stress	5	4	3	6	5
Don't know	1	1	1	1	1
Base = 100%	*1987*	*605*	*1000*	*1594*	*2592*

* Respondents were classified as having good health if they reported their general health as 'very good' or 'good'.
† Includes limiting and non-limiting long-standing illnesses.

Table 8.13 Self-reported effect of stress on health by self-reported stress and sex
Adults aged 16–74, reporting stress in the last 12 months

Self-reported stress	Small amount	Moderate amount	Large amount	Total
Self-reported effect of stress on health	%	%	%	%
Men				
Very harmful	1	2	20	6
Quite harmful	16	43	56	37
Not harmful	82	52	24	55
Don't know	1	3	1	2
Base = 100%	*620*	*754*	*505*	*1879*
Women				
Very harmful	1	3	27	11
Quite harmful	20	52	59	45
Not harmful	77	45	13	43
Don't know	1	1	1	1
Base = 100%	*678*	*950*	*854*	*2452*
All				
Very harmful	1	3	24	9
Quite harmful	18	47	57	41
Not harmful	80	48	18	49
Don't know	1	2	1	1
Base = 100%	*1298*	*1674*	*1359*	*4331*

Table 8.14 Respondents' assessment of whether they lead a healthy life by age and sex
Adults aged 16–74

Age	16–24	25–34	35–44	45–54	55–64	65–74	Total	Total HEMS 1995
Respondents' assessment of whether they lead a healthy life	%	%	%	%	%	%	%	%
Men								
Leads a very healthy life	19	13	10	19	20	26	17	16
Leads a fairly healthy life	72	78	80	71	71	68	74	73
Leads a not very healthy life	9	8	9	10	8	5	8	9
Leads an unhealthy life	0	1	1	1	1	1	1	1
Don't know	-	0	-	-	1	0	0	0
Base = 100%	*224*	*436*	*396*	*367*	*308*	*308*	*2042*	*2119*
Women								
Leads a very healthy life	9	10	12	13	24	31	15	14
Leads a fairly healthy life	78	82	78	81	66	64	76	77
Leads a not very healthy life	13	7	9	6	7	4	8	7
Leads an unhealthy life	0	1	1	1	2	1	1	1
Don't know	0	-	0	-	1	1	0	0
Base = 100%	*266*	*586*	*533*	*392*	*361*	*460*	*2598*	*2547*
All								
Leads a very healthy life	14	12	11	16	22	29	16	15
Leads a fairly healthy life	75	80	79	75	68	66	75	75
Leads a not very healthy life	11	7	9	8	8	4	8	8
Leads an unhealthy life	0	1	1	1	1	1	1	1
Don't know	0	0	0	-	1	1	0	0
Base = 100%	*490*	*1022*	*929*	*760*	*669*	*770*	*4640*	*4666*

Table 8.15 Respondents' assessment of whether they lead a healthy life by social class based on own current or last job, age and sex
Adults aged 16–74

Social class	I & II	III(NM)	III(M)	IV & V	Total*
Age	\multicolumn{5}{c}{Percentage leading a fairly or very healthy life}
Men					
16–44	91	90	90	89	91
45–64	91	93	88	91	90
65–74	97	94	94	91	94
All	91	91	90	90	91
Bases = 100%					
16–44	394	116	257	187	1055
45–64	278	48	201	117	676
65–74	111	31	103	62	310
All	783	195	561	366	2041
Women					
16-44	92	91	87	91	90
45-64	94	93	91	88	92
65-74	93	96	97	95	94
All	92	92	90	91	91
Bases = 100%					
16–44	386	463	111	314	1385
45–64	195	240	63	226	753
65–74	96	159	49	140	459
All	677	862	223	680	2597

* Members of the Armed Forces, persons in inadequately described occupations and persons who have never worked are not shown as separate categories but are included in the figures for all persons.

Table 8.16 Age-standardised ratios for respondents' assessment of whether they lead a healthy life* by social class based on own current or last job and sex
Adults aged 16–74

Social class†	I & II	III(NM)	III(M)	IV & V
Percentage leading a healthy life*				
Men				
Observed %	91	91	90	90
Expected %**	91	90	91	90
Standardised ratio††	101	101	99	99
Standard error of the ratio	0.6	1.4	0.8	1.0
Base = 100%	783	195	561	366
Women				
Observed %	92	92	90	91
Expected %**	92	92	92	92
Standardised ratio††	101	101	98	99
Standard error of the ratio	0.7	0.6	1.6	0.8
Base = 100%	677	862	223	680

* Respondents reporting a large or moderate amount of stress.
† Excludes members of the Armed Forces, persons in inadequately described occupations and persons who have never worked.
** Calculations of the expected numbers used age-specific rates for having self-reported good general health for all men and all women. The age-groups used were 16–24, 25–34, 35–44, 45–54, 55–64, and 65–74.
†† The standardised ratio is given as the observed rate divided by the expected rate and the ratio multiplied by 100. A 2-tailed test was used to show whether the ratio was significantly different from 100. The resulting figure was multiplied by the square root of the mean of the weight to allow for weighting.

Table 8.17 Respondents' assessment of what is currently good for their health by age and sex
Adults aged 16–74

Age	16–24	25–34	35–44	45–54	55–64	65–74	Total
Factors which are good for their health			Percentage choosing each factor				
Men							
Relationships, family	42	56	61	65	56	50	56
What I eat	43	54	51	58	57	63	54
The exercise I do	63	54	49	44	44	45	50
My income, standard of living	27	39	43	42	31	35	37
My work	26	29	26	26	22	4	23
My alcohol consumption	18	14	12	13	10	20	14
None of these	9	6	9	7	13	15	9
*Base = 100%**	*224*	*436*	*396*	*368*	*309*	*307*	*2040*
Women							
Relationships, family	51	65	64	69	57	56	61
What I eat	53	59	58	62	55	58	58
The exercise I do	45	48	44	46	39	40	44
My income, standard of living	34	38	43	41	37	35	38
My work	26	22	22	27	19	6	21
My alcohol consumption	7	9	10	11	9	8	9
None of these	12	6	9	8	14	15	10
*Base = 100%**	*266*	*585*	*531*	*391*	*362*	*461*	*2596*
All							
Relationships, family	46	61	63	67	57	54	59
What I eat	48	57	55	60	56	60	56
The exercise I do	54	51	46	45	41	42	47
My income, standard of living	30	38	43	41	34	35	38
My work	26	25	24	26	20	5	22
My alcohol consumption	12	11	11	12	9	13	11
None of these	10	6	9	8	13	15	10
*Base = 100%**	*490*	*1021*	*927*	*759*	*671*	*768*	*4636*

* Percentages add to more than 100% because respondents may have given more than one answer.

Table 8.18 Respondents' assessment of what is currently bad for their health by age and sex
Adults aged 16–74

Age	16–24	25–34	35–44	45–54	55–64	65–74	Total
Factors which are bad for their health			Percentage choosing each factor				
Men							
Pollution	27	32	35	32	27	25	30
Lack of exercise	20	30	30	27	22	18	26
Others' smoking	30	25	25	25	22	22	25
My smoking	36	29	21	21	21	10	24
My weight	11	16	28	32	28	21	23
What I eat	21	15	15	10	8	5	13
Not having a job	12	10	11	10	15	6	11
My alcohol consumption	20	15	10	7	7	3	11
Relationships, family	5	6	6	5	4	2	5
None of these	17	18	19	20	25	34	21
Base = 100%*	*224*	*436*	*396*	*368*	*309*	*310*	*2043*
Women							
Pollution	27	33	32	28	26	19	28
Lack of exercise	37	30	29	28	21	18	28
Others' smoking	32	27	25	30	22	21	26
My smoking	28	23	19	13	14	12	19
My weight	19	27	32	37	40	31	31
What I eat	20	18	12	13	10	6	14
Not having a job	6	10	8	6	8	2	7
My alcohol consumption	17	6	5	4	1	1	6
Relationships, family	7	9	10	9	8	5	8
None of these	15	18	17	21	21	34	21
Base = 100%*	*266*	*586*	*532*	*392*	*362*	*461*	*2599*
All							
Pollution	27	33	33	30	26	22	29
Lack of exercise	29	30	29	28	22	18	27
Others' smoking	31	26	25	27	22	22	26
My smoking	32	26	20	17	17	11	21
My weight	14	22	30	34	34	26	27
What I eat	20	16	14	11	9	6	13
Not having a job	9	10	9	8	11	4	9
My alcohol consumption	19	10	7	6	4	2	8
Relationships, family	6	8	8	7	6	4	6
None of these	16	18	18	20	23	34	21
Base = 100%*	*490*	*1021*	*927*	*759*	*671*	*771*	*4642*

* Percentages add to more than 100% because respondents may have given more than one answer.

Table 8.19 Respondents' assessment of what is currently good for their health by social class based on own current or last job, age and sex
Adults aged 16–74

Social class	I & II	III(NM)	III(M)	IV & V	Total*
Factors which are good for their health	\multicolumn{5}{c}{Percentage choosing each factor}				
Men					
Relationships, family	64	56	52	45	56
What I eat	59	56	51	50	54
The exercise I do	51	55	45	48	50
My income, standard of living	46	40	32	26	37
My work	22	20	25	27	23
My alcohol consumption	16	18	12	12	14
None of these	7	9	12	11	9
Base = 100%†	783	193	560	367	2039
Women					
Relationships, family	69	62	57	57	61
What I eat	66	57	54	52	58
The exercise I do	50	44	41	37	44
My income, standard of living	52	40	31	29	38
My work	27	20	24	18	21
My alcohol consumption	12	9	5	7	9
None of these	6	9	14	14	10
Base = 100%†	676	861	224	678	2594

* Members of the Armed Forces, persons in inadequately described occupations and persons who have never worked are not shown as separate categories but are included in the figures for all persons.
† Percentages add to more than 100% because respondents may have given more than one answer.

Table 8.20 Respondents' assessment of what is currently bad for their health by social class based on own current or last job, age and sex
Adults aged 16–74

Social class	I & II	III(NM)	III(M)	IV & V	Total*
Factors which are bad for their health	\multicolumn{5}{c}{Percentage choosing each factor}				
Men					
Pollution	31	27	31	32	30
Lack of exercise	31	24	24	20	26
Others' smoking	26	24	26	24	25
My smoking	17	25	27	29	24
My weight	25	21	24	21	23
What I eat	12	12	14	15	13
Not having a job	6	11	11	16	11
My alcohol consumption	9	12	10	14	11
Relationships, family	5	5	4	6	5
None of these	22	20	21	18	21
Base = 100%†	783	195	561	367	2042
Women					
Pollution	33	26	23	27	28
Lack of exercise	30	30	24	24	28
Others' smoking	29	26	23	24	26
My smoking	13	19	24	21	19
My weight	31	29	32	34	31
What I eat	13	15	10	12	14
Not having a job	5	5	8	8	7
My alcohol consumption	6	5	3	4	6
Relationships, family	8	8	9	8	8
None of these	19	21	24	22	21
Base = 100%†	677	862	224	679	2597

* Members of the Armed Forces, persons in inadequately described occupations and persons who have never worked are not shown as separate categories but are included in the figures for all persons.
† Percentages add to more than 100% because respondents may have given more than one answer.

Health in England 1996 : What people know, what people think, what people do

Table 8.21 Whether having good health is the most important thing in life by age and sex
Adults aged 16–74

Age	16–24	25–34	35–44	45–54	55–64	65–74	Total	Total HEMS 1995
Whether agrees	%	%	%	%	%	%	%	%
Men								
Strongly agrees	26	26	40	47	50	56	39	42
Agrees	49	53	47	46	44	42	48	46
Neither agrees nor disagrees	12	14	6	5	4	1	8	4*
Disagrees	13	7	6	2	2	1	6	8
Strongly disagrees	-	1	-	-	-	-	0	0
Base = 100%	224	436	396	368	309	309	2042	2120
Women								
Strongly agrees	24	37	44	50	53	55	43	46
Agrees	55	49	48	42	42	41	47	48
Neither agrees nor disagrees	13	9	5	4	4	2	6	2*
Disagrees	9	5	2	3	2	2	4	4
Strongly disagrees	-	0	-	0	-	0	0	0
Base = 100%	266	586	532	392	361	460	2597	2548
All								
Strongly agrees	25	31	42	48	51	56	41	44
Agrees	52	51	48	44	43	41	47	47
Neither agrees nor disagrees	12	11	6	5	4	2	7	3*
Disagrees	11	6	4	2	2	1	5	6
Strongly disagrees	-	0	-	0	-	0	0	0
Base = 100%	490	1022	928	760	670	769	4639	4669

* 'Don't know' in 1995.

Table 8.22 Whether it is sensible to do exactly what the doctors say by age and sex
Adults aged 16–74

Age	16–24	25–34	35–44	45–54	55–64	65–74	Total	Total HEMS 1995
Whether agrees	%	%	%	%	%	%	%	%
Men								
Strongly agrees	12	7	11	14	12	17	12	15
Agrees	59	56	50	57	57	61	56	55
Neither agrees nor disagrees	21	25	22	18	15	16	20	15*
Disagrees	7	11	16	11	15	6	11	14
Strongly disagrees	0	1	0	0	1	-	0	1
Base = 100%	*223*	*436*	*396*	*368*	*309*	*308*	*2040*	*2121*
Women								
Strongly agrees	10	10	12	13	15	16	12	14
Agrees	52	47	48	55	60	64	53	54
Neither agrees nor disagrees	20	29	25	20	16	12	21	15*
Disagrees	16	14	15	11	9	7	12	16
Strongly disagrees	2	1	0	0	1	0	1	1
Base = 100%	*265*	*586*	*533*	*391*	*362*	*460*	*2597*	*2547*
All								
Strongly agrees	11	9	12	13	13	17	12	15
Agrees	56	52	49	56	58	63	55	55
Neither agrees nor disagrees	20	27	24	19	15	14	21	15*
Disagrees	11	12	15	11	12	7	12	15
Strongly disagrees	1	1	0	0	1	0	1	1
Base = 100%	*488*	*1022*	*929*	*759*	*671*	*768*	*4637*	*4668*

* 'Don't know' in 1995.

Table 8.23 Whether health is generally a matter of luck by age and sex
Adults aged 16–74

Age	16–24	25–34	35–44	45–54	55–64	65–74	Total	Total HEMS 1995
Whether agrees	%	%	%	%	%	%	%	%
Men								
Strongly agrees	0	3	1	4	3	3	2	2
Agrees	14	15	21	24	29	38	22	24
Neither agrees nor disagrees	20	19	12	15	14	14	16	10*
Disagrees	54	55	56	51	50	42	52	54
Strongly disagrees	11	8	10	6	5	4	8	10
Base = 100%	224	436	396	368	307	308	2039	2121
Women								
Strongly agrees	1	1	3	3	2	2	2	2
Agrees	17	17	20	28	30	35	23	24
Neither agrees nor disagrees	19	21	19	16	17	17	19	14*
Disagrees	58	57	50	46	46	41	50	55
Strongly disagrees	5	5	9	6	4	4	6	6
Base = 100%	266	586	529	389	360	459	2589	2548
All								
Strongly agrees	1	2	2	3	2	2	2	2
Agrees	15	16	20	26	30	36	23	24
Neither agrees nor disagrees	20	20	16	16	16	16	17	12*
Disagrees	56	56	53	49	48	41	51	54
Strongly disagrees	8	7	9	6	4	4	7	8
Base = 100%	490	1022	925	757	667	767	4628	4669

* 'Don't know' in 1995.

Table 8.24 Whether you are more likely to be ill if you think too much about your health by age and sex
Adults aged 16–74

Age	16–24	25–34	35–44	45–54	55–64	65–74	Total	Total HEMS 1995
Whether agrees	%	%	%	%	%	%	%	%
Men								
Strongly agrees	3	4	3	5	5	10	5	5
Agrees	31	38	44	55	63	69	48	46
Neither agrees nor disagrees	31	23	22	13	13	10	19	14*
Disagrees	31	30	26	23	19	12	25	31
Strongly disagrees	4	4	4	4	0	0	3	4
Base = 100%	224	436	396	365	308	310	2039	2121
Women								
Strongly agrees	4	5	6	5	11	14	7	7
Agrees	41	42	49	62	62	65	52	52
Neither agrees nor disagrees	21	21	21	17	12	8	17	13*
Disagrees	32	30	22	15	14	13	22	25
Strongly disagrees	2	3	2	1	2	0	2	3
Base = 100%	266	586	531	392	361	458	2594	2547
All								
Strongly agrees	4	4	5	5	8	12	6	6
Agrees	36	40	47	58	62	67	50	49
Neither agrees nor disagrees	26	22	21	15	13	9	18	14*
Disagrees	31	30	24	19	16	12	23	28
Strongly disagrees	3	4	3	2	1	0	2	3
Base = 100%	490	1022	927	757	669	768	4633	4668

* 'Don't know' in 1995.

Table 8.25 Whether respondents have to be very ill before they go to the doctor by age and sex
Adults aged 16–74

Age	16-24	25-34	35-44	45-54	55-64	65-74	Total	Total HEMS 1995
Whether agrees	%	%	%	%	%	%	%	%
Men								
Strongly agrees	11	16	18	13	15	14	15	16
Agrees	38	52	52	56	53	57	51	48
Neither agrees nor disagrees	9	11	9	9	8	7	9	4*
Disagrees	33	20	19	20	24	21	22	28
Strongly disagrees	8	1	3	1	1	2	3	3
Base = 100%	224	436	396	368	307	310	2041	2120
Women								
Strongly agrees	12	15	17	19	16	19	16	17
Agrees	33	45	52	50	53	50	47	49
Neither agrees nor disagrees	13	9	7	6	7	8	8	3*
Disagrees	38	29	23	24	22	22	26	28
Strongly disagrees	4	2	1	1	1	1	2	3
Base = 100%	266	586	533	392	359	459	2595	2548
All								
Strongly agrees	12	16	18	16	16	17	16	17
Agrees	36	48	52	53	53	53	49	48
Neither agrees nor disagrees	11	10	8	8	7	7	9	4*
Disagrees	36	24	21	22	23	22	24	28
Strongly disagrees	6	1	2	1	1	1	2	3
Base = 100%	490	1022	929	760	666	769	4636	4668

* 'Don't know' in 1995.

Table 8.26 Whether respondents don't really have time to think about their health by age and sex
Adults aged 16–74

Age	16–24	25–34	35–44	45–54	55–64	65–74	Total	Total HEMS 1995
Whether agrees	%	%	%	%	%	%	%	%
Men								
Strongly agrees	0	2	2	2	0	3	2	2
Agrees	16	27	26	26	25	28	25	24
Neither agrees nor disagrees	22	22	17	18	17	18	19	9*
Disagrees	53	46	51	50	57	49	51	60
Strongly disagrees	9	3	4	4	1	2	4	6
Base = 100%	*224*	*436*	*396*	*367*	*306*	*307*	*2036*	*2120*
Women								
Strongly agrees	3	2	6	4	5	3	4	4
Agrees	17	27	33	36	35	38	31	32
Neither agrees nor disagrees	20	20	18	19	13	17	18	8*
Disagrees	55	48	41	40	43	41	45	52
Strongly disagrees	4	3	2	1	3	2	2	4
Base = 100%	*266*	*586*	*531*	*391*	*362*	*458*	*2594*	*2546*
All								
Strongly agrees	2	2	4	3	3	3	3	3
Agrees	17	27	30	31	30	33	28	28
Neither agrees nor disagrees	21	21	18	18	15	17	19	8*
Disagrees	54	47	46	46	50	45	48	55
Strongly disagrees	7	3	3	3	2	2	3	5
Base = 100%	*490*	*1022*	*927*	*758*	*668*	*765*	*4630*	*4666*

* 'Don't know' in 1995.

Health in England 1996 : What people know, what people think, what people do

Table 8.27 Consultations with GPs and other health professionals in the last 12 months by age and sex
Adults aged 16–74

Age	16–24	25–34	35–44	45–54	55–64	65–74	Total	Total HEMS 1995
	\multicolumn{8}{c}{Percentage consulting a GP or other health professional in the last 12 months}
Men								
Consulted doctor at surgery	48	52	59	62	70	76	60	60
Consulted doctor at home	2	3	2	2	3	3	2	2
Talked to doctor on telephone	-	1	0	-	-	-	0	0
Talked to other health professional	3	2	2	4	4	4	3	3
Talked to doctor and/or other health professional	53	58	64	66	75	81	65	63
Base = 100%	*224*	*436*	*396*	*368*	*309*	*310*	*2043*	*2120*
Women								
Consulted doctor at surgery	71	73	73	74	77	72	73	71
Consulted doctor at home	2	2	1	1	3	4	2	2
Talked to doctor on telephone	-	0	0	1	-	0	0	0
Talked to other health professional	3	3	5	5	5	5	4	4
Talked to doctor and/or other health professional	75	78	78	80	85	80	79	75
Base = 100%	*266*	*586*	*533*	*392*	*362*	*461*	*2600*	*2548*

Table 8.28 Consultations with GPs and other health professionals in the last 12 months by social class and sex
Adults aged 16–74

Social class	I & II	III (NM)	III (M)	IV & V	Total*
	\multicolumn{5}{c	}{Percentage consulting a GP or other health professional in the last 12 months}

	I & II	III (NM)	III (M)	IV & V	Total*
Men					
16–44					
Consulted doctor at surgery	58	54	49	54	53
Talked to other health professional	2	1	3	4	3
45–64					
Consulted doctor at surgery	69	57	64	57	65
Talked to other health professional	4	7	3	3	4
65–74					
Consulted doctor at surgery	75	78	79	72	76
Talked to other health professional	7	2	4	1	4
All					
Consulted doctor at surgery	64	57	58	57	60
Talked to other health professional	3	2	3	3	3
Bases = 100%					
16–44	394	116	257	187	1055
45–64	278	48	201	118	677
65–74	111	31	103	62	310
All	783	195	561	367	2042
Women					
16–44					
Consulted doctor at surgery	73	77	63	67	72
Talked to other health professional	5	3	5	4	4
45–64					
Consulted doctor at surgery	69	78	79	76	75
Talked to other health professional	7	4	-	7	5
65–74					
Consulted doctor at surgery	72	73	64	72	72
Talked to other health professional	4	5	13	3	5
All					
Consulted doctor at surgery	72	76	68	71	73
Talked to other health professional	6	3	5	5	2
Bases = 100%					
16–44	386	463	111	314	1385
45–64	195	240	63	226	753
65–74	96	159	50	140	460
All	677	862	224	680	2598

* Members of the Armed Forces, persons in inadequately described occupations and persons who have never worked are not shown as separate categories but are included in the figures for all persons.

Health in England 1996 : What people know, what people think, what people do

Table 8.29 Age-standardised ratios for consultations with GPs and other health professionals by social class based on own current or last job and sex
Adults aged 16–74

Social class*	I & II	III (NM)	III (M)	IV & V
Consultations with GPs and other health professionals in the last 12 months				
Men				
Observed %	69	62	64	61
Expected %†	66	63	66	64
Standardised ratio**	105***	99	97	95
Standard error of the ratio	1.3	3.3	1.7	2.3
Base = 100%	*783*	*195*	*561*	*367*
Women				
Observed %	79	81	74	77
Expected %†	79	79	79	79
Standardised ratio**	100	103	93	98
Standard error of the ratio	1.3	1.0	2.7	1.3
Base = 100%	*677*	*862*	*224*	*680*

* Excludes members of the Armed Forces, persons in inadequately described occupations and persons who have never worked.
† Calculations of the expected numbers used age-specific rates for having self-reported good general health for all men and all women. The age-groups used were 16–24, 25–34, 35–44, 45–54, 55–64, and 65–74.
**The standardised ratio is given as the observed rate divided by the expected rate and the ratio multiplied by 100. A 2-tailed test was used to show whether the ratio was significantly different from 100. The resulting figure was multiplied by the square root of the mean of the weight to allow for weighting.
*** Significant at the 95% level.

Table 8.30 Consultations with GPs and other health professionals in the last 12 months by a) self-reported general health b) self-reported long-standing illness or disability and sex
Adults aged 16–74

	Self-reported general health		Self-reported long-standing illness		Total
	Good*	Not good	Long-standing illness†	No long-standing illness	
	Percentage consulting a GP or other health professional in the last 12 months				
Men					
Consulted doctor at surgery	55	78	79	49	60
Consulted doctor at home	2	3	3	2	2
Talked to doctor on telephone	0	1	0	0	0
Talked to other health professional	3	2	3	3	3
Talked to doctor and/or other health professional	61	82	84	54	65
Base = 100%	*1602*	*436*	*754*	*1287*	*2041*
Women					
Consulted doctor at surgery	70	85	86	66	73
Consulted doctor at home	2	2	2	2	2
Talked to doctor on telephone	0	-	0	0	0
Talked to other health professional	4	5	4	4	4
Talked to doctor and/or other health professional	76	90	91	72	79
Base = 100%	*1989*	*609*	*1003*	*1597*	*2600*

* Respondents were classified as having good health if they reported their general health as 'very good' or 'good'.
† Includes limiting and non-limiting long-standing illnesses.

Table 8.31 Discussions with GPs or other health professionals about health behaviours in the last 12 months
Adults aged 16–74, who had spoken to a doctor or other professional in the last 12 months

Health behaviour	Smoking*	Drinking†	Activity	Diet
Whether had spoken to GP or other health professional	%	%	%	%
Men				
Spoken to GP at surgery	27	11	15	14
Spoken to GP elsewhere	0	0	0	0
Spoken to other professional	2	1	2	3
Not spoken to anyone	70	87	82	83
Base = 100%	445	1334	1357	1356
Whether found it helpful				
Helpful	31	48	57	66
Unhelpful	22	8	12	11
Neither helpful nor unhelpful	46	44	30	22
Don't know	1	-	1	1
Who raised the subject				
Respondent	23	24	41	33
Doctor or health professional	74	73	51	60
Both	2	1	6	7
Can't remember	1	1	2	0
Base = 100%	132	183	234	234
Women				
Spoken to GP at surgery	33	5	14	13
Spoken to GP elsewhere	1	0	1	0
Spoken to other professional	2	1	2	4
Not spoken to anyone	64	94	83	82
Base = 100%	632	1966	2074	2072
Whether found it helpful				
Helpful	22	46	61	61
Unhelpful	26	6	10	10
Neither helpful nor unhelpful	51	47	28	28
Don't know	1	1	-	1
Who raised the subject				
Respondent	23	35	52	45
Doctor or health professional	76	62	42	50
Both	1	1	5	4
Can't remember	-	1	1	1
Base = 100%	224	124	353	386

* Current and ex-smokers who gave up less than a year ago.
† Current and ex-drinkers.

Table 8.32 Discussions with GPs or other health professionals about health behaviours in the last 12 months by selected characteristics

Adults aged 16–74, who had spoken to a doctor or other professional in the last 12 months

Health behaviour	Discussed with GP or health professional %	Base= 100%	Respondent raised the subject %	Whether found it helpful %	Base= 100%
Smoking*					
Number of cigarettes a day					
0–9	23	285	26	41	69
10–19	36	398	17	20	140
20 or more	37	322	22	22	119
Whether wants to give up smoking					
Yes	32	655	28	31	220
No	32	312	9	17	98
Drinking†					
Weekly alcohol consumption (units)					
Less than 1	5	647	22	49	32
Men 1–21, Women 1–14	9	1889	30	48	163
Men 22–50, Women 15–35	12	572	24	48	76
Men 51 or more, Women 36 or more	19	135	34	43	32
Frequency of drinking					
Less than once a week	5	1067	20	46	49
1–2 days a week	8	1032	26	50	82
3–6 days a week	10	645	34	45	67
Almost every day	23	399	30	45	95
Whether wants to cut down					
Drinks the right amount	10	1713	27	50	180
Would like to cut down	17	346	39	39	62
Physical activity					
Number of occasions of moderate activity per week					
Less than one	18	1069	46	65	196
1–2	16	1066	42	55	170
3–4	15	525	39	64	82
5 or more	19	771	58	55	139
Whether would like to take more exercise					
Yes	19	2207	46	59	439
No	11	1080	51	61	117
Diet					
Attitude to own diet					
Never felt any need to change	11	945	36	62	102
Already changed as much as is likely to	22	1164	40	66	274
Ought to make changes, but probably won't	16	659	42	62	106
Likely to make changes in the future	20	650	40	59	137
Whether would like diet to be healthier					
Yes	19	1738	43	62	343
No	13	881	30	61	120
Don't know	19	67	[4]	[10]	13

* Current and ex-smokers who gave up less than a year ago.

† Current and ex-drinkers.

Health in England 1996 : What people know, what people think, what people do

Table A.1 The sample of addresses and households

	No.
Selected addresses	**8000**
Ineligible addresses	*942*
Demolished or derelict	49
Used solely for business purposes	198
Used for temporary accommodation only	82
Empty	412
Institution	14
Address not traced	97
Other ineligible	90
Addresses at which interviews were sought	*7058*
Number of extra households sampled at multi-household addresses	94
Total number of households	7152
Household with no-one aged 16-74	842
Total eligible sample of households	**6310**

Table A.2 Response of adults at interview stage

Response	No.	%
Set sample of households	**6310**	**100**
Fully co-operating adults	4640	74
Partially co-operating adults	5	0
Proxy interview carried out	145	2
Non-responding households/adults	*1520*	*24*
Refusal:	1094	17
direct to HQ	89	1
at sampling stage	316	5
by sampled person	689	11
Non-contact:	367	6
at sampling stage	216	3
with sampled person	151	2
No proxy interview possible	59	1

Table A.3 Response of adults aged 16–54 to the self-completion module

Response	No.	%
Adults aged 16–54	**3203**	**100**
Co-operated with self-completion:	3150	98
completed drugs section only	9	0
completed sexual health only	7	0
completed by respondent	2769	86
completed by interviewer	385	11
Self-completion refused	50	2
Did not complete main interview	3	0

Table A.4 Weights for household size

Household size	Weight
1 adult aged 16–74	1
2 adults aged 16–74	2
3 adults aged 16–74	3
4 adults aged 16–74	4
5 adults aged 16–74	5
6 adults aged 16–74	6
7 adults aged 16–74	7
8 adults aged 16–74	8

Table A.5 Distribution of responders to HEMS compared with Labour Force Survey (LFS) estimates for England by age and sex

	Men HEMS* %	Men LFS† %	Women HEMS* %	Women LFS† %	Total HEMS* %	Total LFS† %
Age group						
16–19	7.0	6.5	4.5	6.1	5.6	6.3
20–24	8.6	9.1	8.4	8.6	8.5	8.9
25–29	9.9	11.1	10.5	10.6	10.2	10.9
30–34	10.4	11.7	11.1	11.2	10.8	11.4
35–39	10.1	10.1	10.5	9.9	10.3	10.0
40–44	8.5	9.1	11.1	9.0	9.9	9.0
45–49	10.2	9.9	8.7	9.8	9.4	9.8
50–54	8.0	8.1	8.7	8.1	8.3	8.1
55–59	7.6	7.1	6.9	7.1	7.2	7.1
60–64	7.0	6.4	6.2	6.6	6.6	6.5
65–69	6.8	5.9	7.1	6.6	7.0	6.2
70–74	6.0	5.1	6.3	6.4	6.1	5.7
Base = 100%	2,044	17,393,607	2,601	17,500,137	4,645	34,893,744

* HEMS proportions are reweighted for number of adults in household.
† LFS survey estimates are weighted and grossed to the population estimates for England.

Table A.6 Distribution of responders to HEMS compared with Labour Force Survey (LFS) estimates for England by standard region

	Males HEMS* %	Males LFS† %	Females HEMS* %	Females LFS† %	Total HEMS* %	Total LFS† %
Standard region						
North	5.8	6.3	6.8	6.4	6.4	6.4
Yorkshire and Humberside	11.1	10.4	11.7	10.3	11.4	10.4
North West	13.2	13.0	13.9	13.1	13.6	13.0
East Midlands	9.2	8.5	9.2	8.5	9.2	8.5
West Midlands	10.5	10.9	11.2	10.8	10.9	10.9
East Anglia	4.1	4.4	4.8	4.4	4.5	4.4
Greater London	12.6	14.4	11.7	14.5	12.1	14.4
South East	22.8	22.3	21.3	22.3	22.0	22.3
South West	10.7	9.8	9.3	9.8	9.9	9.8
Base = 100%	2,044	17,393,607	2,601	17,500,137	4,645	34,893,744

* HEMS proportions are reweighted for number of adults in household.
† LFS survey estimates are weighted and grossed to the population estimates for England.

Table A.7 Distribution of responders to HEMS compared to GHS 1994 by marital status

	Men HEMS*	Men GHS 1994	Women HEMS*	Women GHS 1994	All HEMS*	All GHS 1994
Marital status	%	%	%	%	%	%
Married	59.5	60.5	58.0	57.3	58.7	58.9
Cohabiting	7.6	7.5	8.1	7.4	7.9	7.4
Single	25.0	24.5	18.5	19.1	21.5	21.7
Widowed	2.4	2.3	7.1	7.4	4.9	5.0
Divorced	3.9	3.8	5.8	6.3	4.9	5.1
Separated	1.3	1.3	2.5	2.5	2.0	1.9
Base = 100%	2044	6946	2601	7433	4645	14379

* HEMS proportions are reweighted for number of adults in household.

Table A.8 Distribution of responders to HEMS compared with Labour Force Survey (LFS) by ethnic origin and sex

	Men HEMS*	Men LFS†	Women HEMS*	Women LFS†	All HEMS*	All LFS†
Ethnic origin	%	%	%	%	%	%
White	94.4	93.9	94.7	94.0	94.5	94.0
Indian	1.1	1.8	1.2	1.7	1.4	1.7
Pakistani	0.7	0.9	0.5	0.9	0.6	0.9
Bangladeshi	0.5	0.4	0.1	0.3	0.3	0.3
Black-Caribbean	0.6	0.9	1.2	1.1	0.9	1.0
Other ethnic group	2.7	2.0	1.9	2.0	2.2	2.0
Base = 100%	2,043	17,388,346	2,043	17,496,583	4,640	34,884,930

* HEMS proportions are reweighted for number of adults in household.
† LFS survey estimates are weighted and grossed to the population estimates for England

Table A.9 Age-sex-region weights

	LFS population totals	LFS proportion	Total responding in sample	Sample proportion	Age-sex-region weight
		%		%	
South East					
Men					
16–24	986,922	2.8	84	2.7	1.04
25–39	2,234,842	6.4	256	5.3	1.21
40–54	1,711,435	4.9	193	4.3	1.14
55–74	1,469,791	4.2	191	3.9	1.08
Women					
16–24	949,075	2.7	76	2.1	1.29
25–39	2,170,318	6.2	307	6.2	1.00
40–54	1,726,800	4.9	218	5.1	0.97
55–74	1,607,741	4.6	262	4.5	1.02
Not South East					
Men					
16–24	1,761,543	5.0	140	4.4	1.14
25–39	3,501,364	10.0	399	8.6	1.16
40–54	3,002,100	8.6	353	7.9	1.09
55–74	2,779,219	7.9	428	8.6	0.92
Women					
16–24	1,664,237	4.8	190	4.9	0.97
25–39	3,384,445	9.7	558	11.2	0.86
40–54	2,991,626	8.5	429	10.3	0.83
55–74	3,049,249	8.7	561	9.9	0.88
Base = 100%	34,990,707	100	4645	100	

Table A.10 The effects of weighting for non-response on survey estimates

Survey estimate	Weighted only for probability of selection %	Weighted for probability of selection and for non-response %
Smoking status		
Current cigarette smokers	30	30
Ex-regular cigarette smokers	24	24
Never or only occasionally smoked cigarettes	46	46
Alcohol consumption		
Men		
Non-drinker	7	7
Under one	7	7
1–10	31	31
11–21	24	24
22–35	17	17
36–50	7	7
51 or over	7	7
Women		
Non-drinker	10	10
Under one	17	17
1–7	39	39
8–14	17	17
15–25	11	11
26–35	3	3
36 or over	3	3
Physical activity		
Participates in moderate-intensity activity lasting at least 30 minutes at least five times a week	35	36
Nutrition		
Eats foods containing fibre and starchy carbohydrates daily	38	39
Eats low-fat varieties of foods	22	22
Skin cancer		
Has had sunburn in the last 12 months	25	26
Drugs		
Has used drugs in the last 12 months	13	14
General health		
Has limiting long-standing illness	20	19
Base = 100%	8915	8928

Table A.11 Social class based on own current or last job by age and sex
Adults aged 16–74

Age	16–24	25–34	35–44	45–54	55–64	65–74	Total
Social class	%	%	%	%	%	%	%
Men							
I & II	14	38	43	46	36	36	36
III (NM)	18	10	9	5	8	10	10
III (M)	22	25	26	27	34	34	27
IV & V	23	18	16	18	17	20	18
Unclassifiable*	23	9	6	3	6	1	8
Base = 100%	224	436	396	368	309	310	2043
Women							
I & II	12	29	32	30	21	21	25
III (NM)	37	35	33	33	32	35	34
III (M)	8	8	8	6	11	11	9
IV & V	25	21	21	26	33	30	25
Unclassifiable*	18	7	5	5	3	3	7
Base = 100%	266	586	533	393	361	460	2599

* Members of the Armed Forces, persons in inadequately described occupations and persons who had never worked.

Table A.12 Age by social class based on own current or last job, and sex
Adults aged 16–74

Social class	I & II	III (NM)	III (M)	IV & V	Unclassifiable*	Total
Age	%	%	%	%	%	%
Men						
16–24	6	29	13	19	44	16
25–34	23	23	20	21	25	22
35–44	23	17	19	17	14	20
45–54	24	10	18	18	7	18
55–64	13	10	16	12	9	13
65–74	11	11	14	12	1	11
Base = 100%	783	195	561	367	137	2043
Women						
16–24	7	16	14	15	39	15
25–34	25	22	21	18	21	21
35–44	27	20	19	18	16	21
45–54	20	16	12	17	11	16
55–64	11	12	17	17	6	13
65–74	11	14	17	16	7	13
Base = 100%	677	862	224	680	156	2599

* Members of the Armed Forces, persons in inadequately described occupations and persons who had never worked.

Table A.13 Social class of HOH based on HOH's current or last job by respondent's social class based on own current or last job, and sex
Adults aged 16–74

Respondent's social class Social class of HOH	I & II %	III (NM) %	III (M) %	IV & V %	Unclassifiable* %	Total %
Men						
I & II	95	11	3	8	11	39
III (NM)	1	78	2	3	6	10
III (M)	2	7	89	6	14	28
IV & V	1	2	4	83	8	17
Unclassifiable*	1	1	2	1	62	6
Base = 100%	*783*	*195*	*561*	*367*	*137*	*2043*
Women						
I & II	69	32	19	18	23	36
III (NM)	7	29	7	6	12	15
III (M)	15	24	52	29	14	25
IV & V	6	11	15	41	16	18
Unclassifiable*	3	3	6	6	34	6
Base = 100%	*675*	*862*	*224*	*679*	*156*	*2596*

* Members of the Armed Forces, persons in inadequately described occupations and persons who have never worked.

Table A.14 Highest qualification level by age and sex
Adults aged 16–74

Age Highest qualification level	16–24 %	25–34 %	35–44 %	45–54 %	55–64 %	65–74 %	Total %
Men							
'A' level or above	32	50	49	41	24	19	38
Other qualifications	56	39	35	29	38	30	38
No qualifications	12	11	16	30	37	51	24
Base = 100%	*223*	*434*	*395*	*367*	*309*	*309*	*2037*
Women							
'A' level or above	40	34	35	23	15	14	28
Other qualifications	50	53	40	37	32	27	41
No qualifications	9	12	25	40	52	60	31
Base = 100%	*264*	*586*	*533*	*392*	*360*	*460*	*2595*

Table A.15 Highest qualification level by social class based on own current or last job, and sex
Adults aged 16–74

Social class	I & II	III (NM)	III (M)	IV & V	Total*
Highest qualification level	%	%	%	%	%
Men					
'A' level or above	64	35	22	16	38
Other qualifications	27	47	44	42	38
No qualifications	9	18	35	43	24
Base = 100%	*781*	*195*	*561*	*365*	*2037*
Women					
'A' level or above	63	19	14	9	28
Other qualifications	28	56	42	36	41
No qualifications	10	25	43	54	31
Base = 100%	*677*	*861*	*224*	*679*	*2593*

* Includes members of the Armed Forces, persons in inadequately described occupations and persons who had never worked.

Table A.17 Housing tenure status by social class based on own current or last job, and sex
Adults aged 16–74

Social class	I & II	III (NM)	III (M)	IV & V	Total*
Tenure status	%	%	%	%	%
Men					
Owner occupied	84	79	72	55	72
Rented from Local Authority or Housing Association	5	7	18	29	14
Privately rented	10	14	10	16	14
Base = 100%	*783*	*195*	*561*	*366*	*2040*
Women					
Owner occupied	82	78	66	56	70
Rented from Local Authority or Housing Association	4	11	20	32	16
Privately rented	14	11	14	12	13
Base = 100%	*675*	*862*	*224*	*679*	*2595*

* Includes members of the Armed Forces, persons in inadequately described occupations and persons who had never worked.

Table A.16 Economic activity status by social class based on own current or last job, and sex
Adults aged 16–74

Social class	I & II	III (NM)	III (M)	IV & V	Total*
Economic activity status	%	%	%	%	%
Men					
Working	80	76	72	67	70
Unemployed	2	2	4	8	6
Economically inactive	18	21	24	25	24
Base = 100%	*783*	*195*	*561*	*367*	*2042*
Women					
Working	71	60	56	54	58
Unemployed	2	2	2	3	3
Economically inactive	27	37	42	43	39
Base = 100%	*677*	*862*	*224*	*680*	*2599*

* Includes members of the Armed Forces, persons in inadequately described occupations and persons who had never worked.

Table A.18 Gross household income by social class based on own current or last job, and sex
Adults aged 16–74

Social class	I & II	III (NM)	III (M)	IV & V	Total*
Gross household income	%	%	%	%	%
Men					
Under £5,000	4	3	6	10	6
£5,000–£9,999	7	16	21	29	16
£10,000–£15,000	23	37	40	38	32
£20,000 or more	66	45	34	23	45
Base = 100%	*759*	*184*	*540*	*350*	*1958*
Women					
Under £5,000	5	9	12	19	11
£5,000–£9,999	8	17	23	34	20
£10,000–£15,000	25	34	39	31	31
£20,000 or more	62	40	26	17	38
Base = 100%	*657*	*828*	*215*	*640*	*2483*

* Includes members of the Armed Forces, persons in inadequately described occupations and persons who had never worked.

Health in England 1996 : What people know, what people think, what people do

Table A.19 Characteristics of respondents interviewed face-to-face and by proxy
Adults aged 16–74

Characteristic	Face-to-face respondents %	Respondents interviewed by proxy %
Sex		
Male	46	62
Female	54	38
Base = 100%	*4645*	*145*
Age		
16–24	14	18
25–34	21	24
35–44	20	21
45–54	18	19
55–64	14	10
65–74	13	8
Base = 100%	*4645*	*145*
Marital status		
Single	21	26
Married, cohabiting	67	68
Widowed, divorced or separated	12	6
Base = 100%	*4645*	*145*
Highest qualification level		
'A' level or above	32	25
GCSE Grade A–G or equivalent	40	36
No qualifications	28	39
Base = 100%	*4632*	*145*
Social class		
I & II	30	33
III (NM)	23	10
III (M)	17	14
IV & V	22	23
Unclassified*	7	20
Base = 100%	*4642*	*145*
Tenure status		
Owner occupied	71	68
Rented from Local Authority or Housing Association	16	13
Privately rented	13	19
Base = 100%	*4637*	*145*
Type of accommodation		
Detached house	24	17
Semi-detached house	37	26
Terraced house	28	41
Purpose-built flat	8	9
Flat in a converted house	2	6
Caravan, mobile home	0	1
Other	1	1
Base = 100%	*4643*	*145*

Table A.19 – *continued*

Characteristic	Face-to-face respondents %	Respondents interviewed by proxy %
Standard region		
North	6	8
Yorkshire and Humberside	11	10
North West	14	13
East Midlands	9	2
West Midlands	11	8
East Anglia	4	7
Greater London	12	26
Outer Metropolitan and Outer South East	22	18
South West	10	9
Base = 100%	*4645*	*145*

* Members of the Armed Forces, persons in inadequately described occupations and persons who have never worked.

Proportions are reweighted for number of adults in household.

Table A.20 Selected estimates for respondents interviewed face-to-face and by proxy
Adults aged 16–74

Type of behaviour	Face-to-face respondents	Respondents interviewed by proxy
	Percentage reporting each behaviour	
Working last week	59	62
Good general health	79	78
Long-standing illness	37	39
Limiting long-standing illness	20	20
Spoken to doctor in the last 12 months	70	63
Sunburnt in the last 12 months	25	17
Current cigarette smoker	30	29
Drinks alcohol at last 1–2 times a week	68	69
Very or fairly physically active at work	66	75
At least one walk of 1–2 miles in the last four weeks	66	50
Participated in sports or exercise in the last four weeks	59	45
Eats wholemeal bread	22	21
Eats fruit and vegeatables every day	67	71
Drinks skimmed or semi-skimmed milk	71	62
Base = 100%	*4645*	*145*

Proportions are reweighted for number of adults in household.

Table A.21 Type of accommodation occupied by respondents interviewed face-to-face and by proxy and at non-responding addresses
Sampled households

Type of accommodation	Face-to-face respondents %	Interview carried out by proxy %	Non-responding addresses %
Detached house	22	16	16
Semi-detached house	35	24	30
Terraced house	29	41	31
Purpose-built flat	11	10	16
Flat in a converted house	3	7	6
Caravan, mobile home	0	1	0
Other	1	1	1
Base = 100%	*4643*	*145*	*1417*

Table A.22 Standard errors and 95% confidence intervals for socio-demographic variables

Base	Characteristic	%(p)	Sample size	Standard error of p	95% confidence interval	Deft
	Age					
Men	16–24	15.7	2044	1.07	13.6 – 17.8	1.33
	25–34	22.0	2044	1.01	20.0 – 24.0	1.10
	35–44	19.5	2044	0.86	17.8 – 21.2	0.98
	45–54	18.5	2044	0.95	16.6 – 20.4	1.10
	55–64	13.0	2044	0.80	11.4 – 14.6	1.08
	65–74	11.3	2044	0.69	9.9 – 12.7	0.99
Women	16–24	15.0	2601	0.93	13.2 – 16.8	1.33
	25–34	21.3	2601	0.90	19.5 – 23.1	1.12
	35–44	20.8	2601	0.91	19.0 – 22.6	1.15
	45–54	16.4	2601	0.81	14.8 – 18.0	1.12
	55–64	13.2	2601	0.76	11.7 – 14.7	1.15
	65–74	13.3	2601	0.69	11.9 – 14.7	1.03
	Social class of respondent					
Men	I & II	36.2	2043	1.31	33.6 – 38.8	1.23
(excluding armed	III NM	9.9	2043	0.70	8.5 – 11.3	1.06
forces, never worked	III M	27.4	2043	1.26	24.9 – 29.9	1.27
and not known)	IV & V	18.4	2043	1.00	16.4 – 20.4	1.16
Women	I & II	25.3	2599	0.92	23.5 – 27.1	1.08
(excluding armed	III NM	34.1	2599	1.11	31.9 – 36.3	1.19
forces, never worked	III M	8.5	2599	0.65	7.2 – 9.8	1.18
and not known)	IV & V	25.3	2599	0.99	23.4 – 27.2	1.16
	Highest qualification level					
Men	'A' level or above	38.4	2037	1.37	35.7 – 41.1	1.27
	Other qualifications	38.0	2037	1.24	35.6 – 40.4	1.15
	No qualifications	23.5	2037	1.07	21.4 – 25.6	1.14
Women	'A' level or above	28.2	2595	1.21	25.8 – 30.6	1.37
	Other qualifications	41.1	2595	1.12	38.9 – 43.3	1.16
	No qualifications	30.7	2595	1.09	28.6 – 32.8	1.20
	Marital status					
Men	Married	58.9	2044	1.26	56.4 – 61.4	1.16
	Cohabiting	8.1	2044	0.63	6.9 – 9.3	1.04
	Single	25.6	2044	1.16	23.3 – 27.9	1.20
	Widowed/separated/divorced	7.3	2044	0.48	6.4 – 8.2	0.83
Women	Married	56.6	2601	1.19	54.3 – 58.9	1.23
	Cohabiting	8.2	2601	0.63	7.0 – 9.4	1.18
	Single	20.0	2601	0.98	18.1 – 21.9	1.24
	Widowed/separated/divorced	15.1	2601	0.62	13.9 – 16.3	0.89

Table A.23 Standard errors and 95% confidence intervals for smoking variables

Base	Characteristic	%(p)	Sample size	Standard error of p	95% confidence interval	Deft
	Cigarette smoking status					
Men	Heavy smoker	11.4	2042	0.67	10.1 – 12.7	0.96
	Moderate smoker	11.5	2042	0.88	9.8 – 13.2	1.26
	Light smoker	7.9	2042	0.66	6.6 – 9.2	1.11
	Ex-regular smoker	27.8	2042	1.14	25.6 – 30.0	1.15
	Never smoked regularly	41.1	2042	1.23	38.7 – 43.5	1.13
Women	Heavy smoker	7.0	2600	0.56	5.9 – 8.1	1.12
	Moderate smoker	12.1	2600	0.72	10.7 – 13.5	1.12
	Light smoker	9.4	2600	0.65	8.1 – 10.7	1.13
	Ex-regular smoker	19.7	2600	0.93	17.9 – 21.5	1.20
	Never smoked regularly	51.6	2600	1.24	49.2 – 54.0	1.26
	When smokers intend to give up smoking					
Men: smokers	Within the next month	6.4	628	1.13	4.2 – 8.6	1.15
	Within the next six months	13.1	628	1.65	9.9 – 16.3	1.23
	Within the next year	16.0	628	1.60	12.9 – 19.1	1.12
	Intends to give up but not in the next year	18.6	628	1.63	15.4 – 21.8	1.05
	Unlikely to give up smoking	46.0	628	2.03	42.0 – 48.8	1.02
Women: smokers	Within the next month	6.2	751	0.99	4.3 – 8.1	1.12
	Within the next six months	8.9	751	1.10	6.7 – 11.1	1.05
	Within the next year	14.0	751	1.54	11.0 – 17.0	1.21
	Intends to give up but not in the next year	26.7	751	1.81	23.2 – 30.2	1.12
	Unlikely to give up smoking	44.2	751	2.00	40.3 – 48.1	1.08
	Attitudes to children smoking					
Men	Does not want them to smoke	93.5	267	1.42	90.7 – 96.3	0.94
	It is up to them whether they smoke	6.5	267	1.42	3.7 – 9.3	0.94
Women	Does not want them to smoke	90.6	424	1.57	87.5 – 93.7	1.11
	It is up to them whether they smoke	9.4	424	1.60	6.3 – 12.5	1.11

Table A.24 Standard errors and 95% confidence intervals for drinking variables

Base	Characteristic	Sample size	Standard error of p	95% confidence interval	Deft
	Mean alcohol consumption level (units per week)				
	Mean				
Men	18.0	2042	0.56	16.9 – 19.1	1.13
Women	7.7	2600	0.35	7.0 – 8.4	1.31
	When respondent intends to cut down on drinking				
	%(p)				
Men	Within the next month 22.8	266	2.54	17.8 – 27.8	0.99
	Within the next six months 11.1	266	2.00	7.2 – 15.0	1.04
	Within the next year 11.5	266	1.81	8.0 – 15.0	0.92
	Intends to cut down, but not in the next year 12.0	266	2.31	7.5 – 16.5	1.16
	Unlikely to cut down 42.6	266	3.00	36.7 – 48.5	0.99
Women	Within the next month 16.3	209	2.61	11.2 – 21.4	1.02
	Within the next six months 14.1	209	2.70	8.8 – 19.4	1.12
	Within the next year 11.4	209	2.49	6.5 – 16.3	1.13
	Intends to cut down, but not in the next year 8.9	209	3.29	2.5 – 15.3	1.67
	Unlikely to cut down 49.2	209	4.43	40.5 – 57.9	1.28
	Attitude to changes in sensible drinking levels				
Men	I haven't heard anything about the changes 25.3	2035	1.11	23.1 – 27.5	1.15
	I feel confused about the changes 14.1	2035	0.84	12.5 – 15.7	1.08
	I don't feel confused about the changes 24.8	2035	1.02	22.8 – 26.8	1.06
	It is of no interest to me 35.8	2035	1.19	33.5 – 38.1	1.11
Women	I haven't heard anything about the changes 28.2	2590	1.11	26.0 – 30.4	1.26
	I feel confused about the changes 14.3	2590	0.82	12.7 – 15.9	1.18
	I don't feel confused about the changes 19.9	2590	0.92	18.1 – 21.7	1.17
	It is of no interest to me 37.5	2590	1.16	35.2 – 39.8	1.22

Table A.25 Standard errors and 95% confidence intervals for physical activity variables

Base	Characteristic	%(p)	Sample size	Standard error of p	95% confidence interval	Deft
	Number of days and length of time people should be physically active					
Men	30 minutes or more on at least five days a week	25.3	1994	1.10	23.1 – 27.5	1.13
	20 minutes or more on at least three days a week	63.2	1994	1.15	60.9 – 65.5	1.06
	Fewer than three occasions or less than 20 minutes	31.9	1994	1.11	29.7 – 34.1	1.06
Women	30 minutes or more on at least five days a week	24.5	2529	0.99	22.6 – 26.4	1.16
	20 minutes or more on at least three days a week	63.6	2529	1.20	61.2 – 66.0	1.25
	Fewer than three occasions or less than 20 minutes	32.2	2529	1.16	29.9 – 34.1	1.25
	When intends to take more exercise					
Men	Within the next month	25.2	1984	1.13	23.0 – 27.4	1.16
	Within the next six months	19.1	1984	1.05	17.0 – 21.2	1.18
	Within the next year	9.8	1984	0.74	8.3 – 11.3	1.11
	Intends to take more exercise but not in the next year	3.0	1984	0.42	2.2 – 3.8	1.10
	Unlikely to take more exercise	42.9	1984	1.25	40.5 – 45.4	1.13
Women	Within the next month	25.5	2515	1.01	23.4 – 27.5	1.16
	Within the next six months	21.6	2515	0.95	19.7 – 23.5	1.16
	Within the next year	9.4	2515	0.61	8.2-10.6	1.05
	Intends to take more exercise but not in the next year	4.2	2515	0.42	3.4 – 5.0	1.06
	Unlikely to take more exercise	39.4	2515	1.06	37.6 – 41.5	1.09
	Frequency of moderate-intensity activity for 30 minutes					
Men	Less than one day a week (sedentary)	24.0	2043	1.03	22.0 – 26.0	1.09
	1-2 days a week	23.5	2043	1.03	21.5 – 25.5	1.10
	3-4 days a week	11.7	2043	0.88	10.0 – 13.4	1.23
	5 or more days a week	40.8	2043	1.10	38.6 – 43.0	1.02
Women	Less than one day a week (sedentary)	25.7	2599	1.05	23.6 – 27.8	1.22
	1-2 days a week	29.6	2599	0.94	27.8 – 31.4	1.05
	3-4 days a week	14.0	2599	0.82	12.4 – 15.6	1.21
	5 or more days a week	30.8	2599	1.06	28.7 – 32.9	1.17

Table A.26 Standard errors and 95% confidence intervals for nutrition variables

Base	Characteristic	%(p)	Sample size	Standard error of p	95% confidence interval	Deft
	Eats bread; fruit, vegetables and salad; and potatoes, pasta or rice daily					
Men		35.8	2042	1.20	33.4 – 38.2	1.13
Women		39.8	2598	1.12	37.6 – 42.0	1.18
	Uses low-fat varieties of milk, cooking fat and spread, and eats chips less than once a week					
Men		16.6	1934	0.91	14.8 – 18.4	1.08
Women		27.2	2474	1.10	25.0 – 29.4	1.23
	Intentions to change diet					
Men	Intends to change in next month	13.3	937	1.29	10.8 – 15.8	1.16
	Intends to change in next 6 months	24.5	937	1.60	21.4 – 27.6	1.14
	Intends to change in next year	12.6	937	1.19	10.3 – 14.9	1.10
	Wants to change but thinks it unlikely	49.6	937	1.67	46.3 – 52.9	1.02
Women	Intends to change in next month	21.6	1359	1.27	19.1 – 24.1	1.14
	Intends to change in next 6 months	23.6	1359	1.05	21.5 – 25.7	0.91
	Intends to change in next year	10.8	1359	0.96	8.9 – 12.7	1.14
	Wants to change but thinks it unlikely	44.0	1359	1.43	41.2 – 46.8	1.06
	Whether agrees that 'experts never agree about what foods are good for you'					
Men	Strongly agrees	14.0	2030	0.94	12.2 – 15.8	1.22
	Agrees	53.4	2030	1.23	51.0 – 55.8	1.10
	Neither agrees nor disagrees	17.5	2030	0.96	15.6 – 19.4	1.14
	Disagrees	13.3	2030	0.87	11.6 – 15.0	1.16
	Strongly disagrees	1.8	2030	0.31	1.2 – 2.4	1.06
Women	Strongly agrees	12.6	2581	0.92	10.8 – 14.4	1.40
	Agrees	57.0	2581	1.15	54.7 – 59.3	1.18
	Neither agrees nor disagrees	15.3	2581	0.82	13.7 – 16.9	1.16
	Disagrees	14.2	2581	0.77	12.7 – 15.7	1.11
	Strongly disagrees	0.8	2581	0.22	0.4 – 1.2	1.22

Table A.27 Standard errors and 95% confidence intervals for drugs variables

Base	Characteristic	%(p)	Sample size	Standard error of p	95% confidence interval	Deft
	Whether had ever used any drug					
Men		38.0	1398	1.45	35.2 – 40.8	1.12
Women		26.4	1745	1.25	24.0 – 28.9	1.19
	Whether had used any drug in the last year					
Men		17.4	1398	1.20	15.0 – 19.8	1.19
Women		10.7	1745	0.95	8.8 – 12.6	1.29
	Whether had used any drug in the last month					
Men		11.9	1398	1.01	9.9 – 13.9	1.17
Women		6.4	1745	0.69	5.0 – 7.8	1.18
	Whether agrees that 'all use of drugs is wrong'					
Men	Strongly agrees	40.3	1398	1.53	37.3 – 43.3	1.16
	Agrees	25.9	1398	1.36	23.2 – 28.6	1.16
	Neither agrees nor disagrees	13.9	1398	1.11	11.7 – 16.1	1.20
	Disagrees	16.1	1398	1.03	14.1 – 18.1	1.05
	Strongly disagrees	3.7	1398	0.56	2.6 – 4.8	1.11
Women	Strongly agrees	45.1	1742	1.55	42.1 – 48.1	1.30
	Agrees	28.5	1742	1.36	25.8 – 31.2	1.26
	Neither agrees nor disagrees	12.6	1742	0.94	10.8 – 14.4	1.19
	Disagrees	12.0	1742	0.96	10.1 – 13.9	1.23
	Strongly disagrees	1.8	1742	0.38	1.1 – 2.5	1.21

Health in England 1996 : What people know, what people think, what people do

Table A.28 Standard errors and 95% confidence intervals for sexual health variables

Base	Characteristic	%(p)	Sample size	Standard error of p	95% confidence interval	Deft
	Number of sexual partners in the last 12 months					
Men	None	14.4	1375	0.92	12.6 – 16.2	0.97
	One	69.2	1375	1.52	66.2 – 72.2	1.22
	Two or more	16.3	1375	1.14	14.1 – 18.5	1.14
Women	None	12.1	1716	0.79	10.6 – 13.6	1.01
	One	78.3	1716	1.07	76.2 – 80.4	1.08
	Two or more	9.7	1716	0.78	8.2 – 11.2	1.09
	Whether would use a condom if in the 'near future' did have sex with a new partner					
Men	Would always use a condom	57.5	1392	1.70	54.2 – 60.8	1.28
	It would depend	31.2	1392	1.48	28.3 – 34.1	1.19
	Would never use a condom	1.3	1392	0.29	0.7 – 1.9	0.96
	Wouldn't contemplate having sex	10.0	1392	0.98	8.1 – 11.9	1.26
Women	Would always use a condom	66.9	1729	1.39	64.2 – 69.6	1.23
	It would depend	16.9	1729	1.27	14.4 – 19.4	1.41
	Would never use a condom	1.1	1729	0.22	0.7 – 1.5	0.90
	Wouldn't contemplate having sex	15.2	1729	1.02	13.2 – 17.2	1.18
	Used a condom with a new partner					
Men		60.3	315	2.82	54.8 – 65.8	1.02
Women		63.2	287	3.35	56.6 – 69.8	1.17

Table A.29 Standard errors and 95% confidence intervals for behaviour in the sun variables

Base	Characteristic	%(p)	Sample size	Standard error of p	95% confidence interval	Deft
	Whether uses a suncream					
Men	Yes	61.5	2042	1.34	58.9 – 64.1	1.25
	No	37.7	2042	1.28	35.2 – 40.2	1.20
	Never goes out in the sun	0.8	2042	0.20	0.4 – 1.2	1.01
Women	Yes	74.4	2600	1.00	72.4 – 76.4	1.17
	No	23.1	2600	1.02	21.1 – 25.1	1.23
	Never goes out in the sun	2.5	2600	0.34	1.8 – 3.2	1.11
	Whether agrees that 'having a suntan makes me feel healthier'					
Men	Agrees	40.8	1798	1.32	38.2 – 43.4	1.14
	Disagrees	40.7	1798	1.50	37.8 – 43.6	1.27
	Neither agrees nor disagrees	18.4	1798	1.05	16.3 – 20.5	1.15
Women	Agrees	48.6	2346	1.11	46.4 – 50.8	1.08
	Disagrees	38.5	2346	1.15	36.2 – 40.8	1.14
	Neither agrees nor disagrees	13.0	2346	0.82	11.4 – 14.6	1.18
	Whether agrees that 'having a suntan makes me look more attractive'					
Men	Agrees	40.2	1795	1.20	37.8 – 42.6	1.04
	Disagrees	33.5	1795	1.27	31.0 – 36.0	1.14
	Neither agrees nor disagrees	26.2	1795	1.13	24.0 – 28.4	1.08
Women	Agrees	49.2	2344	1.33	46.6 – 51.8	1.29
	Disagrees	33.4	2344	1.13	31.2 – 35.6	1.16
	Neither agrees nor disagrees	17.4	2344	0.80	15.8 – 19.0	1.03

Table A.30 Standard errors and 95% confidence intervals for general health variables

Base	Characteristic	%(p)	Sample size	Standard error of p	95% confidence interval	Deft
	Self-reported effect of stress on health					
Men	Very harmful	5.9	2039	0.57	4.8 – 7.0	1.08
	Quite harmful	34.7	2039	1.11	32.5 – 36.9	1.05
	Not harmful	50.7	2039	1.13	48.4 – 52.8	1.02
	Completely free of stress	7.1	2039	0.64	5.8 – 8.4	1.12
Women	Very harmful	10.0	2594	0.68	8.7 – 11.3	1.16
	Quite harmful	43.1	2594	1.18	40.8 – 45.4	1.22
	Not harmful	40.9	2594	1.24	38.9 – 42.9	1.03
	Completely free of stress	4.8	2594	0.51	3.8 – 5.8	1.20
	Consultations with GP in last 12 months					
Men	Consulted doctor at surgery	59.5	2043	1.33	56.9 – 62.1	1.23
	Consulted doctor at home	2.3	2043	0.35	1.6 – 3.0	1.03
	Talked to doctor on telephone	0.2	2043	0.13	-0.1 – 0.5	1.29
	Not consulted a GP	37.9	2043	1.31	35.3 – 40.5	1.22
Women	Consulted doctor at surgery	73.1	2600	1.14	70.9 – 75.3	1.31
	Consulted doctor at home	2.0	2600	0.28	1.4 – 2.5	1.01
	Talked to doctor on telephone	0.2	2600	0.11	0 – 0.4	1.22
	Not consulted a GP	24.7	2600	1.11	22.5 – 26.9	1.31

Appendix A Sample design, response to the survey, weighting, characteristics of the responding sample and sampling errors

A.1 Introduction

This appendix gives details of the sample design used for the 1996 Health Education Monitoring Survey (HEMS), and of response to the survey. It also describes the weighting procedure applied to the data and presents information on the characteristics of the responding sample, including those interviewed by proxy, and the sampling errors associated with the estimates shown in this report.

A.2 The sample design

The sample design is the same as that used for the 1995 survey; it follows the recommendations of a previous consultancy carried out by ONS for the Health Education Authority (HEA) in Summer 1994 which considered the optimum design for health surveys[1]. It concluded that the Postcode Address File (PAF) is the most complete sampling frame available for general population surveys, and recommended that the sample design incorporate socio-economic as well as regional stratifiers.

A.2.1 Requirements of the sample

The sample selection process was designed to yield a representative sample of approximately 5,000 interviews with adults aged 16–74 living in private households in England. One person in this age-group was interviewed in each eligible household.

The sample was geographically clustered to give areas of a realistic size for interviewers to cover.

A.2.2 Selection of households

Since no suitable frame of households exists, a sample of addresses was selected from the Postcode Address File (PAF). In order to select the appropriate number of addresses a stratified multi-stage random probability design was used. The stages in the selection of the sample were as follows:

(i) The chosen primary sampling units (PSUs) were postcode sectors, which are similar in size to wards. Two hundred were selected by a systematic sampling method from a stratified list of postcode sectors. For this purpose all postcode sectors in England were stratified first by standard region, then according to the proportion of households in rented accommodation, then by the proportion of heads of household in socio-economic groups 1 to 5 and 13, i.e. professionals. Postcode sectors within the resulting strata were ranked by the proportion of households with a car. The regional stratification differentiated between metropolitan and non-metropolitan areas within standard regions. The other stratifying information was based on 1991 Census data.

(ii) A random selection of postcode sectors was then made, with the chance of selection of each postcode sector being proportional to the total number of delivery points in the sector. From each of the 200 postcode sectors, 40 addresses were randomly selected, to give a total of 8,000 addresses.

A.2.3 Ineligible addresses

Since the requirement was for a sample of adults living in private households, business addresses and institutions were excluded at the sample selection stage as far as possible by using the PAF small users' file as the sampling frame. Twelve per cent (942) of the selected addresses did not contain a private household and were excluded from the set sample of addresses. These ineligible addresses included demolished or permanently empty addresses, addresses used only on an occasional basis and business premises and institutions where there was no resident private household. (Table A.1)

A.2.4 Conversion of addresses to households

The PAF is a list of delivery points for mail so most households within multi-occupied addresses are separately listed on the frame. It is estimated, however, that a small proportion (less than 2%) of addresses on the PAF contain more than one private household.

Since each address listed on the PAF was given only one chance of selection for the HEMS sample, additional procedures were carried out in the field by interviewers at addresses found to contain more than one household in order to ensure that all households were given a chance of selection. Where the sampled address contained more than one private household, interviewers were asked to interview at all households up to a maximum of three. In the rare event that an address contained more than three households, the interviewer was instructed to list the households systematically and then three were chosen at random by reference to a selection table. In order to limit workloads a maximum of four extra households per quota of addresses was allowed on this survey. In total, 94 extra households were identified in this way for inclusion in the survey, resulting in 7,152 households to be approached by interviewer. Twelve per cent (842) of these households contained no-one aged 16–74. Thus the total eligible sample of households was 6,310.

A.3 Sampling individuals within households

As noted above, one adult aged 16–74 was interviewed in each eligible household. This was done in preference to interviewing all eligible adults because it helped interviewers to carry out interviews in private and obtain more reliable information. It also ensured that respondents' answers, particularly to the attitudinal questions, were not contaminated by hearing other household members' answers. Finally, individuals in households tend to be similar to one another and where households differ markedly from one another, the resultant clustering can lead to a substantial increase in the standard error around survey estimates. This is particularly true in a topic area such as health behaviours where household members may influence each other.

In households where there was more than one person aged 16–74, the interviewer selected one person at random for interview, ensuring that all household members in the eligible age range had the same chance of being selected.

The selection procedure carried out at the household was a standard Social Survey Division procedure and was as follows:

(i) The interviewers listed everyone in the household on a selection sheet. They then numbered those aged 16 to 74 in order of age, eldest first.

(ii) The person to be interviewed was then defined by reference to a selection table which was printed on a set of reference cards.

(iii) The cards indicated which one of the eligible people should be selected for a given address, depending upon the serial number of the address and the number of eligible people in the household.

The selection table was based on those designed by Kish, which gave a close approximation to the proper fractional representation of each eligible adult in the household for up to six adults[2]. For this survey, selection tables for up to 8 eligible adults were used and a different set of possible selections was shown for each of the 40 addresses in each postcode sector.

In theory this meant that in households with nine or more eligible people some people would not get a chance of selection. In practice no households as large as this were found on the survey.

Often the person who had been selected for interview was not the person who had given the interviewer the household details, and so interviewers made arrangements to interview the selected person.

A.4 Response to the survey

Table A.2 shows the outcome for the sample of eligible individuals to the interviewer visit. Seventy four per cent of adults selected agreed to take part in the survey. An additional 2% of eligible individuals were interviewed by proxy. Seventeen per cent refused to take part, either before the interviewer visited the address (1%), at the sampling stage (5%) or at the main interview stage (11%). Interviewers were unable to contact 3% of households, and were not able to contact the sampled person in another 2%. In 1% of cases, the selected person was unable to be interviewed, either in person or by proxy, because he or she was too ill or absent for the whole field period or because of language difficulties. (**Table A.2**)

Adults aged 16–54 were eligible for the self-completion module on drugs and sexual health. A small number (3) had terminated the interview before reaching this module. The overwhelming majority (98%) of eligible respondents agreed to take part in the self-completion. As the interview was conducted using Computer-Assisted Interviewing (CAI), 86% recorded their own answers on the laptop, while 11% asked the interviewer to key their answers in for them. Nine respondents completed the drugs section but refused the sexual health section and seven completed the sexual health section but refused to answer questions on the drugs section. (**Table A.3**)

A.5 Non-response and weighting

This section describes the reweighting procedures used to compensate for differing probabilities of selection and non-response bias in the sample.

A.5.1 Weighting for probability of selection

There were two steps to the weighting. Firstly, weights were applied to take account of the different probabilities of selecting respondents in differently sized households. Secondly, all respondents were weighted up to represent the age-sex-region structure of the total national population of England living in private households.

Sample weights to allow for the different probabilities of selecting a respondent in differently sized households are shown in Table A.4, and correspond to the number of members of the household aged 16–74. (**Table A.4**)

A.5.2 Weighting for non-response bias

As noted above, the response rate for the face-to-face interviews was 74%. An additional 2% (145 cases) were interviewed by proxy; the proxy data are looked at in more detail in Section A.6.6. The weighting for non-response was applied to the full and partial interviews only as only these cases were used for analysis. The cases where interviews were carried out by proxy were therefore given a weight of one for non-response so that in effect they were only re-weighted for probability of selection.

The age, sex, regional, marital status and ethnic origin distributions of the responding sample on HEMS were compared with other national estimates, having first been reweighted for household size.

Estimates of age, sex, region and ethnic origin were taken from the December 1995 to February 1996 quarter of the Labour Force Survey (LFS) for England only. The LFS is a large sample survey carried out quarterly; the data are weighted and grossed to represent the total population. The 1995 mid-year population estimates which are based on the 1991 Census were also looked at but because these estimates include individuals living in institutions it was decided that the LFS estimates were more appropriate for comparison with HEMS. Estimates for marital status were taken from the 1994 General Household Survey (GHS)[3] as the categories for marital status used by the LFS differ from those used by HEMS. HEMS and the GHS use the same categories.

The HEMS sample under-represented men as a whole, although among men the age breakdown was similar to the LFS. The HEMS sample under-represented women aged 16–19 and over-represented women aged 40–44. The sample also under-represented people, particularly women, living in Greater London. **(Tables A.5–A.6)**

There were no significant differences between the proportions of GHS and HEMS respondents in different marital statuses. It should be noted that although the GHS results are themselves estimates and therefore subject to bias, Foster et al[4] conclude that evidence from the 1991 Census-linked study of the GHS sample showed that the non-response bias was relatively modest. **(Table A.7)**

With regard to ethnic origin the HEMS sample slightly under-represented Bangladeshi women. It was decided not to re-weight for this, however, as the numbers were too small to use for weighting and ethnic origin was not used in the analysis. **(Table A.8)**

It was decided to reweight the HEMS sample to give the correct proportions for age, sex and region. When the number of men and women living in London was broken down by age the numbers in some of the cells were too small to use for weighting so it was decided to create a new regional variable; those living in the South East and those not living in the South East and to weight by this. The age-sex-region weights were produced by dividing the population proportion by the sample proportion. The weights are shown in Table A.9. Categories with weights of less than 1.0 were over-represented in the HEMS responding sample and those with weights of more than 1.0 were under-represented. **(Table A.9)**

A.5.3 Creating a final weight

The final weight applied to the sample is the product of these two sets of weights. For example, applying the product of the two weights would give a weight of 3.87 for a female aged 16–24 living in the South East in a household containing three eligible people (1.29 x 3). Table A.10 shows the difference weighting for non-response made to some of the HEMS estimates. They show that, for behaviours associated with younger age-groups such as the prevalence of sunburn or use of drugs, weighting increases the proportion. **(Table A.10)**

The tables in the main body of the report present weighted proportions, and unweighted bases.

A.6 Characteristics of the responding sample

A.6.1 Age

The previous section discussed the age, sex and regional distribution of the responding sample. In general, this report shows results for six age-groups:

16–24
25–34
35–44
45–54
55–64
65–74

As the module on drugs and sexual health was only addressed to respondents aged 16–54, results for that part of the questionnaire are shown only for the first four age-groups.

When age has been cross-tabulated with other variables it has sometimes been necessary to collapse these 10 year age-groupings into broader groups because of small numbers in each age-group. Where the whole sample (aged 16–74) is covered, three groupings are used:

16–44
45–64
65–74

In the sexual health chapter, two age-groups are used:

16–34
35–54

and in the drugs chapter three age-groups are used:

16–24
25–34
35–54

A.6.2 Social class as defined by occupation

Respondents were assigned to a social class on the basis of their own current or last job, using the Standard Occupational Classification[5]. Social class has been presented throughout the report in four categories. Because of the small number of respondents in Social Classes I, II, IV and V, classes I and II, and IV and V have been combined. The four categories used are:

I and II	Professional, managerial and technical occupations
III Non-Manual	Skilled non-manual occupations
III Manual	Skilled manual occupations
IV and V	Unskilled occupations

Respondents who were members of the Armed Forces, whose occupation had been inadequately described or who had never worked were not allocated a social class.

Tables A.11–A.12 show the distribution by sex and age of respondents' social class. They show that men were more likely than women, and those aged 45–54 more likely than other age-groups, to be in the professional and managerial groups. Not surprisingly, the youngest age-groups were most likely to be in the 'unclassifiable' group. (Tables A.11–A.12)

The tables in the report show respondents' own social class. Fifty per cent of respondents were classified as the 'head of household' according to SSD's current definition[6]; where this was not the case, information regarding occupation was also collected for the head of household. The majority (81%) of male respondents were themselves the head of household; only 21% of female respondents were the head of household. Table A.13 shows the relationship between respondents' own social class and that of the head of household.

The overwhelming majority of men were, of course, classified to the same social class as the head of household. The proportion of women belonging to the same social class as the head of household varied from 29% of women in Social Class III (Non-Manual) to 69% of those categorised as belonging to Social Classes I and II. (Table A.13)

A.6.3 Highest qualification level

Respondents were asked if they had any qualifications. Those who had were shown a card and asked to indicate their highest qualification from a list of educational qualifications (See Appendix E). In common with other surveys[4,7], men in the HEMS sample were more likely than women to be qualified at 'A' level or above, and older people were more likely than younger people to report no qualifications. (Tables A.14–A.15)

A.6.4 Other socio-demographic characteristics

Men in the HEMS sample were more likely than women to be working, and to report higher gross household annual incomes. A higher proportion of women than of men were classified as 'economically inactive' and were living in Local Authority or Housing Association accommodation. (Tables A.16–A.18)

A.6.5 Social class and other characteristics

The analysis presented in the report has concentrated on sex, age and social class. Other characteristics have usually only been reported on when they have been of particular interest; previous studies have shown, for example, a strong association between marital status and sexual behaviour, so this characteristic was reported on in the chapter on sexual health.

Tables A.15–A.18 show the association between social class on the one hand, and highest qualification level, economic activity status, housing tenure status and income on the other. A higher proportion of respondents belonging to Social Classes I and II than of those categorised to other groups were qualified to 'A' level or above, were working, living in owner-occupied accommodation and receiving a gross annual household income of £20,000 or more. Conversely, those in Social Classes IV and V were most likely to have no qualifications, to live in accommodation rented from a Local Authority or Housing Association and to report an annual income of under £5,000. A higher proportion of men in these groups were unemployed. (Tables A.15–A.18)

A.6.6 Respondents interviewed by proxy

In households where it proved impossible to interview the selected person, a limited amount of information was collected from a proxy informant. (This was not done in 1995.) Proxy interviews were considerably shorter than full interviews, lasting 10–15 minutes. With a few exceptions, the questions concentrated on behaviour and proxies were not asked any knowledge or attitude questions. In total, 145 selected people were interviewed by proxy; in 23% of cases, the selected person was present at the interview. The main reason for taking a proxy interview was the absence of the selected person during the fieldwork period; this accounted for 65% of proxy interviews. Other reasons were language difficulties (21%) and illness (19%)[8]. Almost three fifths (59%) of proxy interviews were given by the spouse or partner of the selected person; other informants were a child (10%), a parent (12%) or sibling (6%) of the selected person. Eleven per cent of proxy informants did not live in the sampled household.

Tables A.19–A.20 show selected characteristics of respondents interviewed face-to-face and those interviewed by proxy. The data in these tables have been weighted for the probability of selection, but not for non-response. A higher proportion of those interviewed by proxy than of face-to-face respondents were male; 62%, compared with 46%. People interviewed by proxy were more likely than face-to-face respondents to live in Greater London (where, as noted earlier, response tended to be lower) and to live in a terraced house. They were less likely to be widowed, divorced or separated; to report any qualifications; to live in the East Midlands, or to live in a semi-detached house. There were no significant differences between the two groups in age or housing tenure status. A comparison of information provided by proxies and by informants themselves for the LFS[9] found that that there were more missing answers in proxy interviews for questions requiring detailed information; an example was the detailed description of respondents' jobs which is needed to code occupation and which is used to derive social class on the HEMS surveys; Table A.19 shows that a higher proportion of those interviewed by proxy than of face-to-face respondents were coded to the 'unclassified' group. (Table A.19)

Selected estimates for the two groups are shown in Table A.20. There were very few significant differences between them; respondents interviewed by proxy were less likely than face-to-face respondents to report being sunburnt in the last year, and to have undertaken a walk of 1–2 miles or participated in sports or exercise in the last four weeks. The LFS study showed that information collected by proxy was most accurate for demographic variables, but less reliable for estimates such as the number of hours worked. It is possible that HEMS proxy informants were unaware of all the walks, sports or exercise engaged in by the selected person and that the differences between respondents interviewed face-to-face and those interviewed by proxy arise, at least in part, from the method of data collection. The lack of significant difference between the two groups on other reported behaviours suggests that no systematic bias was introduced into the estimates presented in the report by not being able to conduct a full interview with these particular selected respondents. Because proxy informants were only asked a limited set of questions, the data were not included in Tables 1.1 to Figure 9.3. (Table A.20)

A.6.7 Non-responding addresses

Very little information is available about the people who did not respond at all to the survey, but interviewers were able to code the type of accommodation at 1,417 of the addresses at which the residents either refused to take part or could not be contacted. The proportions of responding and non-responding addresses in different types of accommodation are shown in Table A.21. (No information is available about the number of people aged 16–74 living in the majority of non-responding addresses; the data are therefore unweighted.) Non-responding addresses were less likely than responding addresses to be detached or semi-detached houses, and more likely to be terraced houses or flats. **(Table A.21)**

A.7 The accuracy of the survey results

Like all estimates based on samples, the results of the HEMS survey are subject to variations and errors. The total error associated with any survey estimate is the difference between the estimate derived from the data collected and the true value for the population. The total error can be divided into two main types of error: systematic error and random error.

Systematic error is often referred to as bias. Bias can arise because the sampling frame is incomplete, because of variation in the way interviewers ask questions and record answers, or because non-respondents to the survey have different characteristics to respondents. When designing surveys considerable effort is made to minimise systematic error; these include training interviewers to maximise response rates and to ask questions in a standard way, and carrying out pilot work to test questions and survey procedures and to assess whether the interview and individual questions are understood by and acceptable to respondents. Nonetheless, some systematic error is likely to remain.

Random error occurs because survey estimates are based not on the whole population but only a sample of it. There may be chance variations between such a sample and the whole population. If a number of repeats of the same survey were carried out, this error could be expected to average to zero. The variations depend on both the size of the sample and its design.

Statistical theory, however, enables estimates to be made of how close the survey results are to the true population values for each characteristic. A statistical measure of variation, the standard error, can be estimated from the values obtained for the sample, and provides a measure of the statistical precision of the survey estimate. This allows confidence intervals to be calculated around the sample estimate which give an indication of the range in which the true population value is likely to fall. The confidence interval generally used in survey research is the 95% confidence interval; it comprises the range of values from two standard errors below the estimate to two standard errors above the estimate.

For results based on simple random samples, without clustering or stratification, the estimation of standard errors is straightforward. When, as in the case of the HEMS and most other surveys, the sample design is not a simple random sample, a more complex calculation, using a formula which takes account of the random variation of the denominator and the stratification and clustering of the sample design, is necessary[10]. Stratification tends to reduce the standard error, while clustering tends to increase it.

In a complex sample design, the size of the standard error depends on how the characteristic of interest is spread within and between primary sampling units and between strata. So, for example, characteristics likely to be associated with the primary sampling unit, postcode sectors, will tend to have larger standard errors.

Tables A.22–A.30 show the standard error and 95% confidence intervals for selected survey estimates. They also show the design factor, or deft; the ratio of the standard error to the standard error that would have resulted had the survey design been a simple random sample of the same size. This is often used to give a broad indication of the degree of clustering. The tables do not cover all the topics discussed in the report; where possible, estimates for attitudes and behaviour are presented for each chapter. Standard errors were calculated for a different set of estimates from those used in 1995.

Design factors of less than 1.2 are considered to be small and indicate that the characteristic is not markedly clustered. However, substantial design factors of 1.2 or more were recorded for a number of characteristics, and this is reflected in being able to make less precise estimates for these characteristics than for other survey measures. A higher design factor indicates that the characteristic is more clustered geographically.

Among the sample characteristics covered in Table A.22, design factors of 1.2 or higher were found for the youngest age-groups, for those qualified to 'A' level or above and for single women. The design factors were also high for men in Social Classes I and II and Social Class III (Non-Manual). There were also high design factors for GP consultations. Very few of the other health-related characteristics covered in the tables had design factors of 1.2 or more and most of the occurrences were for single categories of a variable of interest. **(Tables A.22–A.30)**

Notes and references

1. Elliot D. *Optimising sample designs for surveys of health and related behaviour and attitudes*. Unpublished paper (1994).

2. Kish L. *Survey Sampling*. J Wiley & Sons Ltd (London 1965).

3. The data from the 1995 GHS were not available at the time the HEMS weighting was carried out.

4. Foster K et al. *General Household Survey 1993*. HMSO (London 1995).

5. OPCS. *Standard Occupational Classification Volume 3*. HMSO (London 1991).

6. The current definition of 'head of household' used by SSD is as follows:

    The member of the household in whose name the accommodation is owned or rented *except in the case of a married or cohabiting couple where the male partner takes precedence over the female*.

    If two people who are not a couple are jointly responsible for the accommodation, the oldest is taken if they are of the same sex, *but the male is taken if they are of different sex*.

    See McCrossan L. *A handbook for interviewers*. HMSO (London 1991).

    SSD is continuing methodological work to investigate whether the concept of 'head of household' should be replaced by a 'household reference person'. See Martin J. Defining a household reference person, *Survey Methodology Bulletin*, vol. 37, 1995, pp1–7, and Martin J and Barton J. The effect of changes in the definition of the household reference person, *Survey Methodology Bulletin*, vol. 38, 1996, pp1–8.

7. Bennett N et al. *Health Survey for England 1993*. HMSO (London 1995).

8. Percentages total more than 100% as interviewers could code more than one reason for taking a proxy interview.

9. Dawe F and Knight I. A study of proxy response on the Labour Force Survey. *Survey Methodology Bulletin*, 1997, vol 40, pp. 21–27.

10. For a full description of the method used to calculate standard errors for complex survey design, see Butcher B and Elliot D. A Sampling Errors Manual. HMSO (London 1992).

Appendix B Monitoring Frameworks and Health Promotion Indicators
by Antony Morgan and Mary Hickman – *Health Education Authority*

B.1 Introduction and background

The Health Education Authority (HEA) is concerned to improve assessment of national needs and outcomes as they relate to the targets set out in the *Health of the Nation*, as well as other wider health goals. It is committed to:

- providing serial measures of public awareness, knowledge, attitudes and behaviour towards specific health issues at national level; and

- monitoring both exposure and response to factors known or thought to influence behaviour change in these areas.

The HEA has a long history of carrying out health-related surveys. Recent published surveys include the National Fitness Survey (published jointly with the Sports Council), the Health and Lifestyle Survey 1992, Health and Lifestyles in England: Black and Minority Ethnic Groups 1993, as well as two surveys of young people aged 9–15 and 16–19 (published as *Tomorrow's Young Adults* and *Today's Young Adults* respectively). The publication of *Health in England 1995: What people know, what people think, what people do* in 1996 provided for the first time at national level available statistics placed within a framework for monitoring movements towards health targets. *Health in England 1996* provides the first update of these data.

B.2 Monitoring Frameworks

During 1996, the HEA continued to develop its series of monitoring frameworks which support the HEA's ability to contextualise its work in relation to a series of agreed health promotion objectives and interventions. Monitoring frameworks have now been prepared for adults in the areas of smoking, alcohol, sexual health, nutrition, skin cancer, immunisation, drugs and folic acid, and for young people in the areas of alcohol, drugs, mental health, nutrition, skin cancer, teenage pregnancy, teenage smoking, sexual health and oral health. Each monitoring framework contains a number of health promotion indicators which can be used as interim measures of progress towards HON targets.

Through analysis of data from a number of surveys, approximately 80 health promotion indicators were identified for possible inclusion in the monitoring frameworks. These indicators have been compiled into an internal document mirroring the format of the 'Specification of National Indicators' giving details of:

The HON Area/ Target of Relevance
Indicator Title
Indicator Definition
Years for which baseline data are available
Area
Source of Information
Monitoring Frequency

Essentially, the HEA's monitoring frameworks enable us systematically to identify:

- the organisation's *overall* objective in relation to a particular *Health of the Nation* target;

- a series of more *specific* objectives which will secure the achievement of the overall objective;

- the interventions that are necessary to achieve the specific objectives; and

- the information, in the form of health promotion indicators, which can be used as proxy measures of success in the achievement of objectives.

The first HEMS report provided baseline data for the indicators that have been developed on knowledge, attitudes and behaviour (KAB) of the individual. The HEA recognises the importance of monitoring trends in health-related knowledge, attitudes, behaviours and beliefs, norms and perceptions of risk, and risk taking among individuals, and therefore is committed to carrying out this survey at regular intervals.

Monitoring frameworks so far have described health promotion objectives in relation to the KAB paradigm as a valid model of individual behaviour change. Health promotion indicators contained within these frameworks are largely individually focused. Health promotion research contributes further understanding of health-related behaviour change, risk and risk perception within the wider social, economic, cultural and political contexts within which human behaviour occurs. It is increasingly recognised that community-based approaches to health promotion are among the most effective approaches in reducing risk factors, increasing life expectancy and reducing morbidity in non-communicable diseases. Community-based approaches also go beyond increasing the autonomy, knowledge and/or skills of individuals. Monitoring frameworks will therefore continue to be developed to reflect this wider view of the contribution health promotion can make to the achievement of wider health goals.

B.3 Other related work

B 3.1 Health Behaviour of School Aged Children Survey (HBSC)

This survey is a WHO Cross-National Survey initiated in 1982. The study has three main aims. Firstly to gain new insights into and increase understanding of young people's health attitudes and behaviour; secondly, to increase understanding of how young people perceive health itself; thirdly to develop national information systems on health and lifestyles of each country's young people. The HBSC is administered to school-aged young people at regular intervals, at least every four years, in a growing number of countries. England, as represented by the HEA, was accepted as an associate member of the project in 1995. It was decided to run the first survey in the autumn of 1995, based on the questionnaire used by other countries during the 1993–4 school year. The HEA commissioned BMRB International to carry out the work in 1995. The first report was published earlier this year.

This survey is complimentary to the HEMS, since it will be used to track some of the health promotion indicators identified in the young people's monitoring frameworks described above.

B 3.2 Health and Lifestyles Guide to Sources CDROM

Those working in the areas of health education and promotion need to be aware of information sources which might inform their work. Health and lifestyle surveys which investigate attitudes as well as behaviour are of particular value, but there is no easy way of identifying which surveys exist. This CDROM, published in January 1997, was developed in response to a need for a reference tool to access health education related sources of information, particularly those covering the five Key Areas of the *Health of the Nation*.

This resource is not intended to present data in terms of survey results although, where available, key findings are presented. More particularly, it highlights quantitative surveys of sound methodological design available at national level, including those carried out by and on behalf of the HEA in the last six years. It presents details of these surveys, indicating information which could be usefully collected at local level and used to support policy development and planning.

The Guide was initially developed as a paper-based document at the HEA to assist researchers and planners in identifying what information exists at a national level and to assist in day-to-day problems of questionnaire content and design. It was recognised that this document would be useful to many others working in health education and promotion and the CDROM format was found to be the most appropriate way of presenting the information contained within the document.

The HEA intends to update this guide on an annual basis. Although it contains details of the major surveys which exist nationally it is not comprehensive. Some surveys which appeared in the original internal paper version are not included in the CDROM because some originators of the survey questionnaires would not give their permission.

B 3.3 Reviews of Effectiveness

Over the last few years there has been increasing pressure on health authorities to provide evidence of effectiveness to support decision making processes in the delivery of health care. *The Health of the Nation* Strategy reinforced this need in relation to health promotion and disease prevention, stating that resources should be concentrated on areas where action is more likely to be effective.

The Cochrane Centre (UKCC), established in 1992 to facilitate systematic reviews of effectiveness of health care and prevention and provide a co-ordinated focus for collation of the findings on randomised controlled trials, provides a coherent foundation for the development of evidence-based medicine. The UKCC has spawned the Cochrane Collaboration comprising review groups on a wide range of topics serviced by a volunteer network of international researchers with the task of extending the evidence for health care interventions.

In seeking to establish a similarly sound basis for evidence-based health promotion, the HEA has commissioned a series of literature reviews of effectiveness.

The HEA is currently publishing its series of reviews, which aim to support purchasers and providers of health promotion by meeting an increased need for information on how limited resources might be used in the most effective way.

Reviews published to date are :

- health promotion in older people for the prevention of coronary heart disease and stroke.
- health promotion in childhood and young adolescence for the prevention of unintentional injuries.
- effectiveness of videos in health education

Forthcoming reviews will be in the areas of :

- mental health
- young people and substance abuse
- young people and alcohol
- healthy eating
- oral health

Each review :

- pulls together the scientific knowledge base to date
- identifies the main collective recommendations for policy developers and purchasers about planning effective interventions
- identifies directions for further research

This work will feed directly into the further development of monitoring frameworks by identifying those interventions which have been found to be most effective.

Appendix C Physical activity – Energy intensity categories and frequency measures for different types of activity

by Alison Walker

C.1 The indicators of participation in physical activity

Physical activity as measured by the Health Education Monitoring Survey included:

- 'home' activities, (housework, gardening and DIY)
- walking
- sports and exercise activities including cycling
- activity at work

Stair climbing and caring activities were not included.

Two HEA indicators of participation were used, based on the intensity and frequency of activity. Both indicators included an element of duration; activities in the sports and recreational category were included in the first summary only if they had lasted at least 30 minutes and in the second if they had lasted at least 20 minutes.

> HEA suggested health promotion indicator: Percentage active at moderate or vigorous level for 30 minutes or more, five times a week

The first summary measure is based on occasions of 'moderate or vigorous' intensity activity, defined as having an energy cost of at least 5 kcals/min. This included:

- 'heavy' housework and 'heavy' gardening or DIY
- walks of 1–2 miles at a fast or brisk pace
- sports and exercise activities (including cycling) defined as having an energy cost of at least 5 kcal/min - see below
- occupational activity defined as involving at least moderate intensity activity – see below

A duration threshold of at least 30 minutes was applied to sports activities, and walking was included only if the walk was of 1–2 miles or more. All other types of activity were included irrespective of duration.

> HEA suggested health promotion indicator: Percentage of adults 16–74 active at a vigorous level for 20 minutes three times a week

The second summary measure of activity is based on occasions of 'vigorous' intensity activity, defined as having an energy cost of at least 7.5 kcals/min. By definition, sports and exercise activities and occupational activity were the only categories which could be classified as 'vigorous' activity – see section C.2.

A duration threshold of at least 20 minutes was applied to sports activities.

C.2 Energy intensity categories and frequency measures

C.2.1 Home activities: Energy cost

Moderate   'Heavy' housework and 'heavy' gardening/DIY were both classified as moderate-intensity activities. Respondents were shown cards giving the following examples:

Walking with heavy shopping for more than 5 minutes, moving heavy furniture, spring cleaning, scrubbing floors with a scrubbing brush, cleaning windows, or other similar heavy housework.

Digging, clearing rough ground, building in stone/bricklaying, mowing large areas with a hand mower, felling trees, chopping wood, mixing/laying concrete, moving heavy loads, refitting a kitchen or bathroom or any similar heavy manual work.

C.2.2 Home activities: Frequency

Number of days in the past four weeks on which informant did 'heavy' housework plus number of days on which did 'heavy' gardening/DIY.

C.2.3 Occupational activity: Energy cost

Vigorous   Considers self 'very physically' active in job and is in one of the following occupations defined as involving heavy work, including:

fishermen/women, furnace operators, rollermen, smiths, forgers, faceworking coal-miners, construction workers, fire service officers, metal plate workers, shipwrights, riveters, steel erectors, benders, fitters, galvanisers, tin platers, dip platers, plasterers, roofers, glaziers, general building workers, road surfacers, stevedores, dockers, goods porters, refuse collectors.

Moderate Considers self 'very physically' active in job and is **not** in occupation groups listed above
OR
considers self 'fairly physically' active in job and is in one of the occupations listed above

C.2.4 Occupational activity: Frequency

Not collected for occupational activity.

C.2.5 Sports and exercise activities: Energy cost

Vigorous

    a) All occasions of running/jogging, squash, boxing, kick boxing, skipping, trampolining

    b) Sports coded as vigorous intensity if they had made the respondent breathe heavily or sweat a lot, but otherwise coded as moderate intensity including: cycling, aerobics, keep fit, gymnastics, dance for fitness, weight training, football, rugby, swimming, tennis, badminton

Moderate

    a) See 'vigorous' category (b), but where the activity did not make the respondent breathe heavily or sweat a lot

    b) All occasions of a large number of sports including: basketball, canoeing, fencing, field athletics, hockey, ice skating, lacrosse, netball, roller skating, rowing, skiing, volleyball

    c) Sports coded as moderate intensity if they had made respondent breathe heavily or sweat a lot, but otherwise coded as light intensity, including: exercises (press-ups, sit-ups etc), dancing

C.2.6 Sports and exercise activities: Frequency

Number of days in past four weeks.
Time usually spent per day of activity.

C.2.7 Walking: Energy cost

Moderate Walks of 1–2 miles or more with a brisk or fast pace.

C.2.8 Walking: Frequency

Number of walks of 1–2 miles or more in the past four weeks.

C.3 Reference period

A four-week reference period was used in the interview. Frequency of activity during the four-week period is expressed in the results as an average frequency per week, based on the following conversion:

Frequency of activity in past four weeks	Average frequency per week
0–3 occasions	Less than once a week
4–11 occasions	1–2 times a week
12–19 occasions	3–4 times a week
20+ occasions	5+ times a week

C.4 Changes to the physical activity questions between 1995 and 1996

There is always a dilemma in conducting repeated surveys as to whether it is more important to maintain total comparability from year to year or whether it is better to attempt to improve/modify the questions where necessary.

The questions on physical activity have been slightly modified in 1996 to be more closely aligned with the content of the HEA indicator based on participation in at least moderate-intensity activity. This indicator refers to **30 minutes** of activity on five or more **days** a week. Two changes have been made.

Previously, information relating to frequency and duration of participation in sports and exercise activities referred to 'occasions' of participation. The questions now refer to the number of 'days' and the time spent per day. Information on home activities has always referred to participation per day.

The definition of minimum walking distance has also been changed to be more closely aligned with the 30 minutes of activity specified in the indicator. Previous HEMS' analyses have been based on walks of two miles or more. This has been changed in 1996 to walks of 1–2 miles or more. This change has been made on the basis of a walking speed of at least three mph.

C.5 Effect of the changes

C.5.1 Use of 'days' for sports and exercise participation

In HEMS 96 the unit of participation for sports and exercise activities was changed from an 'occasion' to a 'day'. There is the possibility that this could affect the measure of frequency of participation if respondents tended to participate on more than one occasion per day. In order to investigate this effect, if any, the results of a recent methodological study were examined.

As part of the development work for the 1997 Health Survey for England, the Department of Health conducted a study to investigate various aspects of the collection of data relating to physical activity (DH 1996 unpublished). One method of data collection referred to 'days' as the basic unit of participation but subdivided 'days' into 'occasions'. This allows a comparison of frequency measures for participation in sports and exercise activities based on these two units of participation. Both 'days' and 'occasions' included the 30 minute minimum duration. Table C.1 shows that there was no significant difference between the frequency distribution based on 'days' compared with that based on 'occasions'. Further investigation within age-groups also showed no differences between the two distributions.

C.5.2 Walking

The definition for walks for inclusion in the activity summary was changed in 1996 to a 'walk of 1–2 miles or more'. Previously walks had been included if they were of '2 miles or more'. (The pace requirement was maintained unchanged as 'fast or brisk'.) A possible effect of this change would be to increase the numbers of respondents who reported such walks and therefore increase the overall frequency of participation in activity.

The walking data for HEMS 96 was compared with those for HEMS 95 to investigate the effect of this change on the reported frequency of walking. Table C.2 shows that the proportion of men and women walking less than once a week (at the appropriate pace) was significantly lower in 1996 than in 1995 and the proportion of men and women who reported walking five times a week or more was higher in 1996. Although it is not possible to say conclusively that this does not represent a genuine population change in walking behaviour, it seems more likely that most of this difference is attributable to the change in definition. The size of the increase would also serve to explain the apparent increase between the two years in overall participation in at least moderate-intensity activity, shown in Table 3.1.

Table C.1 Weekly frequency of participation in at least moderate-intensity sports and exercise activities lasting 30 minutes or more per unit of participation

	Men — 30 mins per occasion %	Men — 30 mins per day %	Women — 30 mins per occasion %	Women — 30 mins per day %
Less than once per week	66	65	75	75
1–2 per week	15	15	15	15
3–4 per week	7	7	5	5
5+ per week	12	13	5	5
Base	898		1096	

Unpublished data from Department of Health methodological survey.

Table C.2 Frequency of walking 2+ miles compared with 1–2+ miles (both at a fast or brisk pace)

	Men HEMS 95 2+ miles %	Men HEMS 96 1–2+ miles %	Women HEMS 95 2+ miles %	Women HEMS 96 1–2+ miles %
Less than once per week	85	80	90	86
1–4 per week	12	13	7	9
5+ per week	3	7	3	5
Base	2122	2044	2550	2601

Appendix D Technical appendix

D.1 Logistic regression

Logistic regression is a multivariate statistical technique which has been used in a number of chapters in this report. It predicts the outcome of a dependent variable which only has two possible outcomes, for example being a current smoker and not being a current smoker, from a set of independent variables. Variables with only two possible outcomes are also known as dichotomous variables or binary variables. Logistic regression was developed specifically for dichotomous variables and makes more appropriate assumptions about the underlying distributions and the range of possible proportions than the more familiar multiple linear regression method.

Most of the tables in the HEMS report (for example Table 2.1) are based on crosstabulations. These tables show the proportion of people with a given characteristic who display the behaviour of interest; an example would be the proportion of people aged 16-24 who smoke. What such tables do not show, however, is how much other factors may interrelate with the independent variable; for example, how much social class and sex may interrelate with age to influence whether or not a person smokes. Logistic regression looks at how different independent variables interrelate by looking at the odds of the behaviour occurring for different combinations of the independent variables. Odds refers to the ratio of the probability that the event will occur to the probability that the event will not occur. The odds can be converted into a probability (p) using the following formula:

$$p = \frac{odds}{1 + odds}$$

Logistic regression can therefore be used to predict the probability of a behaviour occurring given a combination of characteristics, for example, it can be used to model the probability of a person being either a smoker or a non-smoker given their age, sex and social class.

The logistic regression model can be written as:

$$Prob(event) = \frac{e^z}{1 + e^z}$$

where e is the base of the natural logarithms. Logistic regression actually models independent variables against the log odds (the natural logarithm of the odds) of an event because this forms a linear relationship:

$$Z = B_0 + B_1X_1 + \ldots\ldots B_pX_p,$$

where the Xs are the independent variables, Bs are the model parameters and B_0 is the baseline odds. The odds of engaging in behaviour can then be calculated by multiplying the baseline odds by the appropriate factors.

Before carrying out the logistic regression analysis data are crosstabulated to give an indication of which independent variables should be included in the regression. One of the categories of each of the independent variables is then defined as a reference category (with a value of 1); the reference category is the group least likely to display the behaviour of interest. For each of the independent variables included in the regression a coefficient is produced which represents the factor by which the odds of a person taking part in the behaviour increases if the person has that characteristic. The odds produced by the regression are relative odds, that is they are relative to the reference category. Taking the example above, where smoking is the dependent variable, the age group 65–74 would be defined as the reference category as this is the group least likely to smoke and the odds given by the model would be relative to this; so it would be possible to say how much greater the odds were of a person aged 16–24 being a smoker than the odds of a person aged 65–74 being a smoker.

There are different methods of including independent variables in the logistic regression model. The method used in the HEMS analysis was forward stepwise selection which is where the model starts off only containing the constant and then at each step the independent variable which is the most highly significant is added in. Variables are then examined and the coefficients which make the observed results 'most likely' are selected while the others are removed using either the Wald statistic or the Likelihood-Ratio test. The Likelihood-Ratio test was used in the HEMS analysis.

The odds ratios produced by the regression are presented in the report as 'multiplying factors' and they are shown with the 95% confidence intervals. If the confidence interval does not include 1.00 then the odds ratio is likely to be significantly different from the reference category.

For a more detailed description of logistic regression analysis see Chapter 2 of *SPSS Advanced Statistics User's Guide* (SPSS Inc. 1990).

D.2 Age-standardisation

The association between age and health and many health-related behaviours is well-documented. It is therefore important to take age into account when investigating the relationship between health and other characteristics such as social class and marital status. One commonly-used method is the presentation of three-way tables such as Tables 8.2 and 8.5, which tabulate the prevalence of self-reported good general health and self-reported long-standing illness by social class for a number of age-groups. The resulting tables may, however, be difficult to interpret and suffer from small cell sizes; in both tables, for example, there are only 31 men aged 65–74 in Social Class III (Non-Manual).

Alternatives are the use of modelling techniques, such as logistic regression, which is discussed above and has been used in a number of chapters in the report, or age standardisation, which presents the data in tabular format. The method of standardisation used in this report, in Chapters 3 and 8, is that of indirect standardisation; this is considered more appropriate for survey data than the direct method of standardisation which is used in medical statistics. Direct standardisation involves applying age-specific rates for the whole population of men or women to the age distribution in the sub-group (for example, the social class) of interest. The method does not make use of the rates observed for age-groups within social classes which are likely to be based on small sample totals and to be affected by substantial sampling error.

The age-standardised ratios shown in tables such as Tables 8.3 and 8.6 were calculated by dividing the observed proportions reporting good health by the expected proportion and then multiplying by 100. An age-standardised ratio of more than 100 indicates a greater likelihood of reporting a particular characteristic or behaviour than would be expected in that group on the basis of age distribution alone. Conversely, a ratio of less than 100 indicates that the members of the group are less likely to report the characteristic or behaviour under consideration than would be expected from the age composition of the group. Since standardised ratios are calculated from survey data, they are subject to sampling error and a more precise assessment of their deviation from 100 involves the use of the standard error of the ratio in a conventional test of statistical significance. To take Table 8.3 as an example, the standard error of the ratio for men in Social Classes I and II is 0.9; multiplying this by 1.96 (the 95% level of significance) gives 1.76; as the difference between 106 (the standardised ratio for this group) and 100 is greater than the resulting figure, this difference is taken to be significant.

As explained in Appendix A, however, because the sample for the HEMS survey was a multi-stage probability sample involving both stratification and clustering, standard errors assuming a simple random sample will tend to be underestimates. One way of dealing with this is to adjust the standard error by the design factor (deft) to allow for the complex sample design. Table A.20 in the 1995 HEMS report (this estimate is not presented in the 1996 report) shows that the deft for self-reported good general health was 1.04 for men and 1.11 for women; multiplying the standard error for men in Social Classes I and II by this deft gives 1.83, still significant.

A final stage is needed to take account of the weighting which was applied to the sample to compensate for non-response. The standard error was multiplied by the square root of the mean weight (1.5 for men and 1.3 for women) to allow for the fact that the standardised ratios were calculated on weighted data. In the example of men in Social Classes I and II discussed above, the final calculation was as follows:

$$0.9 \times 1.96 \times 1.04 \times 1.5 = 2.75$$

The standardised ratio for this group was 106; as the difference between this and 100 is larger than 2.75, it can be concluded that the ratio was higher than expected at the 95% level of significance.

For a more detailed description of the indirect method of standardisation see Foster K. The use of standardisation in survey analysis. *Survey Methodology Bulletin*, OPCS, vol. 33, 1993, pp. 19–27.

Appendix E Fieldwork Documents

The survey was carried out using computer-assisted interviewing. This is a copy of the questions.

HEALTH EDUCATION MONITORING SURVEY 1996

HOUSEHOLD BOX

Interviewer code

IntType   Code whether interview is full or proxy

     1   Full
     2   Proxy

Ask all respondents

Npersons   I would like to start by asking you about yourself and your household. How many people normally live in this household?
INCLUDE ALL PERSONS, INCLUDING THOSE AGED 75 AND OVER

     1...14

Ask about everyone in the household

Name   START WITH SELECTED PERSON
ASK THE FOLLOWING QUESTIONS OF EVERY ONE IN THE HOUSEHOLD. IF INFORMANT IS MARRIED/COHABITING, ENTER SPOUSE/ PARTNER AS PERSON 2.

     Name or other identifier

Sex   INTERVIEWER: CODE NAME's SEX.

     1   Male
     2   Female

Ask about selected person only

DoB   INTERVIEWER: CODE NAME's DATE OF BIRTH

Ask about everyone in the household

Age   What was NAME's age last birthday?
IF AGE NOT GIVEN, PROBE FOR AN ESTIMATE

Ask if household member is aged 16 or over

Marstat   Are you

     1   married
     2   living as married
     3   single/never married
     4   widowed
     5   divorced
     6   or separated?
     7   SPONTANEOUS living with a same sex partner

Ask about everyone in the household

RelToInf   ASK OR CODE RELATIONSHIP TO SELECTED PERSON

     1   Informant
     2   Spouse\partner (incl. same-sex partner)
     3   Son\daughter (include adopted/step-child)
     4   Foster child
     5   Son-in-law\daughter-in-law
     6   Parent\step-parent
     7   Parent-in-law
     8   Brother\sister(incl. adopted)
     9   Brother-in-law\sister-in-law
     10   Grandchild
     11   Grandparent
     12   Other (related)
     13   Other (not related)

Ask if household member is aged 16 or over

WhoHOH   IS THIS PERSON THE HOH?
REMEMBER THAT WHERE A PROPERTY IS OWNED\RENTED IN THE NAME OF A WOMAN WHO IS MARRIED\COHABITING WITH A MAN, THEN BY DEFINITION, THE MAN IS THE HOH.

     1   Yes
     2   No

Ask all respondents

NAdults   ASK OR CODE
Number of adults aged 16-74 in the household

1...14

Ask respondents who are married, living as married, or living with a same sex partner

Livtgthr   How long have you and your husband/wife/partner been living together as a couple?
INCLUDE ANY TIME SPENT COHABITING BEFORE MARRIAGE.
ENTER TIME IN YEARS. IF LESS THAN ONE YEAR, ENTER 0

Ask respondents who are single, widowed, divorced or separated and aged 16-54

Partner   May I just check, do you have a regular partner who does not live in the household?

1   Yes
2   No

Ask all respondents

WorkLast   Did you do any paid work in the week ending last Sunday, either as an employee or as self-employed?

1   Yes
2   No

If working last week

Fullpart   In your present job do you work

1   full-time
2   or part-time?

Ask all respondents

Ownorent   Does your household own or rent this accommodation?
CODE FIRST THAT APPLIES

1   Buying with a mortgage
2   Owned outright
3   Rented from Local Authority/New Town
4   Rented from Housing Association
5   Rented unfurnished
6   Rented furnished
7   Rented from employer
8   Other with payment
9   Rent-free

AccomType   INTERVIEWER CODE TYPE OF ACCOMMODATION

1   Detached house
2   Semi-detached house
3   Terraced/end of terrace house
4   Purpose-built flat
5   Flat in a converted house
6   Caravan, mobile home or houseboat
7   Other type of accommodation

Car   Is there a car or van **normally** available for use by you or any members of your household?

1   Yes
2   No

GENERAL HEALTH

Ask all respondents

Genhlth   [*] Now I would like to ask you some questions about your health.
How is your health in general? Would you say it was..
RUNNING PROMPT

1   very good
2   good
3   fair
4   bad
5   or very bad?

Illness   [*] Do you have any long-standing illness, disability or infirmity? By long-standing I mean anything that has troubled you over a period of time or that is likely to affect you over a period of time?

1   Yes
2   No

Ask respondents who have a long-standing illness, disability or infirmity (Illness = Yes)

Lmatter   [*] What is the matter with you?

Limitact   [*] Does this illness or disability (Do any of these illnesses or disabilities) limit your activities in any way?

1   Yes
2   No

Ask all respondents

Goodhlth   [*] Here is a list of factors that could affect your health, which, if any, currently have a good effect on your health?
SHOW CARD A

1   Relationships,family
2   My work
3   My income/standard of living
4   My alcohol consumption
5   The exercise I do
6   What I eat
7   None of these

Badhlth   [*] Now I would like you to look at this card. Which of these, if any, currently have a bad effect on **your** health?
SHOW CARD B

1   Not having a job
2   Relationships, family
3   Pollution
4   My smoking
5   Others' smoking

	6 My alcohol consumption
	7 Lack of exercise
	8 What I eat
	9 My weight
	10 None of these
Doctalk	During the past year, that is since (today's date) 1995, apart from any visit to a hospital, have you talked to a GP either in person or by telephone, about your health? CODE FIRST THAT APPLIES 1 Yes, at surgery 2 Yes in person at home 3 Yes by telephone 4 No

Ask respondents who answered 2-4 to Doctalk

OthProf	During the past year, that is since (today's date) 1995, have you talked to another health professional, for example a nurse or health visitor etc at the surgery or health centre. 1 Yes 2 No

Ask of women aged 16-49

Pregnant	May I just check, are you pregnant at the moment? 1 Yes 2 No 3 Don't know

Ask of married or cohabiting men, or same-sex cohabiting women, with a partner aged 16-49

Pregnt2	May I just check, is your wife/partner pregnant at the moment? 1 Yes 2 No 3 Don't know

Ask all respondents

Hlthlife	[*] On the whole, would you say that you lead ... RUNNING PROMPT 1 a very healthy life 2 a fairly healthy life 3 a not very healthy life 4 or an unhealthy life? 5 Don't know
HlthIntr	Here are are some things people have said about health. I'd like you to say how far you agree with each statement, choosing your answer from this card.
Hlthimp	SHOW CARD C [*] To have good health is the most important thing in life. 1 Strongly agree 2 Agree 3 Neither agree nor disagree 4 Disagree 5 Strongly disagree
Docsay	SHOW CARD C [*] It's sensible to do exactly what the doctors say. 1 Strongly agree 2 Agree 3 Neither agree nor disagree 4 Disagree 5 Strongly disagree
Hlthluck	SHOW CARD C [*] Generally health is a matter of luck. 1 Strongly agree 2 Agree 3 Neither agree nor disagree 4 Disagree 5 Strongly disagree
Toomuch	SHOW CARD C [*] If you think too much about your health you are more likely to be ill. 1 Strongly agree 2 Agree 3 Neither agree nor disagree 4 Disagree 5 Strongly disagree
Illdoc	SHOW CARD C [*] I have to be very ill before I go to the doctor. 1 Strongly agree 2 Agree 3 Neither agree nor disagree 4 Disagree 5 Strongly disagree
Dontthnk	SHOW CARD C [*] I don't really have time to think about my health. 1 Strongly agree 2 Agree 3 Neither agree nor disagree 4 Disagree 5 Strongly disagree
Stress	[*]Looking at this card, which of these statements best describes the amount of stress or pressure you experienced in the past 12 months, that is since (today's date) 1995. SHOW CARD D 1 Completely free of stress 2 Small amount of stress 3 Moderate amount of stress 4 Large amount of stress 5 Don't know

Ask respondents who answered 2-4 to stress

Harm	How harmful would you say the amount of stress and pressure you have experienced in the last 12

months has been to your physical and mental health? Has it been...
RUNNING PROMPT

1　very harmful
2　quite harmful
3　or not harmful at all?
4　Don't know

SKIN CANCER

Ask all respondents

IntroSoc　There's been a lot of publicity recently about skin cancer. I would like to ask you a few questions about this.

Creamsun　Do you ever wear a suncream?

1　Yes
2　No
3　Never go out in the sun

Ask if Creamsun = Yes

Whencrem　When do you use a suncream?
Please choose your answers from this card.
SHOW CARD E
CODE ALL THAT APPLY

1　Sunbathing abroad
2　Outdoors abroad, but not sunbathing
3　Sunbathing in this country
4　Outdoors in this country doing something else

Factor　Which factor level of suncream do you use most regularly?

1　2-5
2　6-10
3　11-16
4　17 or over
5　Don't know

Ask all respondents

SunBurn　During the last 12 months, that is since (today's date) 1995, have you had sunburn causing redness and soreness of the skin lasting for at least 1-2 days?

1　Yes
2　No
3　Can't remember

Ask if Sunburn = Yes

FreqBurn　How many times?

1　Once
2　Twice
3　Three times
4　Four or more
5　Not in the last 12 months

Ask all respondents

Skinburn　[*]SHOW CARD F
Now I would like you to look at this card and say which of these statements best describes what happens to your skin when you go out in the sun without protection

1　Always burns and never tans
2　Burns at first and tans with difficulty
3　Burns at first then tans easily
4　Rarely burns and tans easily
5　Never burns and always tans
6　Other
7　Refused

SkinType　[*] SHOW CARD G
Now I would like you to look at this card and say which of these statements best describes your natural skin type

1　White skin
2　Brown skin
3　Black skin
4　Olive skin
5　Other
6　Refused

Ask if answer 1 or 4 at SkinType

SunTan　[*] How important is having a suntan to you personally? Is it..
RUNNING PROMPT

1　very important
2　fairly important
3　or not important?
4　Don't know

SunIntr　Here are some things people have said about having a suntan. I'd like you to say how far you agree with each statement, choosing your answer from this card.

Sunhlth　[*] SHOW CARD H
Having a suntan makes me feel healthier

1　Strongly agree
2　Agree
3　Neither agree nor disagree
4　Disagree
5　Strongly disagree

Attract　SHOW CARD H
[*] Having a suntan makes me look more attractive

1　Strongly agree
2　Agree
3　Neither disagree nor disagree
4　Disagree
5　Strongly disagree

SMOKING

Ask all respondents

Smokintr   The following questions are about smoking;

SmokeSC   INTERVIEWER: 16 AND 17 YEAR-OLDS **MUST** SELF-COMPLETE;
FOR INFORMANTS AGED 18 OR OVER THE QUESTIONS SHOULD BE ASKED BY YOU UNLESS YOU THINK THE INFORMANTS WOULD PREFER TO ANSWER THESE QUESTIONS BY SELF-COMPLETION.

1   Completed by interviewer
2   Self-completion accepted and completed

Ask respondents who accepted self-completion

Smkintr2   I would like you to take the computer and answer the questions yourself. Instructions on how to answer the questions are given on the screen.

WORK THROUGH THE FIRST QUESTION WITH THE INFORMANT. IF THE INFORMANT MAKES A MISTAKE, TAKE THEM BACK TO THE QUESTION AND ALLOW THEM TO KEY IN THE RIGHT ANSWER.

Practice   This is the first time I have used a computer.

1   Yes
2   No
3   Don't want to answer

Ask all respondents

Cigever   Have you ever smoked a cigarette, a cigar or a pipe?

1   Yes
2   No

Ask respondents who have ever smoked a cigarette, cigar or a pipe (Cigever = Yes)

Cignow   Do you smoke cigarettes at all nowadays?

1   Yes
2   No

Ask current cigarette smokers (Cignow = Yes)

Qtywkend   About how many cigarettes **a day** do you usually smoke at weekends?
IF LESS THAN 1, ENTER 0.

Qtywkday   About how many cigarettes **a day** do you usually smoke on weekdays?
IF LESS THAN 1, ENTER 0.

Cigtype   Do you mainly smoke...
RUNNING PROMPT

1   filter-tipped cigarettes
2   plain or untipped cigarettes
3   or hand-rolled cigarettes?

Ask respondents who mainly smoke hand-rolled cigarettes (Cigtype = 3)

QtyTob   How much tobacco do you usually smoke **per week**?
Would you prefer to give your answer in

1   quarter ounces
2   or in grammes?

Ask if QtyTob = Ounces

QtyTob1   ENTER NO. OF **QUARTER** OUNCES PER WEEK.
IF ANSWER GIVEN IN OUNCES, MULTIPLY BY FOUR IF LESS THAN QUARTER OF AN OUNCE, ENTER 0

0...20

Ask if QtyTob = Grammes

QtyTobM   ENTER NO. OF GRAMMES PER WEEK

0...150

Ask current cigarette smokers (Cignow = Yes)

Nosmoke   [*] How easy or difficult do you think you would find it to go without smoking for a whole day. Would you find it...
RUNNING PROMPT

1   very easy
2   fairly easy
3   fairly difficult
4   or very difficult?
5   Don't know

Trystop   Have you ever tried to give up smoking?

1   Yes
2   No

Ask respondents who have ever tried to give up smoking (Trystop = Yes)

Lasttime   Thinking of the last time you tried to give up, how long was it for?

1   Less than a day
2   A day, less than a week
3   A week, less than a month
4   A month, less than 3 months
5   Three months, less than six months
6   Six months, less than a year
7   One year or more

WhenSt   And how long is it since you started smoking again?

1   Within last week
2   Within last month
3   Within last six months
4   Within last year
5   More than a year ago

Ask current cigarette smokers (Cignow = Yes)

Giveup [*] Would you like to give up smoking altogether?

1 Yes
2 No
3 Don't know

Ask respondents who would like to give up smoking altogether (Giveup = Yes)

Stop1 Now I would like you to look at this card, and say which of the statements best describes you.
SHOW CARD I

1 I intend to give up smoking within the next month
2 I intend to give up smoking within the next six months
3 I intend to give up smoking within the next year
4 I intend to give up smoking but not in the next year
5 I'm unlikely to give up smoking

Ask respondents who wouldn't like to give up smoking altogether (Giveup = No or don't know)

Stop2 Now I would like you to look at this card, and say which of the statements best describes you.
SHOW CARD J

1 I'm unlikely to give up smoking
2 I intend to give up smoking within the next month
3 I intend to give up smoking within the next six months
4 I intend to give up smoking within the next year
5 I intend to give up smoking but not in the next year

Ask ex-cigarette smokers (Cignow = No)

CigReg [*] Did you smoke cigarettes..
RUNNING PROMPT

1 regularly, that is, at least one cigarette a day
2 or did you smoke them only occasionally?
3 SPONTANEOUS Never really smoked cigarettes, just tried them once or twice

Ask ex-regular smokers, i.e. those who smoked at least one cigarette a day (CigReg = 1)

CigUsed About how many cigarettes did you smoke in a day when you smoked them regularly?
IF LESS THAN 1, ENTER 0.

CigStop How long ago did you stop smoking cigarettes regularly?
PROMPT AS NECESSARY

1 Less than 6 months ago
2 6 months but less than a year ago
3 1 year but less than 2 years ago
4 2 years but less than 5 years ago
5 5 years or more ago

WhyStop What was the **main** reason for giving up smoking
DO NOT PROMPT

1 Health reasons
2 Cost
3 Family reasons
4 Pregnant
5 Advised to by health professional
6 Did not like it/enjoy it
7 Other: PLEASE SPECIFY

Ask respondents who answered 7 at Whystop

Xwhystop Please specify other reasons for giving up.

Ask current and ex-smokers who gave up less than a year ago, who have spoken to a doctor or another health professional in the last year

Smktlk In the last year, have you discussed smoking with your GP or another member of staff at the surgery?
INCLUDE DISCUSSIONS WITH GP AT HOME OR ON TELEPHONE

1 Yes, with GP at surgery
2 Yes, with GP elsewhere
3 Yes, with other member of staff at surgery
4 No

Ask respondents who answered 1-3 at Smktlk

Smkhelp [*] Did you find this
RUNNING PROMPT

1 helpful
2 unhelpful
3 or neither helpful nor unhelpful?
4 Don't know

Whosmk Who raised the subject?

1 I raised it
2 Person I spoke to raised it
3 Both of us
4 Can't remember

Ask respondents who have tried to give up smoking or used to smoke regularly (Trystop = Yes OR Cigreg = Regular)

Stopaid Here is a list of things that people use to give up smoking.
Which, if any, have you used?

SHOW CARD K
CODE ALL THAT APPLY

1 Nicotine chewing gum
2 Nicotine patch
3 Special clinic or stop smoking group
4 Quitline
5 Will power
6 Advice from a doctor, or other health professional
7 Support from family and friends
8 Other
9 None of these

Health in England 1996 : What people know, what people think, what people do

Ask respondents who have ever smoked a cigarette, cigar or a pipe (Cigever = Yes)

Cigar (May I just check) Do you smoke at least one cigar or cigarello of any kind per month nowadays?

1 Yes
2 No

Ask respondents who had a job last week (WorkLast = Yes)

Worksmk At your workplace are people allowed..
RUNNING PROMPT

1 to smoke anywhere
2 in special areas only
3 or is smoking banned?
4 SPONTANEOUS Work at home
5 Don't know

Ask non-smokers if there is more than one person in the household (Cigever = No OR Cignow = No)

Anysmoke Does anyone in the household smoke at home at all nowadays?

1 Yes
2 No

Ask all respondents

Visitsmk Do you allow visitors to smoke cigarettes in your home?
CODE FIRST THAT APPLIES
SHOW CARD L

1 Yes, can smoke anywhere
2 Not when children are around
3 Yes, in some places only
4 No, smoking not allowed in the house
5 Don't know

Ask current cigarette smokers (Cignow = Yes)

Homesmk Do you ever smoke at home?

1 Yes
2 No

Ask respondents who are married or cohabiting and have someone in the household who smokes at home (Anysmoke = Yes)

Partsmk Does your husband/wife/partner ever smoke at home?

1 Yes
2 No
3 No, not a smoker

Ask if smoking is allowed in the home (Anysmoke = yes or Homesmk = yes or VisitSmk = 1 or 3) AND informant has at least one child under 16 living in the household

Kidshlth How much, if at all, do you think that the health of your child/children is affected by people smoking in your home? Do you think it is ...

1 a great deal
2 quite a lot
3 a little
4 or not at all?
5 Don't smoke at home

Ask parents of 9-15 year olds

Parssmk2 Which of these statements best describes how you feel about your children smoking?

1 I don't want them to smoke
2 It's up to them whether they smoke

DRINKING

Ask all respondents

DrnkIntr I'd now like to ask you some questions about what you drink - that is, if you do drink.

DrinkNow Do you ever drink alcohol nowadays, including drinks you brew at home?

1 Yes
2 No

Ask respondents who do not drink nowadays (DrinkNow = No)

DrinkAny Could I just check, does that mean you never have an alcoholic drink nowadays, or do you have an alcoholic drink very occasionally, perhaps for medicinal purposes or on special occasions like Christmas or New Year?

1 Very occasionally
2 Never

Ask respondents who never drink alcohol (DrinkAny = Never)

TeeTotal Have you always been a non-drinker, or did you stop drinking for some reason?

1 Always a non-drinker
2 Used to drink but stopped

Ask current drinkers (DrinkNow = Yes) or (DrinkAny = Occasionally)

Drtyintr I'd like to ask you whether you have drunk different types of alcoholic drink in the last 12 months. I do not need to know about non-alcoholic or low alcohol drinks.

Shandy SHOW CARD M
How often have you had a drink of SHANDY (exclude bottles/cans) during the last 12 months, that is since (today's date) 1995?

1 Almost every day
2 5 or 6 days a week
3 3 or 4 days a week
4 once or twice a week
5 once or twice a month
6 once every couple of months
7 once or twice a year
8 not at all in the last 12 months

Ask respondents who have drunk shandy in the last 12 months (Shandy = 1-7)

ShandyAm   How much SHANDY (exclude bottles/cans) have you usually drunk on any one day during the last 12 months, that is since (today's date) 1995?
ENTER NUMBER OF **HALF** PINTS.

Ask current drinkers (DrinkNow = Yes) or (Drinkany = Occasionally)

Beer   SHOW CARD M
How often have you had a drink of BEER, LAGER, STOUT, CIDER during the last 12 months, that is since (today's date) 1995?

1   Almost every day
2   5 or 6 days a week
3   3 or 4 days a week
4   once or twice a week
5   once or twice a month
6   once every couple of months
7   once or twice a year
8   not at all in last 12 months

Ask respondents who have drunk beer in the last 12 months (Beer = 1-7)

BeerAm   How many HALF PINTS of ....BEER,LAGER,STOUT,CIDER have you usually drunk on any one day during the last 12 months, that is since (today's date) 1995? ENTER NUMBER OF **HALF** PINTS.
IF YOU NORMALLY DRINK CANS OR BOTTLES, ENTER 97

Ask respondents who normally drink cans or bottles (Beeram = 97)

XBeeram   (Please write in) How many bottles or cans (do) you normally drink on one day. For example, 3 large cans or 2 small cans.

Ask current drinkers (DrinkNow = Yes) or (Drinkany = Occasionally)

Spirits   SHOW CARD M
How often have you had a drink of ... SPIRITS OR LIQUEURS (eg. gin, whisky, rum, brandy, vodka, advocaat) during the last 12 months, that is since (today's date) 1995?

1   Almost every day
2   5 or 6 days a week
3   3 or 4 days a week
4   once or twice a week
5   once or twice a month
6   once every couple of months
7   once or twice a year
8   not at all in last 12 months

Ask respondents who have drunk spirits in the last 12 months (Spirits = 1-7)

SpiritAm   How much .... SPIRITS OR LIQUEURS (eg. gin, whisky, rum, brandy, vodka, advocaat) have you usually drunk on any one day during the last 12 months, that is since (today's date) 1995?
ENTER NUMBER OF SINGLES (COUNT DOUBLES AS TWO SINGLES).

Ask current drinkers (DrinkNow = Yes) or (Drinkany = Occasionally)

Sherry   SHOW CARD M
How often have you had a drink of ... SHERRY OR MARTINI (including port, vermouth, cinzano, dubonnet) during the last 12 months, that is since (today's date) 1995?

1   Almost every day
2   5 or 6 days a week
3   3 or 4 days a week
4   once or twice a week
5   once or twice a month
6   once every couple of months
7   once or twice a year
8   not at all in last 12 months

Ask respondents who have drunk sherry in the last 12 months (Sherry = 1-7)

SherryAm   How much .... SHERRY OR MARTINI (including port, vermouth, cinzano, dubonnet) have you usually drunk on any one day during the last 12 months, that is since (today's date) 1995?
ENTER NUMBER OF SMALL GLASSES

Ask current drinkers (DrinkNow = Yes) or (Drinkany = Occasionally)

Wine   SHOW CARD M
How often have you had a drink of ... WINE (including babycham, champagne) during the last 12 months, that is since (today's date) 1995?

1   Almost every day
2   5 or 6 days a week
3   3 or 4 days a week
4   once or twice a week
5   once or twice a month
6   once every couple of months
7   once or twice a year
8   not at all in last 12 months

Ask respondents who have drunk wine in the last 12 months (Wine = 1-7)

WineAm   How much .... WINE (including babycham, champagne) have you usually drunk on any one day during the last 12 months, that is since (today's date) 1995?
ENTER NUMBER OF GLASSES

Ask current drinkers (DrinkNow = Yes) or (Drinkany = Occasionally)

Lemon   SHOW CARD M
How often have you had a drink of...ALCOHOLIC LEMONADE, ALCOHOLIC COLA OR OTHER ALCOHOLIC SOFT DRINKS during the last 12 months, that is since (today's date) 1995?

1. Almost every day
2. 5 or 6 days a week
3. 3 or 4 days a week
4. once or twice a week
5. once or twice a month
6. once every couple of months
7. once or twice a year
8. not at all in last 12 months

Ask respondents who have drunk alcoholic lemonade/cola or other alcoholic soft drinks in the last 12 months

XlemonAm   How much ...ALCOHOLIC LEMONADE, ALCOHOLIC COLA OR OTHER ALCOHOLIC SOFT DRINKS have you usually drunk on any one day during the last 12 months, that is since (today's date) 1995?
ENTER AMOUNT

Ask current drinkers (DrinkNow = yes or DrinkAny = Occasionally)

Ifother   Have you had any other alcoholic drinks during the last 12 months, that is since (today's date) 1995?

1. Yes
2. No

Ask if Ifother = yes

XIfother   Please say which other kind of drink you have had

Otherd   SHOW CARD M
How often have you had a drink of (other) during the last 12 months, that is since (today's date) 1995?

1. Almost every day
2. 5 or 6 days a week
3. 3 or 4 days a week
4. once or twice a week
5. once or twice a month
6. once every couple of months
7. once or twice a year
8. not at all in last 12 months

Ask respondents who have drunk another type of drink in the last 12 months

OtherAm   How much of ....OTHER have you usually drunk on any one day during the last 12 months, that is since (today's date) 1995?
ENTER AMOUNT IN HALF PINTS, GLASSES OR SINGLES

Ask current drinkers (DrinkNow = Yes) or (Drinkany = Occasionally)

Droften   SHOW CARD M
Now I would like you to think about alcoholic drinks of **all** kinds. How often would you say you had an alcoholic drink of any kind?

1. Almost every day
2. 5 or 6 days a week
3. 3 or 4 days a week
4. once or twice a week
5. once or twice a month
6. once every couple of months
7. once or twice a year
8. not at all in last 12 months

Ask respondents who answered 1-4 at Droften

LikeCut   On the whole would you say that you drink
RUNNING PROMPT

1. about the right amount
2. or would you like to drink less?

Ask respondents who would like to drink less If LikeCut = Less

dStop1   Now I would like you to look at this card, and say which of these statements best describes you
SHOW CARD N

1. I intend to cut down my drinking within the next month
2. I intend to cut down my drinking within the next six months
3. I intend to cut down my drinking within the next year
4. I intend to cut down my drinking but not in the next year
5. I'm unlikely to cut down on my drinking

Ask all respondents

Units   As you may know some drinks contain more alcohol than others. The amount is sometimes measured in terms of units of alcohol.

UnitAlc   Have you heard about measuring alcohol in units?

1. Yes
2. No
3. Don't know

Ask if UnitAlc = Yes

UnitGlas   We are interested to know what people understand by a unit of alcohol.
How many units are there in a glass of wine?
IF LESS THAN ONE, CODE 0

UnitBeer   How many units are there in a pint of normal strength beer?
IF LESS THAN ONE, CODE 0

UnitSprt   How many units are there in a single pub measure of spirits, for example whisky or gin?
IF LESS THAN ONE, CODE 0

Ask all respondents

Nlimit   [*] You may have heard that the recommended sensible drinking levels have recently been changed. Now would you like to look at this card and say which of the statements best applies to you.
SHOW CARD O

1. I haven't heard anything about the changes
2. I feel confused about the changes
3. I don't feel confused about the changes
4. It is of no interest to me

Ask current, occasional drinkers and ex-drinkers, who have spoken to a doctor or another health professional in the last year

Drktlk In the last year, have you discussed drinking alcohol with your GP or another member of staff at the surgery?

INCLUDE DISCUSSIONS WITH GP AT HOME OR ON TELEPHONE

1 Yes, with GP at surgery
2 Yes, with GP elsewhere
3 Yes, with other member of staff at surgery
4 No

Ask respondents who have discussed drinking alcohol with their GP or a member of staff at the surgery (1-3 at Drktalk)

Drkhelp [*] Did you find this
RUNNING PROMPT

1 helpful
2 unhelpful
3 neither helpful nor unhelpful?
4 don't know

Whodrk Who raised the subject

1 I raised it
2 Person I spoke to raised it
3 Both of us
4 Can't remember

Ask respondents who accepted self-completion (SmokeSC = 1)

Thankyou That is the end of this section. Thank you for your help. Please now hand the computer back to the interviewer.

PHYSICAL ACTIVITY

Ask all respondents

ExerIntr I'd like to ask you about some of the things you have done (at work or) in your free time that involve physical activity in the past 4 weeks.
SHOW THE LAST FOUR WEEKS ON THE CALENDAR

Ask respondents who had a job last week (WorkLast = Yes)

Active Thinking about your job in general, (ASK ABOUT MAIN JOB ONLY) would you say that you are ....
RUNNING PROMPT

1 very physically active
2 fairly physically active
3 not very physically active
4 or not at all physically active in your job?

Ask all respondents

HouseWrk (I'd like you to think about physical activities you have done when you were not doing your paid job.) Have you done any housework in the past 4 weeks?

1 Yes
2 No

Ask respondents who have done housework in the past 4 weeks (HouseWrk = Yes)

HWrkList SHOW CARD P
Have you done any housework listed on this card?

1 Yes
2 No

Ask respondents who have done light housework in the past 4 weeks (HwrkList = Yes)

HevyHWrk SHOW CARD Q
Some kinds of housework are heavier than others. This card gives examples of heavy housework, it does not include everything, these are just examples. Was any of the housework you did in the past 4 weeks this kind of heavy housework?

1 Yes
2 No

Ask respondents who have done heavy housework in the past 4 weeks

HeavyDay During the past 4 weeks on how many separate days have you done that kind of heavy housework?

1..28

Ask all respondents

Garden (Apart from at work) Have you done any gardening, DIY or building in the past 4 weeks?

1 Yes
2 No

Ask respondents who have done some gardening, DIY, or building in the past 4 weeks (Garden = Yes)

GardList SHOW CARD R
Have you done any gardening, DIY or building work listed on this card?

1 Yes
2 No

Ask respondents who have done some light gardening, DIY, or building work (Gardlist = Yes)

ManWork SHOW CARD S
Have you done any gardening, DIY or building work from this card, or any similar heavy manual work?

1 Yes
2 No

Ask respondents who have done heavy gardening, DIY, or building work (Manwork = Yes)

ManDays   During the past 4 weeks, on how many days have you done this kind of heavy manual gardening or DIY?

Ask all respondents

WalkPre   I'd like you to think now about all the walking you've done in the past 4 weeks, either locally or away from here. Include any country walks and any walking to and from work, and any other walks that you have done.

WalkB   Have you done any walks of a quarter of a mile or more in the past 4 weeks? That would usually be continuous walking lasting 5 to 10 minutes.

     1   Yes
     2   No
     3   Can't walk at all

Ask respondents who have done a walk of a quarter of a mile or more in the past 4 weeks (WalkB = Yes)

MileWlkB   Did you do any walks of 1-2 miles or more in the past 4 weeks? That would usually be continuous walking for at least 30 minutes.

     1   Yes
     2   No

Ask respondents who have done any walks of 2 miles or more in the past 4 weeks (MileWlk B = Yes)

MileNumB   During the past 4 weeks how many times did you do any walks of 1-2 miles or more?

     1..97

WalkPace   Which of the following best describes your usual walking pace..
RUNNING PROMPT

     1   a slow pace
     2   a steady average pace
     3   a fairly brisk pace
     4   or a fast pace - at least 4 mph?

Ask all respondents

ActAny   SHOW CARD T
Now I'd like you to think about any sports or excercise activities you do. Can you look at this card and tell me if you've done any of these types of activities during the past 4 weeks?

     1   Yes
     2   No

Ask if ActAny = Yes

WhchAc   Which of the activities did you do?
SHOW CARD T
CODE ALL THAT APPLY

     1   Aerobics/keep fit/gymnastics
     2   Bowls/Crown bowls
     3   Circuit training/weight training
     4   Cycling
     5   Excercises
     6   Dancing
     7   Football/Rugby
     8   Golf
     9   Hiking
     10   Hockey/Netball/Ice-skating
     11   Jogging/Running/Athletics
     12   Squash
     13   Swimming
     14   Tennis/Badminton
     15   Any other sport or exercise activity like these
     16   Any other sport or exercise activity like these

Ask if WhchAc = Other 15 or 16

XWhchAc1/   SPECIFY OTHER ACTIVITY
XWhchAc2   (You can specify two extra types)

Ask about any activities which the informant has done

Occ   Can you tell me on how many separate days did you (name of activity) during the past four weeks?

TimeAct   How much time did you usually spend (name of activity) on each day?
ENTER TIME IN MINUTES
IF MORE THAN ONE HOUR, CALCULATE TIME IN MINUTES

Effort   During the past four weeks, was the effort of (name of activity) usually enough to make you feel out of breath **or** sweaty?

     1   Yes
     2   No

Ask all respondents

CompAct   Compared to other people of your age would you describe yourself as..
RUNNING PROMPT

     1   very physically active
     2   fairly physically active
     3   not very physically active
     4   or not at all physically active?

EnufAct   On the whole, do you think you get enough exercise at present to keep you fit?

     1   Yes
     2   No
     3   Can't take exercise

Ask if Enufact = yes or no

LikeMore   [*] Would you like to take more exercise than you do at the moment?

     1   Yes
     2   No

Ask respondents who would like to take more exercise than at present (LikeMore = Yes)

Exermor1   Now I would like you to look at this card, and say which of the statements best describes you.
SHOW CARD U

1   I'm unlikely to take more exercise
2   I intend to take more exercise within the next month
3   I intend to take more exercise within the next six months
4   I intend to take more exercise within the next year
5   I intend to take more exercise, but not in the next year

Ask if Likemore = No or Don't Know

Exermor2   Now I would like you to look at this card, and say which of the statements best describes you.
SHOW CARD V

1   I intend to take more exercise within the next month
2   I intend to take more exercise within the next six months
3   I intend to take more exercise within the next year
4   I intend to take more exercise but not in the next year

Ask all respondents

Stpexer   SHOW CARD W
Here is a list of things that people say stops them getting more exercise. Looking at this card, could you please tell which, if any, apply to you.
CODE ALL THAT APPLY

1   I don't have the time
2   I have an injury or disability that stops me
3   My health is not good enough
4   I don't enjoy physical activity
5   I'm not the sporty type
6   Other
7   None of these

Daysintr   We've talked about (whether you are active at work), housework and gardening, walking and sports. Now I would like to ask you to think about how much physical activity people in general should do for it to be good for their health.

Daysact   [*] On how many days a week do you think people should do physical activity of any type?

1..7
8   **Spontaneous** Does not matter how often
9   **Spontaneous** It depends on the person
10 **Spontaneous** Exercise is/can be bad for you
11 Don't know

Ask if 1-9 at Daysact

Longact   [*] On each of the days someone does physical activity, how long should they do it for it to be good for them?
DO NOT PROMPT

1   Less than 15 minutes
2   15 minutes
3   More than 15 minutes, less than 20 minutes
4   20 minutes
5   More than 20 minutes, less than 30 minutes
6   30 minutes
7   More than 30 minutes, less than an hour
8   One hour or more

Ask respondents who have spoken to a doctor or another health professional in the last year (Doctalk = 1-3 or OthProf = Yes)

Acttlk   In the last year, have you discussed exercise and physical activity with your GP or another member of staff at the surgery?
INCLUDE DISCUSSIONS WITH GP AT HOME OR ON TELEPHONE

1   Yes, with GP at surgery
2   Yes, with GP elsewhere
3   Yes, with other member of staff at surgery
4   No

Ask respondents who have discussed exercise and physical activity with their GP or another member of staff at the surgery (Acttlk = 1-3)

Acthelp   [*] Did you find this
RUNNING PROMPT

1   helpful
2   unhelpful
3   or neither helpful nor unhelpful?
4   Don't know

Whoact   Who raised the subject?

1   I raised it
2   Person I spoke to raised it
3   Both of us
4   Can't remember

NUTRITION

Ask all respondents

IntrDiet   Now I would like to ask you some questions about the foods you eat and buy.

Bread   What kind of bread do you **usually** eat?
SHOW CARD X
CODE ONE ONLY

1   white
2   high fibre white
3   brown, granary, wheatmeal
4   wholemeal
5   pitta bread

6   South Asian breads (chapati, nan, roti, puri etc)
7   or some other type of bread?
    ESTABLISH TYPE AND CODE 1 TO 6 ABOVE
    IF APPROPRIATE OTHERWISE 7.
8   does not eat any type of bread

Ask if respondent eats bread

Spread   What do you usually spread on your bread?

            CODE ONE ONLY FROM CODING LIST

            1   Butter/hard margarine/block margarine
            2   Soft margarine
            3   Reduced fat spread
            4   Low fat spread
            5   **SPONTANEOUS:** Does not have usual type
            6   Don't know
            7   Does not use fat spread on bread

Ask all respondents

CookOil   When you have fried foods, what kind of fat or oil are
            the foods usually cooked in? Is it ...
            RUNNING PROMPT
            CODE ONE ONLY

            1   solid cooking fat (i.e. is it in a packet or a tub)?
                INCLUDE MARGARINE
            2   or oil (i.e. is it in a bottle or a spray)? INCLUDE
                OLIVE OIL
            3   SPONTANEOUS Does not have usual fat/oil
            4   Does not eat fried food
            5   Don't know

Milk   What kind of milk do you usually use for drinks, in tea
            or coffee or in cereals etc?
            Is it..
            CODE ONE ONLY

            1   whole
            2   semi-skimmed
            3   skimmed
            4   or some other kind of milk?
            5   **SPONTANEOUS** does not drink milk

DietIntr   SHOW CARD Y

            I would like to ask you about some foods which you
            may eat.
            Can you tell me about how often on average you eat
            each of these foods by choosing your answer from
            this card.

Rolls   How often do you eat bread or rolls?

            1   More than once every day
            2   Once every day
            3   5-6 days a week
            4   3-4 days a week
            5   1-2 days a week
            6   At least once a month
            7   Less often than once a month
            8   Rarely or never

Starch   How often do you eat potatoes or rice or pasta?

            1   More than once every day
            2   Once every day
            3   5-6 days a week
            4   3-4 days a week
            5   1-2 days a week
            6   At least once a month
            7   Less often than once a month
            8   Rarely or never

Chips   How often do you eat chips and other fried foods?
            EXCLUDE OVEN CHIPS

            1   More than once every day
            2   Once every day
            3   5-6 days a week
            4   3-4 days a week
            5   1-2 days a week
            6   At least once a month
            7   Less often than once a month
            8   Rarely or never

Veges   How often do you eat any fruit, vegetables or salad?

            1   More than once every day
            2   Once every day
            3   5-6 days a week
            4   3-4 days a week
            5   1-2 days a week
            6   At least once a month
            7   Less often than once a month
            8   Rarely or never

Sweets   How often do you eat confectionery, eg. sweets or
            chocolate?

            1   More than once every day
            2   Once every day
            3   5-6 days a week
            4   3-4 days a week
            5   1-2 days a week
            6   At least once a month
            7   Less often than once a month
            8   Rarely or never

Biscuits   How often do you eat biscuits or cakes?

            1   More than once every day
            2   Once every day
            3   5-6 days a week
            4   3-4 days a week
            5   1-2 days a week
            6   At least once a month
            7   Less often than once a month
            8   Rarely or never

ChngeHab   SHOW CARD Z
            [*] Which one of these statements best describes
            how you feel about the sorts of food you eat
            nowadays?

            1   I have never felt any need to change what I eat
            2   I have already changed as much as I am going
                to
            3   I feel that I ought to make changes but probably
                won't
            4   I am likely to make changes in the future.

ExamIngr　When you go shopping, how often do you look at the list of ingredients or nutrition information? Do you..
RUNNING PROMPT..

1　always look
2　sometimes look
3　never look
4　or never go shopping for food?
5　Don't know

Ask respondents who always or sometimes look at the list of ingredients or nutrition information when shopping for food (ExamIngr = 1-2)

WhatLook　What do you look for?
CODE ALL THAT APPLY

1　Total fat content/low fat
2　Sugar
3　Salt
4　Calories/energy content
5　E-numbers, additives
6　Cholesterol
7　Suitable for vegetarians
8　Fibre content
9　Something else

Ask all respondents

vHdiet　In a few words, how would you describe a healthy diet?
ENTER VERBATIM AT THIS QUESTION AND CODE AT FOLLOWING QUESTION.
DO NOT PROMPT

Hdiet　PLEASE CODE DESCRIPTION OF A HEALTHY DIET
CODE ALL THAT APPLY

1　Eat a balanced diet
2　Eat everything in moderation
3　Eat lots of fruit, vegetables or salad
4　Cut down on fatty or fried foods, eat grilled food
5　Eat lots of starch, carbohydrates, potatoes, pasta or rice
6　Cut down on sugar, cakes and confectionary
7　Eat lots of fibre, cereals, wholemeal food
8　Cut down on salt
9　Drink lots of water, fruit juice, liquid
10　Avoid red meat, eat white meat, fish
11　Eat lots of meat, eggs, cheese, drink lots of milk
12　Other

If Hdiet = Other

SpHdiet　Please specify

Ask all respondents

Agrehlth　Now I am going to read you a list of statements. I would like you to say whether you agree or disagree with them, choosing your answer from this card
SHOW CARD AA

HlthFood　SHOW CARD AA
[*] Eating healthy food is expensive.

1　Strongly agree
2　Agree
3　Neither agree nor disagree
4　Disagree
5　Strongly disagree

Tasty　SHOW CARD AA
[*] The tastiest foods are the ones that are bad for you.

1　Strongly agree
2　Agree
3　Neither agree nor disagree
4　Disagree
5　Strongly disagree

EnjyHlth　SHOW CARD AA
[*] Healthy foods are enjoyable.

1　Strongly agree
2　Agree
3　Neither agree nor disagree
4　Disagree
5　Strongly disagree

WhatHlth　SHOW CARD AA
[*] I get confused over what's supposed to be healthy and what isn't.

1　Strongly agree
2　Agree
3　Neither agree nor disagree
4　Disagree
5　Strongly disagree

DontCare　SHOW CARD AA
[*] I don't really care what I eat.

1　Strongly agree
2　Agree
3　Neither agree nor disagree
4　Disagree
5　Strongly disagree

ExpertOp　SHOW CARD AA
[*] Experts never agree about what foods are good for you.

1　Strongly agree
2　Agree
3　Neither agree nor disagree
4　Disagree
5　Strongly disagree

Fashion　SHOW CARD AA
[*] Healthy eating is just another fashion.

1　Strongly agree
2　Agree
3　Neither agree nor disagree
4　Disagree
5　Strongly disagree

ExerEat　SHOW CARD AA
[*] As long as you take enough exercise you can eat whatever foods you like.

	1	Strongly agree
	2	Agree
	3	Neither agree nor disagree
	4	Disagree
	5	Strongly disagree

Diet [*] Thinking overall the things that you eat would you say that your diet is..
RUNNING PROMPT..

1. as healthy as it could be
2. quite good but it could improve
3. or not very healthy?
4. Don't know

Ask respondents who answered 2-4 at Diet

HlthDiet [*] Would you like to eat a healthier diet than you do at the moment?

1. Yes
2. No
3. Don't know

If yes at HlthDiet

ChDiet Now I would like you to look at this card and say which of the statements best describes you.
SHOW CARD BB

1. I intend to change my diet within the next month
2. I intend to change my diet within the next six months
3. I intend to change my diet within the next year
4. I'm unlikely to change my diet

Ask respondents who have spoken to a doctor or another health professional in the last year (Doctalk = 1-3 or OthProf = Yes)

Diettlk In the last year, have you discussed diet or healthy food with a member of staff at the surgery (or with a doctor GP at home or on the telephone)?

1. Yes with GP at surgery
2. Yes with GP elsewhere
3. Yes with other health professional at a surgery
4. No

Ask respondents who have discussed diet or healthy food with a member of staff at the surgery or with a doctor GP at home or on the telephone

HelpTalk Did you find this
RUNNING PROMPT

1. helpful
2. unhelpful
3. or neither helpful nor unhelpful?
4. Don't know

Whodiet Who raised the subject?

1. I raised it
2. Person I spoke to raised it
3. Both of us
4. Can't remember

CLASSIFICATION

Ask all respondents

Demintr Now I would like to ask you a few more questions about yourself.

Quals1 May I just check, have you ever passed any exams?

1. Yes
2. No

Ask respondents who have passed any exams (Quals1 = Yes)

Quals2 SHOW CARD CC
Please look at this card and tell me the first exam you come to that you have passed.

1. Degree or equivalent
2. Teaching or other higher qualification
3. A level or equivalent
4. GCSE, O level or equivalent
5. CSE or equivalent
6. CSE ungraded
7. Other qualifications

Ask all respondents

Origin SHOW CARD DD
[*] To which of the groups on this card do you consider you belong?

1. White
2. Black Caribbean
3. Black African
4. Black Other
5. Indian
6. Pakistani
7. Bangladeshi
8. Chinese
9. None of these

Ask women aged under 63 and men aged under 65 who were not in paid work last week

Scheme You said earlier that you were not in paid work last week, can I just check, were you on a government scheme for employment training?

1. Yes
2. No

Ask if scheme = No OR female aged 63 or over or male aged 65 or over (and not in paid work)

JBAway (You said earlier that you were not in paid work last week)
Did you have a job or business you were away from?

1. Yes
2. No
3. **SPONTANEOUS:** Waiting to take up a new job/ new business already obtained

Ask if JBAway = No

UnPaid — Did you do any unpaid work in that week for any business that you own?

    1   Yes
    2   No

Ask if UnPaid = No

Rel — ...or that a relative owns

    1   Yes
    2   No

Ask if Rel = No

Start4 — Thinking of the four weeks ending last Sunday were you looking for any kind of paid work or government training scheme at any time in those four weeks?

    1   Yes
    2   No

Ask if Start4 = Yes

Start2 — If a job or a place on a government scheme had been available in the week ending last Sunday would you have been able to start work within two weeks?

    1   Yes
    2   No

Ask if Start4 = No or Start2 = No

NoLook — What was the main reason you did not seek any work in the last four weeks/ would not be able to start in the next two weeks?

    1   Student
    2   Looking after family/home
    3   Temporarily sick or injured
    4   Long-term sick or disabled
    5   Retired from paid work
    6   Other reasons

Ask if not working last week, but not retired and not a student

Everpaid — (Apart from the job you are waiting to take up) Have you ever been in paid employment?

    1   Yes
    2   No

Ask if working last week, has ever worked or retired or has a job he/she was away from or does unpaid work for a business owned by self or relative, or is on a government scheme

IndD — What does/did the firm/organisation you work/ed for mainly make or do (at the place where you worked)?

DESCRIBE FULLY PROBE MANUFACTURING or PROCESSING or DISTRIBUTION ETC. AND MAIN GOODS PRODUCED, MATERIALS USED WHOLESALE OR RETAIL ETC.

IndT — ENTER A TITLE FOR THE INDUSTRY

OccT — What is/was your (main) job in the week ending last Sunday?
ENTER JOB TITLE

OccD — What did/do you mainly do in your job?
CHECK SPECIAL QUALIFICATIONS/ TRAINING NEEDED TO DO THE JOB

Stat — Are/were you working as an employee or are/were you self-employed?

    1   Employed
    2   Self-employed

Ask respondents who are/were working as an employee (Stat = 1)

Manage — ASK OR RECORD
Did/do you have any managerial duties, or are/were you supervising any other employees?

    1   Manager
    2   Foreman/supervisor
    3   Not manager/supervisor

EmpNo — How many employees are/were there at the place where you work/ed?

    1   1-24
    2   25 or over

Ask respondents who are/were self-employed at any time in the last 4 weeks (Stat = 2)

Solo — ASK OR RECORD
Are/were you working on your own or did you have employees?

    1   On own/with partner(s) but no employees
    2   With employees

Ask if has employees (Solo=2)

SENo — How many people did/do you employ at the place where you work/ed?

    1   1-24
    2   25 or over

Ask if informant is not HOH

HOHIntro — I would now like to talk about HOH's employment

Hworklst — May I just check, did HOH do any paid work in the week ending last Sunday, either as an employee or as self-employed?

    1   Yes
    2   No

Ask about female HOH aged under 63 and male HOH aged under 65 who were not in paid work last week

Hscheme   Was HOH on a government scheme for employment training?

   1   Yes
   2   No

Ask if HScheme = No OR if HOH is female and aged 63 or over or male and aged 65 or over (and not in paid work)

HJBAway   Did HOH have a job or business he/she was away from?

   1   Yes
   2   No
   3   **SPONTANEOUS** Waiting to take up a new job/ new business already obtained

Ask if HJBAway = No

HUnPaid   Did HOH do any unpaid work in that week for any business that he/she owns?

   1   Yes
   2   No

Ask if HUnPaid = no

Hrel   or that a relative owns?

   1   Yes
   2   No

Ask if HRel = No

HStart4   Thinking of the four weeks ending last Sunday was HOH looking for any kind of paid work or government training scheme at any time in those four weeks?

   1   Yes
   2   No

Ask if HStart4 = Yes

HStart2   If a job or a place on a government scheme had been available in the week ending last Sunday would HOH have been able to start work within two weeks?

   1   Yes
   2   No

Ask if HStart4 = No or HStart2 = No

HNoLook   What was the main reason HOH did not seek any work in the last four weeks/ would not be able to start in the next two weeks?

   1   Student
   2   Looking after family/home
   3   Temporarily sick or injured
   4   Long-term sick or disabled
   5   Retired from paid work
   6   Other reasons

Ask if HOH was not working last week or was not retired or not a student

HEverpd   (Apart from the job he/she is waiting to take up) Has HOH ever been in paid employment?

   1   Yes
   2   No

Ask if HOH was working last week has ever had a job or has a job he/she was away from last week does unpaid work for a business owned by self or a relative if on a government scheme

HIndD   What does/did the firm/organisation HOH work/ed for mainly make or do (at the place where HOH worked)?
DESCRIBE FULLY - PROBE MANUFACTURING or PROCESSING or DISTRIBUTION ETC. AND MAIN GOODS PRODUCED, MATERIALS USED, WHOLESALE OR RETAIL ETC

HIndT   ENTER A TITLE FOR THE INDUSTRY

HOccT   What is/was HOH's (main) job (in the week ending last Sunday?
ENTER JOB TITLE

HOccD   What does HOH mainly do in his/her job?
CHECK SPECIAL QUALIFICATIONS/ TRAINING NEEDED TO DO THE JOB

Hstat   Was HOH working as an employee or was he/she self-employed?

   1   Employed
   2   Self-employed

Ask respondents who are/were working as an employee (HStat = 1)

HManage   ASK OR RECORD
Did HOH have any managerial duties, or was he/she supervising any other employees?

   1   Manager
   2   Foreman/supervisor
   3   Not manager/supervisor

HEmpNo   How many employees are/were there at the place where HOH work/ed?

   1   1-24
   2   25 or over

Ask respondents who are/were self-employed (HStat = 2)

Hsolo   ASK OR RECORD
Is/was HOH working on his/her own or did he/she have employees?

   1   On own/with partner(s) but no employees
   2   With employees

Ask if (HSolo=2)

HSENo   How many people does/did HOH employ at the place where he/she works/ed?

1. 1-24
2. 25 or over

INCOME

Ask all respondents

Benefits   Are you or anyone else in your household receiving any of the following state benefits?
CODE ALL THAT APPLY

1. Income support
2. Family credit
3. Housing benefit
4. None of these
5. Don't know

TotHhInc   SHOW CARD EE
The next question is on income. Choose the number from this card which represents the group in which you would place your TOTAL HOUSEHOLD INCOME from all sources BEFORE tax and other deductions. (EXPLAIN IF NECESSARY: INCOME FOR LAST TWELVE MONTHS)

Per Year	Per Weeek
1 Under £2,500	Under £50
2 £2,500 - £4,999	£50-£99
3 £5,000 - £9,999	£100-£199
4 £10,000 - £14,999	£200-£299
5 £15,000 - £19,999	£300-£399
6 £20,000 - £29,999	£400-£599
7 £30,000 or more	£600 or more
8 Don't know	
9 SPONTANEOUS: Nothing	
10 SPONTANEOUS: Refused	

DRUG USE

Ask those aged 16-54

Nonresp   The following section is self-completion. I would like you to take the computer and answer the questions yourself.
Instructions on how to answer the questions are given on the screen.
WORK THROUGH THE FIRST QUESTION WITH THE INFORMANT. IF THE INFORMANT MAKES A MISTAKE, TAKE HIM/HER BACK TO THE QUESTION AND ALLOW HIM/HER TO KEY IN THE RIGHT ANSWER

HAS THE INFORMANT ACCEPTED SELF-COMPLETION?

1. Self-completion accepted and completed
2. Completed by interviewer
3. All self-completion refused (drugs and sexual health)
4. Informant refused drugs self-completion but completed sexual health
5. Informant refused sexual health self-completion but completed drugs

Ask if Nonresp = 3-5

Whyrefd   INTERVIEWER-CODE REASON WHY INFORMANT REFUSED

1. Didn't like computer
2. Eyesight problems
3. Other disability
4. Objected to subject
5. Worried about confidentiality
6. Could not read or write
7. Ran out of time
8. Language problems
9. Couldn't be bothered
10. Other- specify at next question

Ask if Whyrefd = 10

XWhyrefd   Specify reasons for refusal

Ask if Nonresp = self-completed and has not already answered this question in the smoking and drinking section

Practice   This is the first time I have used a computer

1. Yes
2. No
3. Don't want to answer

Ask if Nonresp = self-completed or accepted and completed by interviewer

Intro2   The following questions are about drugs.

Please answer them honestly.
THE ANSWERS YOU GIVE ARE COMPLETELY CONFIDENTIAL.
The questions ask whether or not you have ever used drugs. If you are not sure what you have taken, there are a couple of questions at the end that cover this. Please do not include drugs prescribed by a doctor.
To go to the next question now, PRESS for YES and PRESS THE RED BUTTON

DRQ1A   Have you EVER taken AMPHETAMINES (SPEED, UPPERS, WHIZZ, SULPHATE, BILLY) even if it was a long time ago?

1. Yes
2. No
3. Never heard of it
4. Don't want to answer

DRQ2A   Have you EVER taken CANNABIS (MARIJUANA, DOPE, POT, BLACK, GRASS, HASH, GANJA, BLOW, SPLIFFS, JOINTS, DRAW) even if it was a long time ago?

1. Yes
2. No
3. Never heard of it
4. Don't want to answer

DRQ3A   Have you EVER taken COCAINE (COKE, CHARLIE) even if it was a long time ago?

1 Yes
2 No
3 Never heard of it
4 Don't want to answer

DRQ4A   Have you EVER taken CRACK (ROCK, SAND, STONE, PEBBLES) even if it was a long time ago

1 Yes
2 No
3 Never heard of it
4 Don't want to answer

DRQ5A   Have you EVER taken ECSTASY ('E', DENIS THE MENACE) even if it was a long time ago?

1 Yes
2 No
3 Never heard of it
4 Don't want to answer

DRQ6A   Have you EVER taken HEROIN (SMACK, MORPHINE, SKAG, 'H') even if it was a long time ago?

1 Yes
2 No
3 Never heard of it
4 Don't want to answer

DRQ7A   Have you EVER taken LSD (ACID, TABS, TRIPS) even if it was a long time ago?

1 Yes
2 No
3 Never heard of it
4 Don't want to answer

DRQ8A   Have you EVER taken MAGIC MUSHROOMS (PSILOCYBIN) even if it was a long time ago?

1 Yes
2 No
3 Never heard of it
4 Don't want to answer

DRQ9A   Have you EVER taken METHADONE (PHYSEPTONE) **NOT PRESCRIBED BY A DOCTOR** even if it was a long time ago?

1 Yes
2 No
3 Never heard of it
4 Don't want to answer

DRQ10A Have you EVER taken SEMERON (SEM) even if it was a long time ago?

1 Yes
2 No
3 Never heard of it
4 Don't want to answer

DRQ12A Have you EVER taken AMYL NITRATE (POPPERS, NITRATES) even if it was a long time ago?

1 Yes
2 No
3 Never heard of it
4 Don't want to answer

DRQ13A Have you EVER taken ANABOLIC STEROIDS (STEROIDS) **NOT PRESCRIBED BY A DOCTOR**) even if it was a long time ago?

1 Yes
2 No
3 Never heard of it
4 Don't want to answer

DRQ11A Have you EVER taken TRANQUILIZERS (eg TEMAZEPAM, (JELLIES) VALIUM) **NOT PRESCRIBED BY A DOCTOR** even if it was a long time ago?

1 Yes
2 No
3 Never heard of it
4 Don't want to answer

DRQ14A Have you EVER taken GLUES OR SOLVENTS (eg LIGHTER FUEL, PETROL GAS, TIPP-EX) (to sniff or inhale)

1 Yes
2 No
3 Never heard of it
4 Don't want to answer

DRQ17A Apart from anything else that you have already mentioned, have you EVER taken ANYTHING ELSE THAT YOU THOUGHT WAS A DRUG **NOT PRESCRIBED BY A DOCTOR** BUT DIDN'T KNOW WHAT IT WAS?

1 Yes
2 No
3 Don't want to answer

Ask if respondent has ever taken amphetamines

DRQ1B   In the last 12 MONTHS have you taken AMPHETAMINES (SPEED, UPPERS, WHIZZ, SULPHATE, BILLY)?

1 Yes
2 No
3 Don't want to answer

Ask if respondent has ever taken cannabis

DRQ2B   In the last 12 MONTHS have you taken CANNABIS (MARIJUANA, DOPE, POT, BLACK, GRASS, HASH, GANJA, BLOW, SPLIFF)

1 Yes
2 No
3 Don't want to answer

Ask if respondent has ever taken cocaine

DRQ3B   In the last 12 MONTHS have you taken COCAINE(COKE,CHARLIE)?

1 Yes
2 No
3 Don't want to answer

Ask if respondent has ever taken crack

DRQ4B   In the last 12 MONTHS have you taken CRACK (ROCK,SAND, STONE, PEBBLES)?

1 Yes
2 No
3 Don't want to answer

Ask if respondent has ever taken ecstasy

DRQ5B   In the last 12 MONTHS have you taken ECSTASY ('E', DENIS THE MENACE)?

1 Yes
2 No
3 Don't want to answer

Ask if respondent has ever taken heroin

DRQ6B   In the last 12 MONTHS have you taken HEROIN (SMACK, MORPHINE, SKAG,'H')?

1 Yes
2 No
3 Don't want to answer

Ask if respondent has ever taken LSD

DRQ7B   In the last 12 MONTHS have you taken LSD (ACID,TABS,TRIPS)?

1 Yes
2 No
3 Don't want to answer

Ask if respondent has ever taken magic mushrooms

DRQ8B   In the last 12 MONTHS have you taken MAGIC MUSHROOMS(PSILOCYBIN)?

1 Yes
2 No
3 Don't want to answer

Ask if respondent has ever taken methadone

DRQ9B   In the last 12 MONTHS have you taken METHADONE (PHYSEPTONE) **(NOT PRESCRIBED BY A DOCTOR)**?

1 Yes
2 No
3 Don't want to answer

Ask if respondent has ever taken semeron

DRQ10B   In the last 12 MONTHS have you taken SEMERON (SEM)?

1 Yes
2 No
3 Don't want to answer

Ask if respondent has ever taken amyl nitrate

DRQ12B   In the last 12 MONTHS have you taken AMYL NITRATE (POPPERS, NITRATE?)

1 Yes
2 No
3 Don't want to answer

Ask if respondent has ever taken anabolic steroids

DRQ13B   In the last 12 MONTHS have you taken ANABOLIC STEROIDS (STEROIDS) **NOT PRESCRIBED BY A DOCTOR**?

1 Yes
2 No
3 Don't want to answer

Ask if respondent has ever taken tranquilizers

DRQ11B   In the last 12 MONTHS have you taken TRANQUILIZERS (eg TEMAZEPAM, (JELLIES) VALIUM) **NOT PRESCRIBED BY A DOCTOR?**

1 Yes
2 No
3 Don't want to answer

Ask if respondent has ever taken glues or solvents

DRQ14B   In the last 12 MONTHS have you taken GLUES OR SOLVENTS (eg LIGHTER FUEL, PETROL GAS,TIPP-EX) (to sniff or inhale)?

1 Yes
2 No
3 Don't want to answer

Ask if respondent has taken anything else

DRQ17B   Apart from anything else that you have already mentioned, in the last 12 MONTHS have you taken ANYTHING ELSE THAT YOU THOUGHT WAS A DRUG **(NOT PRESCRIBED BY A DOCTOR)** BUT DIDN'T KNOW WHAT IT WAS?

1 Yes
2 No
3 Don't want to answer

Ask if respondent has taken amphetamines in the last 12 months

DRQ1C   In the LAST MONTH have you taken AMPHETAMINES (SPEED, UPPERS, WHIZZ, SULPHATE, BILLY)?

1 Yes
2 No
3 Don't want to answer

Ask if respondent has taken cannabis in the last 12 months

DRQ2C   In the last month have you taken CANNABIS (MARIJUANA, DOPE, POT, BLACK, GRASS, HASH, GANJA, BLOW, SPLIFFS, JOINTS, DRAW) ?

1 Yes
2 No
3 Don't want to answer

Ask if respondent has taken cocaine in the last 12 months

DRQ3C   In the last MONTH have you taken COCAINE (COKE, CHARLIE)?

1 Yes
2 No
3 Don't want to answer

Ask if respondent has taken crack in the last 12 months

DRQ4C   In the last MONTH have you taken CRACK (ROCK, SAND, STONE, PEBBLES)?

1 Yes
2 No
3 Don't want to answer

Ask if respondent has taken ecstasy in the last 12 months

DRQ5C   In the last MONTH have you taken ECSTASY ('E', DENIS THE MENACE)?

1 Yes
2 No
3 Don't want to answer

Ask if respondent has taken heroin in the last 12 months

DRQ6C   In the last MONTH have you taken HEROIN (SMACK, MORPHINE, SKAG, 'H')?

1 Yes
2 No
3 Don't want to answer

Ask if respondent has taken LSD in the last 12 months

DRQ7C   In the last MONTH have you taken LSD (ACID, TABS, TRIPS)?

1 Yes
2 No
3 Don't want to answer

Ask if respondent has taken magic mushrooms in the last 12 months

DRQ8C   In the last MONTH have you taken MAGIC MUSHROOMS (PSILOCYBIN)?

1 Yes
2 No
3 Don't want to answer

Ask if respondent has ever taken methadone in the last 12 months

DRQ9C   In the last MONTH have you taken METHADONE (PHYSEPTONE) **(NOT PRESCRIBED BY A DOCTOR)?**

1 Yes
2 No
3 Don't want to answer

Ask if respondent has taken semeron in the last 12 months

DRQ10C   In the last MONTH have you taken SEMERON (SEM)?

1 Yes
2 No
3 Don't want to answer

Ask if respondent has taken amyl nitrate in the last 12 months

DRQ12C   In the last MONTH have you taken AMYL NITRATE (POPPERS, NITRATES)?

1 Yes
2 No
3 Don't want to answer

Ask if respondent has taken anabolic steroids in the last 12 months

DRQ13C   In the last MONTH have you taken ANABOLIC STEROIDS (STEROIDS) **NOT PRESCRIBED BY A DOCTOR**?

1 Yes
2 No
3 Don't want to answer

Ask if respondent has taken tranquilizers in the last 12 months

DRQ11C   In the last MONTH have you taken TRANQUILIZERS (eg TEMAZEPAM, (JELLIES) VALIUM) **NOT PRESCRIBED BY A DOCTOR?**

1 Yes
2 No
3 Don't want to answer

Ask if respondent has taken glue or solvents in the last 12 months

DRQ14C   In the last MONTH have you taken GLUES OR SOLVENTS(eg LIGHTER FUEL, PETROL GAS,TIPP-EX) (to sniff or inhale)?

1 Yes
2 No
3 Don't want to answer

Ask if respondent has taken anything else in the last 12 months

DRQ17C   Apart from anything else you have already mentioned, in the last MONTH have you taken ANYTHING ELSE THAT YOU THOUGHT WAS A DRUG (**NOT PRESCRIBED BY A DOCTOR**) but didn't know what it was?

1 Yes
2 No
3 Don't want to answer

Ask if respondent has ever taken a drug

Method   Which of these methods of taking drugs have you ever tried? PLEASE PRESS THE NUMBER OF ANY OF THE ANSWERS THAT APPLY. WHEN YOU HAVE FINISHED PRESS THE RED BUTTON

1 Smoked
2 Sniffed
3 Inhaled
4 Swallowed/eaten/drunk
5 Injected
6 Other
7 Don't know

Ask if respondent has injected drugs (Method = 5)

ShareN   Have you ever shared needles/syringes?

1 Yes
2 No
3 Don't want to answer

Ask if informant has used cannabis in last month and Method = Smoked

Cannab   You said you have used cannabis, do you ever smoke it mixed with tobacco?

1 Yes
2 No
3 Never smoked cannabis
4 Don't want to answer

Ask if informant has used two or more drugs in last 12 months

TwoDrug Have you ever used two or more drugs in combination, IN ONE SESSION IN THE LAST 12 MONTHS

1 Yes
2 No
3 Don't want to answer

Ask if informant has used one or more drugs in last 12 months

DrugAlc Have you ever used one or more drugs in combination with alcohol IN ONE SESSION IN THE LAST 12 MONTHS?

1 Yes
2 No
3 Don't want to answer

Ask all those aged under 55

DWrong   Do you agree or disagree with the following statements.
All use of drugs is wrong unless with a doctor's prescription or bought from a chemist

1 Strongly agree
2 Agree
3 Neither agree nor disagree
4 Disagree
5 Strongly disagree

NMind   I don't mind **other** people using drugs

1 Strongly agree
2 Agree
3 Neither agree nor disagree
4 Disagree
5 Strongly disagree

Dsafe   Which **one** of the following statements do you agree with?

1 All drugs are safe to use (as long as you know what you are doing)
2 Some drugs are safe to use (as long as you know what you are doing)
3 No drugs are safe to use
4 I don't know whether drugs are safe to use or not

DFriends Do you know people who use drugs?

1 Yes
2 No
3 Don't know
4 Don't want to answer

Ask those who have used one or more drugs in the last month

LikeStop Which one of the following statements best describes you?

1 I'd like to stop using drugs altogether
2 I see no need to stop using drugs at the moment
3 I don't see the need to ever stop using drugs

Ask if would like to stop using drugs (Likestop = 1)

DrugSt1 Which of these statements best describes you?

1 I intend to stop using drugs within the next month
2 I intend to stop using drugs within the next six months
3 I intend to stop using drugs within the next year
4 I intend to stop using drugs but not in the next year
5 I'm unlikely ever to stop using drugs

Ask if sees no need to stop using drugs at the moment (Likestop = 2)

DrugSt2 Which of these statements best describes you?

1 I'm unlikely ever to stop using drugs
2 I intend to stop using drugs in the next six months

3   I intend to stop using drugs within the next year
4   I intend to stop using drugs but not in the next year

SEXUAL HEALTH

Ask if aged 16-54 and Nonresp= 1, 2 or 4

Sexpart   The following questions are about sexual behaviour. Please answer them honestly. THE ANSWERS YOU GIVE ARE COMPLETELY CONFIDENTIAL. Have you ever had sexual intercourse?
Don't forget to include your husband//wife/ partner

1   Yes
2   No
3   Don't want to answer

Ask if has had sexual intercourse

Tpart   Which one of the following statements applies to you?

1   I have only had sex with the opposite sex
2   I have had sex with both men and women
3   I have only had sex with the same sex

Numparts   Now I would like you to think about the last 12 months, that is since (today's date) 1995. How many sexual partners, in total, have you had intercourse with during that time?
Don't forget to include your husband/wifepartner
PRESS 0 (THE BLUE BUTTON) IF YOU HAVE NOT HAD ANY SEXUAL PARTNERS IN THE LAST 12 MONTHS TYPE IN THE NUMBER THEN PRESS THE RED BUTTON

Ask if Numparts = One

Newpart   Did you have sexual intercourse with this person for the **first** time in the last 12 months? PRESS 1 FOR YES, PRESS 2 FOR NO THEN PRESS THE RED BUTTON

1   Yes
2   No
3   Don't want to answer

Ask if Numparts = Two or more

Newpart2   Have you had a new sexual partner within the last 12 months?
Please include any partner, even if you only had sexual intercourse on one occasion

1   Yes
2   No
3   Don't want to answer

Ask if has had a new partner (Newpart = yes or Newpart2 = yes)

Condnew   Now we would like to think of the last occasion that you **first** had sexual intercourse with **someone new.**
Which if any of the following were used?
PRESS THE NUMBER OF ALL THE ANSWERS THAT APPLY, THEN PRESS THE RED BUTTON

1   Male condom/sheath/durex
2   Female condom
3   The contraceptive pill
4   Emergency ('morning after') contraception
5   Other method of protection, including sterilisation
6   None of thse
7   Can't remember

Ask if used a male or female condom (Condnew = 1,2)

Whycon   Why did you use a condom on that occasion?
PRESS THE NUMBER OF ALL THE ANSWERS THAT APPLY WHEN YOU HAVE FINISHED PRESS THE RED BUTTON

1   For contraception
2   For protection against HIV (the AIDS virus)
3   For protection against other sexually transmitted diseases
4   Other reason
5   Can't remember/Don't know

Ask all respondents completing self-completion

IntrAids   The next two questions are about the risks of getting HIV (the AIDS virus) and other sexually transmitted diseases.
PRESS THE RED BUTTON TO CONTINUE

Aidsrisk   On the whole, the risk of someone like me getting HIV (the AIDS) virus is ..

1   very high
2   quite high
3   low
4   or is there no risk at all?
5   Don't know

Stdrisk   On the whole, the risk of someone like me getting another sexually transmitted disease (STD) is ..

1   very high
2   quite high
3   low
4   or is there no risk at all?
5   Don't know

CondIntr   Please say how much you agree with the following two statements about using condoms. To go to the first statement, PRESS 1 for YES and PRESS THE RED BUTTON

Embarass   I would find it difficult to raise the subject of using a condom with a new partner.

1   Strongly agree
2   Agree
3   Neither agree nor disagree
4   Disagree
5   Strongly disagree

Newcond	If in the near future you did have sex with someone new do you think you would ..

        1   always use a condom
        2   it would depend
        3   never use a condom
        4   or wouldn't you contemplate having sex?

ThankYou	That is the end of the self-completion. Thank you for your help. All the answers you have given are confidential. To finish the interview, PRESS 1 for YES and PRESS THE RED BUTTON.
Laptop	Now hand the computer back to the interviewer.
NumGiv	A few interviews in any survey are checked by Head Office to make sure that people are happy with the way the interview was carried out. In case Head Office needs to contact you, would you mind letting me have your telephone number?

        1   Agree to give number
        2   Does not agree
        3   No telephone

NumIns	Enter telephone number on yellow follow-up card
ReCtct	We may want to contact you again next year. Would this be all right? **Remember to ask for a contact name in case informant moves and enter on yellow card**.

        1   Yes (unconditional)
        2   No (unconditional)
        3   Yes (in certain circumstances)

HEALTH EDUCATION MONITORING SURVEY 1996 - PROXY INTERVIEW

HOUSEHOLD BOX

Ask all proxy informants

NPersons — I would like to start by asking you about yourself and the household. How many people normally live in this household?
INCLUDE ALL PERSONS, INCLUDING THOSE AGED 75 AND OVER

1..14

Ask about everyone in the selected person's household

Name — START WITH THE SELECTED PERSON
ASK THE FOLLOWING QUESTIONS OF EVERY ONE IN THE HOUSEHOLD. IF SELECTED PERSON IS MARRIED\COHABITING, ENTER SPOUSE\PARTNER AS PERSON 2.

Name or other identifier

Sex — INTERVIEWER: CODE NAME's SEX.

1 Male
2 Female

DoB — INTERVIEWER: CODE SELECTED PERSON'S DATE OF BIRTH

Age — What was NAME's age last birthday?
IF AGE NOT GIVEN, PROBE FOR AN ESTIMATE

Ask if household member is aged 16 or over

Marstat — Are you/ is NAME ...

1 married
2 living as married
3 single/never married
4 widowed
5 divorced
6 or separated?
7 SPONTANEOUS living with a same sex partner

ReltoInf — ASK OR CODE RELATIONSHIP TO SELECTED PERSON

1 Informant/sampled person
2 Spouse\partner (incl. same-sex partner)
3 Son\daughter (incl. adopted/step-child)
4 Foster child
5 Son-in-law\daughter-in-law
6 Parent\step-parent
7 Parent-in-law
8 Brother\sister (incl. adopted)
9 Brother-in-law\ sister-in-law
10 Grandchild
11 Grandparent
12 Other (related)
13 Other (not related)

Ask if household member is aged 16 or over

WhoHOH — IS THIS PERSON THE HOH?
REMEMBER THAT WHERE A PROPERTY IS OWNED\RENTED IN THE NAME OF A WOMAN WHO IS MARRIED\COHABITING WITH A MAN, THEN BY DEFINITION, THE MAN IS THE HOH.

1 Yes
2 No

NAdults — ASK OR CODE
Number of adults aged 16-74 in the household

1..14

Ask all proxy informants

SamPP — INTERVIEWER CODE: WAS THE SAMPLED PERSON PRESENT DURING THE PROXY INTERVIEW?

1 Yes
2 No

ProxyNo — INTERVIEWER: PLEASE CODE THE PERSON NUMBER (FROM THE HOUSEHOLD BOX) OF THE PROXY. IF THE PROXY IS A NON-HOUSEHOLD MEMBER CODE AS 20

PWrkLast — May I just check, did .... do any paid work in the week ending last Sunday as an employee or as self-employed?

1 Yes
2 No

Ask if selected person was working last week (PWrkLast = Yes)

PFullPrt — In his/her present job does he/she work

1 full-time
2 or part-time?

Ask all proxy informants

POwnrent — Does ....'s household own or rent this accommodation?
CODE FIRST THAT APPLIES.

1 Buying with a mortgage
2 Owned outright
3 Rented from Local Authority/New Town

	4 Rented from Housing Association
	5 Rented unfurnished
	6 Rented furnished
	7 Rented from employer
	8 Other with payment
	9 Rentfree
PAccomTy	INTERVIEWER CODE TYPE OF ACCOMMODATION
	1 Detached house
	2 Semi-detached house
	3 Terraced/end of terrace house
	4 Purpose-built flat
	5 Flat in a converted house
	6 Caravan, mobile home or houseboat
	7 Other type of accommodation
PCar	Is there a car or van **normally** available for use by .... or any members of his/her household?
	1 Yes
	2 No

GENERAL HEALTH

Ask all proxy informants

PGenhlth	[*] Now I would like to ask you some questions about ....'s health. How is his/her health in general? Would you say it was.. RUNNING PROMPT
	1 very good
	2 good
	3 fair
	4 bad
	5 or very bad?
PIllness	[*] Does .... have any long-standing illness, disability or infirmity? By long-standing I mean anything that has troubled him/her over a period of time or that is likely to affect him/her over a period of time?
	1 Yes
	2 No

Ask if selected person has a long-standing illness (PIllness = Yes)

Pmatter	[*] What is the matter with ....?
PLimitact	[*] Does this illness or disability (Do any of these illnesses or disabilities) limit his/her activities in any way?
	1 Yes
	2 No

Ask all proxy informants

Pdoctalk	During the past year, that is since (today's date) 1995, apart from any visit to a hospital, has ...... talked to a doctor either in person or by telephone, about his/her health? CODE FIRST THAT APPLIES
	1 Yes, at surgery
	2 Yes in person at home
	3 Yes by telephone
	4 No

SKIN CANCER

Ask all proxy informants

PIntoSC	There's been a lot of publicity recently about skin cancer.
PSunBurn	During the last 12 months, that is since (today's date) 1995, has .... had sunburn causing redness and soreness of the skin lasting for at least 1-2 days?
	1 Yes
	2 No
	3 Can't remember

Ask if selected person has had sunburn in the last 12 months (PSunburn = Yes)

PFrqBurn	How many times?
	1 Once
	2 Twice
	3 Three times
	4 Four or more
	5 Not in the last 12 months

SMOKING

Ask all proxy informants

PSmkIntr	The following questions are about smoking.
PCigever	Has .... ever smoked a cigarette, a cigar or a pipe?
	1 Yes
	2 No

Ask if selected person has ever smoked (PCigever = Yes)

PCignow	Does .... smoke cigarettes at all nowadays?
	1 Yes
	2 No

Ask if selected person currently smokes cigarettes (PCignow = Yes)

PQtywknd	About how many cigarettes **a day** does .... usually smoke at weekends? IF LESS THAN 1, ENTER 0
PQtywkdy	About how many cigarettes **a day** does .... usually smoke on weekdays? IF LESS THAN 1, ENTER 0

PCigtype   Does .... mainly smoke...
                  RUNNING PROMPT

                  1   filter-tipped cigarettes,
                  2   plain or untipped cigarettes,
                  3   or hand-rolled cigarettes?

Ask if selected person has ever smoked (PCigever = Yes)

PCigar   (May I just check) Does .... smoke at least one cigar or cigarillo of any kind per month nowadays?

                  1   Yes
                  2   No

Ask if selected person is a non-smoker (PCigever = No OR PCignow = No) and there is more than one person in the household

PAnysmke   Does anyone in the household smoke at home at all nowadays?

                  1   Yes
                  2   No

Ask all proxy informants

PVistsmk   SHOW CARD L
                  Does .... allow visitors to smoke cigarettes in the home?
                  CODE FIRST THAT APPLIES

                  1   Yes, can smoke anywhere
                  2   Not when children are around
                  3   Yes, in some places only
                  4   No, smoking not allowed in the house
                  5   Don't know

Ask if selected person currently smokes cigarettes (PCignow = Yes)

PHomesmk   Does .... ever smoke at home?

                  1   Yes
                  2   No

DRINKING

Ask all proxy informants

PDrnkInt   I'd now like to ask you some questions about how often ....drinks - that is, if he/she does drink.

                  PRESS ENTER TO CONTINUE

PDrnkNow   Does .... ever drink alcohol nowadays, including drinks he/she brews at home?

                  1   Yes
                  2   No

Ask if selected person does not drink nowadays (PDrnknow = No)

PDrnkAny   Could I just check, does that mean he/she never has an alcoholic drink nowadays, or does he/she have an alcoholic drink very occasionally, perhaps for medicinal purposes or on special occasions like Christmas or New Year?

                  1   Very occasionally
                  2   Never

Ask if selected person currently drinks (PDrnknow = Yes or PDrnkAny = Occasionally)

PDrOften   SHOW CARD M
                  How often has .... had an alcoholic drink of any kind during the last 12 months, that is since (today's date) 1995?

                  1   Almost every day
                  2   5 or 6 days a week
                  3   3 or 4 days a week
                  4   once or twice a week
                  5   once or twice a month
                  6   once every couple of months
                  7   once or twice a year
                  8   not at all in last 12 months

PHYSICAL ACTIVITY

Ask all proxy informants

PExrIntr   I'd like to ask you about some of the things ...... has done at work or in his/her free time that involve physical activity in the past 4 weeks, that is from ..... up to yesterday.
                  PRESS ENTER TO CONTINUE

Ask if selected person had a job last week (PWrkLast = Yes)

PActive   Thinking about his/her job in general, would you say that he/she is ....
                  RUNNING PROMPT

                  1   very physically active
                  2   fairly physically active
                  3   not very physically active
                  4   or not at all physically active in his/her job?

Ask all proxy informants

PHseWrk   (I would like you to think about the physical activities .... has done when he/she was not doing his/her paid job). Has ....done any housework in the past 4 weeks?

                  1   Yes
                  2   No

Ask if selected person has done housework in the past four weeks (PHsewrk = Yes)

PHWrkLst SHOW CARD P
Has he/she done any housework listed on this card?

1 Yes
2 No

Ask all proxy informants

PGardLst SHOW CARD R
Has he/she done any gardening, DIY or building work listed on this card?

1 Yes
2 No

PMilWlkB Has he/she done any walks of 1-2 miles or more in the past 4 weeks? That would usually be continuous walking for at least 30 minutes.

1 Yes
2 No
3 Can't walk at all

Ask if selected person has done any walks of 1-2 miles in the past four weeks (PMilwlkB = Yes)

PWlkPace Which of the following best describes his/her usual walking pace..
RUNNING PROMPT

1 a slow pace
2 a steady average pace
3 a fairly brisk pace
4 or a fast pace - at least 4 mph?

Ask all proxy informants

PActAny SHOW CARD T
Can you look at this card and tell me if he/she has done any of these activities during the past 4 weeks.

1 Yes
2 No

NUTRITION

Ask all proxy informants

PIntDiet Now I would like to ask you some questions about the foods .... eats.
PRESS ENTER TO CONTINUE

PBread What kind of bread does .... usually eat?
SHOW CARD X
CODE ONE ONLY

1 white
2 high fibre white
3 brown, granary, wheatmeal
4 wholemeal
5 pitta bread
6 South Asian breads (chapati, nan, roti, puri etc.)
7 or some other type of bread?
ESTABLISH TYPE AND CODE 1 TO 6 ABOVE IF APPROPRIATE. OTHERWISE 7.
8 does not eat any type of bread

Ask if selected person eats bread

PSpread What does ....usually spread on his/her bread?
CODE ONE ONLY FROM CODING LIST F1

1 butter/ hard margarine/ block margarine
2 soft margarine
3 reduced fat spread
4 low fat spread
5 SPONTANEOUS: does not have usual type
6 Don't know
7 Does not use fat spread on bread

Ask all proxy informants

PCookOil When he/she has fried foods, what kind of fat or oil are the foods usually cooked in? Is it ...
CODE ONE ONLY

1 solid cooking fat (ie is it in a packet or a tub) INCLUDE MARGARINE
2 or oil (ie is it in a bottle or a spray)? INCLUDE OLIVE OIL
3 SPONTANEOUS Does not have usual fat/ oil
4 Does not eat fried food
5 Don't know

PMilk What kind of milk does he/she usually use for drinks, in tea or coffee and on cereals etc.? Is it...
CODE ONE ONLY

1 whole
2 semi-skimmed
3 skimmed
4 or some other kind of milk?
5 SPONTANEOUS does not drink milk

PDietInt SHOW CARD Y

Can you tell me about how often on average .... eats each of these foods by choosing your answer from this card
PRESS ENTER TO CONTINUE

PRolls How often does he/she eat bread or rolls?

1 More than once every day
2 Once every day
3 5-6 days a week
4 3-4 days a week
5 1-2 days a week
6 At least once a month
7 Less often than once a month
8 Rarely or never

Health in England 1996 : What people know, what people think, what people do

PStarch | How often does he/she eat potatoes or rice or pasta?

1. More than once every day
2. Once every day
3. 5-6 days a week
4. 3-4 days a week
5. 1-2 days a week
6. At least once a month
7. Less often than once a month
8. Rarely or never

PChips foods? | How often does he/she eat chips and other fried foods?

EXCLUDE OVEN CHIPS

1. More than once every day
2. Once every day
3. 5-6 days a week
4. 3-4 days a week
5. 1-2 days a week
6. At least once a month
7. Less often than once a month
8. Rarely or never

PVeges | How often does he/she eat any fruit, vegetables or salad?

1. More than once every day
2. Once every day
3. 5-6 days a week
4. 3-4 days a week
5. 1-2 days a week
6. At least once a month
7. Less often than once a month
8. Rarely or never

Psweets | How often does he/she eat confectionery eg sweets or chocolate?

1. More than once every day
2. Once every day
3. 5-6 days a week
4. 3-4 days a week
5. 1-2 days a week
6. At least once a month
7. Less often than once a month
8. Rarely or never

Pbiscuit | How often does he/she eat biscuits or cakes?

1. More than once every day
2. Once every day
3. 5-6 days a week
4. 3-4 days a week
5. 1-2 days a week
6. At least once a month
7. Less often than once a month
8. Rarely or never

CLASSIFICATION

Ask all proxy informants

PDemintr | Now I would like to ask you a few more questions about ....
PRESS ENTER TO CONTINUE

Pquals1 | May I just check, has ...... ever passed any exams?

1. Yes
2. No

Ask if selected person has passed any exams (PQuals1 = Yes)

PQuals2 | SHOW CARD CC
Please look at this card and tell me the first exam you come to that he/she has passed.

1. Degree or equivalent
2. Teaching or other higher qualification
3. A level or equivalent
4. GCSE, O level or equivalent
5. CSE or equivalent
6. CSE ungraded
7. Other qualifications

THE PROXY IS THEN ROUTED TO THE ECONOMIC ACTIVITY QUESTIONS AND THE OCCUPATION AND INDUSTRY QUESTIONS (IN THE MAIN QUESTIONNAIRE) WHICH ARE ASKED ABOUT THE INFORMANT AND ABOUT THE HOH

The survey was carried out using computer assisted interviewing. These are copies of the showcards.

HEALTH EDUCATION MONITORING SURVEY 1996

B
1 Not having a job
2 Relationships/family
3 Pollution
4 My smoking
5 Others' smoking
6 My alcohol consumption
7 Lack of exercise
8 What I eat
9 My weight
10 None of these

A
1 Relationships/family
2 My work
3 My income/standard of living
4 My alcohol consumption
5 The exercise I do
6 What I eat
7 None of these

Health in England 1996 : What people know, what people think, what people do 283

C	
1	Strongly agree
2	Agree
3	Neither agree nor disagree
4	Disagree
5	Strongly disagree

D	
1	Completely free of stress
2	Small amount of stress
3	Moderate amount of stress
4	Large amount of stress

E

1 Sunbathing abroad

2 Outdoors abroad, but not sunbathing

3 Sunbathing in this country

4 Outdoors in this country doing something else

F

1 Always burns and never tans

2 Burns at first and tans with difficulty

3 Burns at first then tans easily

4 Rarely burns and tans easily

5 Never burns and always tans

6 Other

H	
1	Strongly agree
2	Agree
3	Neither agree nor disagree
4	Disagree
5	Strongly disagree

G	
1	White skin
2	Brown skin
3	Black skin
4	Olive skin
5	Other

J

1 I'm unlikely to give up smoking

2 I intend to give up smoking within the next month

3 I intend to give up smoking within the next six months

4 I intend to give up smoking within the next year

5 I intend to give up smoking, but not in the next year

I

1 I intend to give up smoking within the next month

2 I intend to give up smoking within the next six months

3 I intend to give up smoking within the next year

4 I intend to give up smoking, but not in the next year

5 I'm unlikely to give up smoking

K	
1	Nicotine chewing gum
2	Nicotine patch
3	Special clinic or stop smoking group
4	Quitline
5	Will power
6	Advice from a doctor, or other health professional
7	Support from family and friends
8	Other
9	None of these

L	
1	Yes, can smoke anywhere
2	Not when children are around
3	Yes, in some places only
4	No, smoking not allowed in the house
5	Don't know

M	
1	Almost every day
2	5 or 6 days a week
3	3 or 4 days a week
4	Once or twice a week
5	Once or twice a month
6	Once every couple of months
7	Once or twice a year
8	Not at all in the last 12 months

N	
1	I intend to cut down my drinking within the next month
2	I intend to cut down my drinking within the next six months
3	I intend to cut down my drinking within the next year
4	I intend to cut down my drinking, but not in the next year
5	I'm unlikely to cut down on my drinking

P

HOUSEWORK

Hoovering

Dusting

Ironing

General tidying

0

1

2

3

4

I haven't heard anything about the changes

I feel confused about the changes

I don't feel confused about the changes

It is of no interest to me

R

GARDENING, DIY AND BUILDING WORK

Hoeing, weeding, pruning

Mowing with a power mower

Planting flowers/seeds

Decorating

Minor household repairs

Car washing and polishing

Car repairs and maintenance

Q

HEAVY HOUSEWORK

Moving heavy furniture

Spring cleaning

Walking with heavy shopping (for more than 5 minutes)

Cleaning windows

Scrubbing floors with a scrubbing brush

T

1. Aerobics/keep fit/gymnastics
2. Bowls/Crown bowls
3. Circuit training/weight training
4. Cycling
5. Exercises
6. Dancing
7. Football/rugby
8. Golf
9. Hiking
10. Hockey/Netball/Ice-skating
11. Jogging/Running/Athletics
12. Squash
13. Swimming
14. Tennis/Badminton
15. Any other sport or exercise activity like these

S

HEAVY MANUAL WORK

Digging, clearing rough ground

Building in stone/bricklaying

Mowing large areas with a hand mower

Felling trees/chopping wood

Mixing/laying concrete

Moving heavy loads

Refitting a kitchen or bathroom

U

1 I intend to take more exercise within the next month

2 I intend to take more exercise within the next six months

3 I intend to take more exercise within the next year

4 I intend to take more exercise, but not in the next year

5 I'm unlikely to take more exercise

V

1 I'm unlikely to take more exercise

2 I intend to take more exercise within the next month

3 I intend to take more exercise within the next six months

4 I intend to take more exercise within the next year

5 I intend to take more exercise, but not in the next year

W	
1	I don't have the time
2	I have an injury or disbility that stops me
3	My health is not good enough
4	I don't enjoy physical activity
5	I'm not the sporty type
6	Other
7	None of these

X	
1	White
2	High fibre white
3	Brown, granary, wheatmeal
4	Wholemeal
5	Pitta bread
6	South Asian breads (chapati, nan, roti, puri etc)
7	Some other type of bread
8	Do not eat any type of bread

Y	
1	More than once every day
2	Once every day
3	5-6 days a week
4	3-4 days a week
5	1-2 days a week
6	At least once a month
7	Less often than once a month
8	Rarely or never

Z	
1	I have never felt any need to change what I eat
2	I have already changed as much as I am going to
3	I feel that I ought to make changes but probably won't
4	I am likely to make changes in the future

AA	
Strongly agree	1
Agree	2
Neither agree nor disagree	3
Disagree	4
Strongly disagree	5

BB	
I intend to change my diet within the next month	1
I intend to change my diet within the next six months	2
I intend to change my diet within the next year	3
I'm unlikely to change my diet	4

CC	
1	Degree (or degree level qualification)
2	Teaching qualification HNC/HND, BRC/TEC Higher, BTEC Higher, City and Guilds Full Technological Certificate, Nursing Qualifications (SRN, SCM, RGN, RM, RHV, Midwife)
3	A levels, SCE Higher, ONC/OND/BTEC/TEC/BTEC not higher City and Guilds Advanced/Final Level
4	O level passes (Grade A-C if after 1975) GCSE (Grades A-C) CSE Grade 1 SCE Ordinary (Bands A-C) Standard Grade (Level 1-3) SLC Lower SUPE Lower or Ordinary School Certificate or Matric City and Guilds Craft/Ordinary Level
5	CSE Grades 2-5 GCE O level (Grades D & E if after 1975) GCSE (Grades D,E,F,G) SCE Ordinary (Bands D & E) Standard Grade (Level 4,5) Clerical or Commercial qualifications
6	CSE Ungraded
7	Other qualifications

DD	
1	White
2	Black Caribbean
3	Black African
4	Black Other
5	Indian
6	Pakistani
7	Bangladeshi
8	Chinese
9	Other

EE		
PER YEAR	PER WEEK	
Under £2,500	Under £50	1
£2,500 - £4,999	£50 - £99	2
£5,000 - £9,999	£100 - £199	3
£10,000 - £14,999	£200 - £299	4
£15,000 - £19,999	£300 - £399	5
£20,000 - £29,999	£400 - £599	6
£30,000 or more	£600 or more	7

FF	
Smoked	1
Sniffed	2
Inhaled	3
Swallowed/eaten/drunk	4
Injected	5
Other	6
Don't know	7

GG

1 Strongly agree

2 Agree

3 Neither agree nor disagree

4 Disagree

5 Strongly disagree

HH

1 All drugs are safe to use (as long as you know what you're doing)

2 Some drugs are safe to use (as long as you know what you're doing)

3 No drugs are safe to use

4 I don't know whether drugs are safe to use or not

Health in England 1996 : What people know, what people think, what people do

JJ

1. I intend to stop using drugs within the next month
2. I intend to stop using drugs within the next six months
3. I intend to stop using drugs within the next year
4. I'm unlikely ever to stop using drugs

II

1. I'd like to stop using drugs altogether
2. I see no need to stop using drugs at the moment
3. I don't see the need to ever stop using drugs

KK

1. I'm unlikely ever to stop using drugs

2. I intend to stop using drugs within the next month

3. I intend to stop using drugs within the next six months

4. I intend to stop using drugs within the next year

LL

1. I have only had sex with people of the opposite sex

2. I have had sex with both men and women

3. I have only had sex with people of the same sex

	MM
Male condom/sheath/durex	1
Female condom	2
The contraceptive pill	3
Emergency ('morning after') contraception	4
Other method of protection, including sterilisation	5
None of these	6
Can't remember	7

List of figures

Chapter 1

		Page
1.1	*Health of the Nation* Key Areas and Risk Factors and topics covered in the HEMS questionnaire in 1995 and 1996	7

Chapter 2

2.1	Prevalence of cigarette smoking by age and sex	15
2.2	Percentage of current smokers who would like to give up smoking by age	15
2.3	How easy or difficult smokers would find it to go without smoking for a whole day by number of cigarettes smoked per day	16
2.4	Percentage of current smokers who have tried to give up smoking by age	16
2.5	Length of time smokers gave up for	16
2.6	Mean weekly consumption of alcohol in units by age	18
2.7	Percentage consuming alcoholic soft drinks in the last 12 months by age and sex	19
2.8	Percentage consuming different types of alcoholic drinks in the last 12 months	19
2.9	Percentage who would like to drink less by the amount of alcohol consumed per week and sex	19
2.10	Percentage who had heard of units of alcohol and correctly identified the number in specified drinks by sex	20
2.11	Percentage who had heard of units of alcohol and correctly identified the number in specified drinks, by alcohol consumption and sex	20
2.12	Attitudes to changes in sensible drinking levels	21
2.13	Odds of an individual smoking and drinking more than 21 units a week (men) or more than 14 units a week (women)	22

Chapter 3

3.1	Level of physical activity by age and sex	26
3.2	Odds of an individual being sedentary	27
3.3	Odds of an individual participating in moderate-intensity activity lasting at least 30 minutes on five or more days a week	28
3.4	Odds of an individual participating in vigorous-intensity activity lasting at least 20 minutes on three or more days a week	28
3.5	Percentage saying people should be physically active for 30+ minutes on 5+ days a week by age and sex	29
3.6	Percentage who would like to take more exercise by age and sex	30
3.7	Percentage who intend to take more exercise in the next six months by age and sex	30
3.8	Barriers to exercise by age and sex	31

Chapter 4

4.1	Percentage of respondents knowing what constitutes a healthy diet	34
4.2	Percentage who examine ingredients when they shop, and what they look for by sex	35
4.3	Percentage eating bread; fruit, vegetables or salad; pasta or rice daily, by age and sex	36
4.4	Percentage drinking semi-skimmed or skimmed milk; using no fat, or low- or reduced- fat spread; using oil for cooking and eating chips less than once a week, by age and sex	37
4.5	Percentage eating confectionery less than once a week by age and sex	37
4.6	Percentage eating biscuits or cakes less than once a week by age and sex	37
4.7	Percentage who thought their diet was as healthy as it could be by age and sex	38
4.8	Percentage agreeing 'I get confused over what's supposed to be healthy and what isn't' by age and sex	38
4.9	Percentage agreeing that 'experts never agree what foods are good for you' by age	39

Chapter 5

5.1	Percentage who had used specific drugs ever, in the past year or in the past month	44

		Page
5.2	Percentage who had ever used specific drugs by age	45
5.3	Ever use of any drug by age and sex	45
5.4	Percentage reporting having ever used drugs by drug category and age	46
5.5	Percentage who had used drugs in the past month by drug category and age	47
5.6	Percentage who had used any drug in the past month, as a proportion of ever users by age and sex	47
5.7	Number of different drugs ever used by recency of use and sex	48
5.8	Percentage of respondents who used cannabis and/or other drugs, by recency of use	48
5.9	Percentage who know people who use drugs by sex and age	48
5.10	Intentions to stop taking drugs by sex	49
5.11	Whether agrees that 'All use of drugs is wrong unless with a doctor's prescription or bought from a chemist'	50
5.12	Whether agrees that 'All use of drugs is wrong unless with a doctor's prescription or bought from a chemist' by drug use	50
5.13	Whether agrees that drugs are safe to use by sex	51
5.14	Whether agrees that drugs are safe to use by drug use	51

Chapter 6

6.1	Percentage reporting two or more sexual partners in the last 12 months by age and sex	53
6.2	Odds of an individual reporting two or more sexual partners in the last year	55
6.3	Percentage who thought there was no risk of 'someone like me getting HIV/the AIDS virus' by age and sex	55
6.4	Percentage who thought there was no risk of 'someone like me getting another sexually transmitted disease' by age and sex	55
6.5	Percentage who would find it difficult to raise the subject of using a condom with a new partner by age and sex	56
6.6	Percentage who would always use a condom with a new partner by age and sex	57

		Page
6.7	Percentage using a condom with a new partner by age and sex	57

Chapter 7

7.1	Percentage who reported being sunburnt in the 12 months prior to interview by age and sex	60
7.2	Percentage using a suncream by age and sex	61
7.3	Percentage who thought it was important to have a suntan by age and sex	62
7.4	Percentage agreeing that 'having a suntan makes me look more attractive' by age and sex	62

Chapter 8

8.1	Self-reported general health by age and sex	64
8.2	Percentage reporting a long-standing illness by age and sex	65
8.3	Percentage reporting a large or moderate amount of stress in the last 12 months by age and sex	66
8.4	Factors which are currently good for respondent's health by sex	67
8.5	Factors which are currently bad for respondents' health by sex	67
8.6	Percentage consulting a GP at the surgery in the last 12 months by age and sex	68

Chapter 9

9.1	Health-related behaviours	75
9.2	Characteristics associated with different levels of knowledge	76
9.3	Attitudes towards health behaviours	77

List of tables

Chapter 1

		Page
1.1	Characteristics of the sample by sex	81

Chapter 2

		Page
2.1	Cigarette smoking status by age and sex	82
2.2	Cigarette smoking status by standard region of residence and sex	83
2.3	Cigarette smoking status by social class based on own current or last job and sex	84
2.4	Mean and median cigarette consumption per smoker by age and sex	85
2.5	Daily cigarette consumption by current regular cigarette smokers and ex-regular cigarette smokers by sex	86
2.6	Whether current smokers would like to give up smoking altogether by age and sex	86
2.7	Proportion of current smokers who would like to give up smoking altogether by how easy they would find it to go without smoking and whether they have ever tried to give up	87
2.8	Proportion of current smokers who would like to give up smoking altogether by age and number of cigarettes smoked per day	87
2.9	How easy or difficult smokers would find it to go without smoking for a whole day by age and sex	88
2.10	How easy or difficult smokers would find it to go without smoking for a whole day by number of cigarettes smoked per day and sex	89
2.11	Percentage of smokers who have tried to give up smoking by age, the number of cigarettes smoked per day and sex	90
2.12	Length of time smokers gave up for by age and sex	91
2.13	Length of time smokers gave up for by number of cigarettes smoked per day and sex	92
2.14	Length of time ex-smokers have stopped smoking by age and sex	93
2.15	Main reason why ex-smokers stopped smoking by age and sex	94
2.16	Main reason why ex-smokers stopped smoking by number of cigarettes they used to smoke per day	94
2.17	Methods smokers used to stop smoking by whether successful or not and number of cigarettes they (used to) smoke per day	95
2.18	When smokers intend to give up smoking by age	95
2.19	When smokers intend to give up smoking by number of cigarettes smoked per day	96
2.20	When smokers intend to give up smoking by whether they want to give up smoking	96
2.21	Extent to which informant thinks the health of his/her children is affected by smoking in the home by age and sex	96
2.22	Extent to which informant thinks the health of his/her children is affected by smoking in the home by social class	96
2.23	Extent to which informant thinks the health of his/her children is affected by smoking in the home by cigarette smoking status and sex	97
2.24	Informant's attitude to his/her children smoking by age and sex	97
2.25	Informant's attitude to his/her children smoking by social class based on own current or last job and sex	97
2.26	Informant's attitude to his/her children smoking by cigarette smoking status and sex	97
2.27	Workplace smoking policy of respondents who had a job in the week before interview by age and sex	98
2.28	Workplace smoking policy of respondents who had a job in the week before interview by social class of job and sex	99
2.29	Workplace smoking policy of respondents who had a job in the week before interview by employment status and size of the establishment and sex	100
2.30	Whether visitors are allowed to smoke cigarettes in respondent's home by age and sex	101
2.31	Whether visitors are allowed to smoke cigarettes in respondent's home by social class based on own current or last job and sex	102

		Page
2.32	Whether visitors are allowed to smoke cigarettes in respondent's home by whether respondent has any children under 16 in the household and sex	102
2.33	Whether visitors are allowed to smoke cigarettes in respondent's home by cigarette smoking status and sex	103
2.34	Alcohol consumption level (AC rating) and mean weekly number of units by age and sex	104
2.35	Alcohol consumption level (AC rating) and mean weekly number of units by social class, based on own current or last job and sex	105
2.36	Frequency and mean weekly consumption of alcoholic soft drinks in the last 12 months by age and sex	106
2.37	Frequency of consuming different types of alcoholic drinks by sex	106
2.38	Mean weekly consumption of 'alcopops' as a proportion of total mean weekly alcohol consumption by age and sex	106
2.39	Percentage who would like to drink less by age and social class based on own current or last job and sex	107
2.40	Percentage who would like to drink less by the amount of alcohol consumed per week and sex	107
2.41	When respondents intend to cut down on drinking by age and sex	108
2.42	When respondents intend to cut down on drinking by social class based on current or last job and sex	108
2.43	When respondents intend to cut down on drinking by the amount of alcohol consumed per week and sex	109
2.44	Percentage who have heard about measuring alcohol in units by age and sex	109
2.45	Percentage who had heard of alcohol units and correctly identified the number in specified drinks by each type of drink	109
2.46	Percentage who had heard of alcohol units and correctly identified the number in specified drinks by age and sex	110
2.47	Percentage who had heard of alcohol units and correctly identified the number in specified drinks by social class based on own current or last job and sex	110

		Page
2.48	Percentage who had heard of alcohol units and correctly identified the number in specified drinks by alcohol consumption and sex	111
2.49	Attitude to changes in sensible drinking levels by age and sex	111
2.50	Attitude to changes in sensible drinking levels by social class based on own current or last job and sex	112
2.51	Attitude to changes in sensible drinking levels by alcohol consumption level	113
2.52	Attitude to changes in sensible drinking levels by whether heard of units of alcohol and sex	114
2.53	Alcohol consumption by smoking status (HEMS 95 and HEMS 96 combined)	114

Chapter 3

3.1	Frequency of at least moderate-intensity activity for 30 minutes or more by age and sex	115
3.2	Frequency of moderate-intensity activity for 30 minutes or more by social class based on last or current job and sex	116
3.3	Age-standardised ratios for at least moderate activity on five or more days a week by social class based on own current or last job and sex	116
3.4	Percentage participating in vigorous activity for 20 minutes or more, at least three times a week by age, social class based on own current or last job and sex	117
3.5	'How long people should be physically active' by age and sex	118
3.6	'How long people should be physically active' by social class based on own current or last job, and sex	119
3.7	Number of days by 'how long people should be physically active', age and sex	119
3.8	Number of days and length of time people should be physically active by age and sex	120
3.9	Number of days and length of time people should be physically active by social class based on own current or last job, and sex	121
3.10	Level of activity 'compared with others of the same age' by age and sex	122

		Page
3.11	Level of activity 'compared with others of the same age' by social class based on own current or last job, and sex	123
3.12	Whether getting enough exercise to keep fit by age and sex	123
3.13	Whether getting enough exercise to keep fit by social class based on own current or last job, and sex	123
3.14	Percentage who would like to take more exercise by age, social class based on own current or last job, and sex	124
3.15	When intends to take more exercise by age and sex	125
3.16	When intends to take more exercise by social class based on own current or last job and sex	126
3.17	When intends to take more exercise by whether would like to take more exercise and sex	126
3.18	When intends to take more exercise by frequency of participation in at least moderate-intensity activity for 30 minutes or more by age and sex	127
3.19	Barriers to exercise by age and sex	128
3.20	Barriers to exercise by social class based on own current or last job and sex	129

Chapter 4

4.1	Knowledge of what constitutes a healthy diet by age and sex	130
4.2	Knowledge of what constitutes a healthy diet by social class based on own current or last job and sex	132
4.3	Whether looks at ingredients when shopping, and what looks for, by age and sex	133
4.4	Whether looks at ingredients when shopping, and what looks for, by social class based on own current or last job, and sex	134
4.5	Whether looks at ingredients when shopping and what looks for, by highest qualification level and sex	134
4.6	What looks for when shopping by sex	135
4.7	Whether looks at ingredients when shopping and what looks for, by number correctly stated of 'eat less fat', eat more fruit', 'eat more starch' and eat more fibre', age and sex	135

		Page
4.8	Consumption of foods containing fibre and starchy carbohydrates by age and sex	136
4.9	Consumption of foods containing fibre and starchy carbohydrates by social class based on own current or last job, and sex	137
4.10	Consumption of foods containing fibre and starchy carbohydrates by highest qualification level and sex	137
4.11	Consumption of foods containing fibre and starchy carbohydrates by standard region and sex	138
4.12	Consumption of foods containing fibre and starchy carbohydrates by number correctly stated of 'eat less fat', 'eat more fruit', 'eat more starch' and 'eat more fibre' and sex	139
4.13	Consumption of fats by age and sex	140
4.14	Consumption of fats by social class based on own current or last job, and sex	141
4.15	Consumption of fats by highest qualification level and sex	141
4.16	Consumption of fats by standard region and sex	142
4.17	Consumption of confectionery and biscuits or cakes by age and sex	143
4.18	Consumption of confectionery and biscuits or cakes by social class based on own current or last job, and sex	143
4.19	Consumption of confectionery and biscuits or cakes by fats by highest qualification level and sex	143
4.20	Consumption of confectionery and biscuits or cakes by standard region and sex	144
4.21	Attitudes to diet by age and sex	144
4.22	Attitudes to diet by frequency of consumption of bread; fruit, vegetables or salad and potatoes; pasta or rice and sex	145
4.23	Attitudes to diet by type of fats consumed and sex	145
4.24	Intentions to change diet by age and sex	146
4.25	Intentions to change diet by social class based on own current or last job, and sex	146
4.26	Whether agrees that 'I get confused over what's supposed to be healthy and what isn't' by age and sex	147

		Page
4.27	Whether agrees that 'I get confused over what's supposed to be healthy and what isn't' by social class based on own current or last job, and sex	148
4.28	Percentage agreeing that 'I get confused over what's supposed to be healthy and what isn't' by number of ways of achieving a healthier diet correctly identified	148
4.29	Percentage agreeing that 'experts never agree what foods are good for you' by age	149
4.30	Percentage 'strongly agreeing' or 'agreeing' that 'eating healthy food is expensive' by selected characteristics	149
4.31	Whether agrees that 'healthy foods' are enjoyable' by age and sex	150
4.32	Percentage 'strongly agreeing' or 'agreeing' that 'healthy foods are enjoyable' by selected characteristics	150
4.33	Percentage 'strongly agreeing' or 'agreeing' that 'the tastiest foods are the ones that are bad for you' by selected characteristics	151

Chapter 5

5.1	Percentage who had ever used drugs, had used drugs in the past year or had used drugs in the past month by sex	152
5.2	Percentage who had ever used drugs by age and sex	152
5.3	Percentage who had ever used drugs, had used drugs in the past year or in the past month, by drug category, age and sex	153
5.4	Whether had ever used drugs by drug category, age and sex	154
5.5	Whether had ever used drugs in the past year by drug category, age and sex	154
5.6	Whether had ever used drugs in the past month by drug category, age and sex	155
5.7	Whether had ever used drugs by drug category, age and sex	155
5.8	Whether had ever used drugs in the last year by drug category, age and sex	156
5.9	Whether had ever used drugs in the last month by drug category, age and sex	156
5.10	Respondents who had used any drug in the past year or in the past month as a proportion of those who had ever used any drug, by age and sex	157

		Page
5.11	Respondents who had used cannabis in the past year or in the past month as a proportion of those who had ever used cannabis, by age and sex	158
5.12	Number of different drugs used, by whether used any drug ever, in the past year or in the past month, and sex	159
5.13	Respondents who had used cannabis and/or other drugs, by recency of use and sex	159
5.14	Whether know people who use drugs by age and sex	160
5.15	Whether respondents know people who use drugs by whether had used a drug in the past month, year, more than a year or never, age and sex	160
5.16	Whether would like to stop using drugs by age and sex	161
5.17	Intentions to stop using drugs by sex	161
5.18	Percentage who had used each method of taking drugs, by age and sex	162
5.19	Percentage who had used drugs in combination by age and sex	162
5.20	Percentage who had used drugs in combination with alcohol by age and sex	162
5.21	Whether agrees that 'All use of drugs is wrong unless with a doctor's prescription or bought from a chemist' by age and sex	163
5.22	Whether agrees that 'All use of drugs is wrong unless with a doctor's prescription or bought from a chemist' by whether had used any drug in the past month, year, longer than a year or never, and sex	163
5.23	Whether agrees that 'I don't mind other people using drugs' by age and sex	164
5.24	Whether agrees that 'I don't mind other people using drugs' by whether had used any drug in the past month, year, longer than a year or never, and sex	164
5.25	Whether agrees that drugs are safe to use by age and sex	165
5.26	Whether agrees that drugs are safe to use by whether had used any drug in the past month, year, more than a year ago or never and sex	166

		Page			Page
5.27	Percentage who had ever used any drug, by selected characteristics	167	6.13	Age-standardised ratios for likelihood of 'someone like me getting another sexually transmitted disease' by number of sexual partners in the last 12 months and sex	179
5.28	Percentage who had used any drug in the past year, by selected characteristics	168	6.14	Whether would find it difficult to raise the subject of using a condom with a new partner by age and sex	180
5.29	Percentage who had used any drug in the past month, by selected characteristics	169	6.15	Percentage 'strongly agreeing' or 'agreeing' that 'it would be difficult to raise the subject of using a condom with a new partner' by selected characteristics	181

Chapter 6

6.1	Number of sexual partners in the last 12 months by age and sex	170	6.16	Whether would use a condom if 'in the near future they did have sex with a new partner' by age and sex	182
6.2	Number of sexual partners in the last 12 months by social class based on own current or last job, age and sex	171	6.17	Whether would use a condom with a new partner by number of sexual partners in the last 12 months and sex	182
6.3	Age standardised ratios for reporting two or more sexual partners in the last year by social class based on own current or last job, and sex	172	6.18	Whether would use a condom with a new partner by whether would find it difficult to raise the subject of using a condom with a new partner, and sex	183
6.4	Number of sexual partners in the last 12 months by marital status, age and sex	173	6.19	Percentage using a condom with a new partner by selected characteristics	184
6.5	Age standardised ratios for reporting two or more sexual partners in the last year by marital status and sex	174			

Chapter 7

6.6	Respondent's assessment of the likelihood of 'someone like me getting HIV (the AIDS virus)' by age and sex	175	7.1	Number of occasions of sunburn in the 12 months prior to interview by age and sex	185
6.7	Respondent's assessment of the likelihood of 'someone like me getting another sexually transmitted disease' by age and sex	176	7.2	Number of occasions of sunburn in the 12 months prior to interview by social class, based on own current or last job and sex	186
6.8	Respondent's assessment of the likelihood of 'someone like me getting HIV (the AIDS virus)' by marital status and sex	177	7.3	Skin type by sex	186
6.9	Respondent's assessment of the likelihood of 'someone like me getting another sexually transmitted disease' by marital status and sex	177	7.4	Number of occasions of sunburn in the 12 months prior to interview by skin type and sex	187
6.10	Respondent's assessment of the likelihood of 'someone like me getting HIV (the AIDS virus)' by number of sexual partners in the last 12 months and sex	178	7.5	Occasions on which respondents use suncream by age and sex	188
			7.6	Occasions on which respondents use suncream by social class based on own current or last job and sex	189
6.11	Respondent's assessment of the likelihood of 'someone like me getting another sexually transmitted disease' by number of sexual partners in the last 12 months and sex	178	7.7	Factor level of suncream used by age and sex	190
			7.8	Factor level of suncream used by sex	190
6.12	Age-standardised ratios for likelihood of 'someone like me getting HIV (the AIDS virus)' by number of sexual partners in the last 12 months and sex	179	7.9	Factor level of suncream used by skin type and sex	191

Health in England 1996 : What people know, what people think, what people do

		Page
7.10	Whether sunburnt in the last 12 months by whether uses a suncream or not and sex	192
7.11	Whether having a suntan is important by age and sex	192
7.12	Whether agrees that 'having a suntan makes me feel healthier' by age and sex	193
7.13	Whether agrees that 'having a suntan makes me feel healthier' by social class based on own current or last job and sex	193
7.14	Whether agrees that 'having a suntan makes me look more attractive' by age and sex	194
7.15	Whether agrees that 'having a suntan makes me look more attractive' by social class, based on own current or last job and sex	194
7.16	Whether agrees that 'having a suntan makes me look more attractive' by skin type and sex	195

Chapter 8

8.1	Self-reported general health by age and sex	196
8.2	Self-reported general health by social class based on own current or last job, age and sex	197
8.3	Age-standardised ratios for self-reported good health by social class based on own current or last job and sex	197
8.4	Self-reported long-standing illness or disability by sex and age: HEMS, GHS 1995 and Health Survey 1994	198
8.5	Self-reported long-standing illness by social class based on own current or last job, age and sex	199
8.6	Age-standardised ratios for self-reported long-standing illness by social class based on own current or last job and sex	200
8.7	Self-reported general health by self-reported long-standing illness or disability, age and sex	201
8.8	Self-reported stress in last 12 months by age and sex	202
8.9	Self-reported stress in last 12 months by by social class based on own current or last job, age and sex	203

		Page
8.10	Age-standardised ratios for self-reported stress by social class based on own current or last job and sex	203
8.11	Self-reported effect of stress on health by age and sex	204
8.12	Self-reported effect of stress on health by a) self-reported general health b) self-reported long-standing illness or disability and sex	204
8.13	Self-reported effect of stress on health by self-reported stress and sex	205
8.14	Respondent's assessment of whether they lead a healthy life by sex and age	205
8.15	Respondent's assessment of whether they lead a healthy life by social class, based on own current or last job, age and sex	206
8.16	Age-standardised ratios for respondents' assessment of whether they lead a healthy life by social class, based on own current or last job, and sex	206
8.17	Respondent's assessment of what is currently good for their health by age and sex	207
8.18	Respondent's assessment of what is currently bad for their health by age and sex	208
8.19	Respondent's assessment of what is currently good for their health by social class, based on own current or last job, age and sex	209
8.20	Respondent's assessment of what is currently bad for their health by social class, based on own current or last job, sex and age	209
8.21	Whether having good health is the most important thing in life by age and sex	210
8.22	Whether it is sensible to do exactly what the doctors say by age and sex	211
8.23	Whether health is generally a matter of luck by age and sex	212
8.24	Whether you are more likely to be ill if you think too much about your health by age and sex	213
8.25	Whether respondents have to be very ill before they go to the doctor by age and sex	214

310 Health in England 1996 : What people know, what people think, what people do

		Page
8.26	Whether respondents don't really have time to think about their health by age and sex	215
8.27	Consultations with GPs and other health professionals in the last 12 months by age and sex	216
8.28	Consultations with GPs and other health professionals in the last 12 months by social class and sex	217
8.29	Age-standardised ratios for consultations with GPs and other health professionals by social class, based on own current or last job, and sex	218
8.30	Consultations with GPs and other health professionals in the last 12 months by a) self-reported general health b) self-reported long-standing illness or disability and sex	219
8.31	Discussions with GPs or other health professionals about health behaviours in the last 12 months	220
8.32	Discussions with GPS or other health professionals about health behaviours in the last 12 months by selected characteristics	221

Appendix A

		Page
A.1	The sample of addresses and households	222
A.2	Response of adults at interview stage	222
A.3	Response of adults aged 16-54 to the self-completion module	222
A.4	Weights for household size	222
A.5	Distribution of responders to HEMS compared with Labour Force Survey (LFS) estimates for England by age and sex	223
A.6	Distribution of responders to HEMS compared with Labour Force Survey (LFS) estimates for England by standard region	223
A.7	Distribution of responders to HEMS compared to GHS 1994 by marital status	224
A.8	Distribution of responders to HEMS compared with Labour Force Survey (LFS) by ethnic origin and sex	224
A.9	Age-sex-region weights	225
A.10	The effects of weighting for non-response on survey estimates	226
A.11	Social class based on own current or last job by age and sex	227
A.12	Age by social class based on own current or last job, and sex	227
A.13	Social class of HOH based on HOH's current or last job by respondent's social class based on own current or last job, and sex	228
A.14	Highest qualification level by age and sex	228
A.15	Highest qualification level by social class based on own current or last job, and sex	229
A.16	Economic activity status by social class based on own current or last job, and sex	229
A.17	Housing tenure status by social class based on own current or last job, and sex	229
A.18	Gross household income by social class based on own current or last job, and sex	229
A.19	Characteristics of respondents interviewed face-to-face and by proxy	230
A.20	Selected estimates for respondents interviewed face-to-face and by proxy	231
A.21	Type of accommodation occupied by respondents interviewed face-to-face and by proxy and at non-responding addresses	231
A.22	Standard errors and 95% confidence intervals for socio-demographic variables	232
A.23	Standard errors and 95% confidence intervals for smoking variables	233
A.24	Standard errors and 95% confidence intervals for drinking variables	234
A.25	Standard errors and 95% confidence intervals for physical activity variables	235
A.26	Standard errors and 95% confidence intervals for nutrition variables	236
A.27	Standard errors and 95% confidence intervals for drugs variables	237
A.28	Standard errors and 95% confidence intervals for sexual health variables	238
A.29	Standard errors and 95% confidence intervals for behaviour in the sun variables	239
A.30	Standard errors and 95% confidence intervals for general health variables	240